Functional and Morphological Ir of the Endocrine System

ENDOCRINE UPDATES

Shlomo Melmed, M.D., Series Editor

---

1. E.R. Levin and J.L. Nadler (eds.): Endocrinology of Cardiovascular Function. 1998. ISBN: 0-7923-8217-X
2. J.A. Fagin (ed.): Thyroid Cancer. 1998. ISBN: 0-7923-8326-5
3. J.S. Adams and B.P. Lukert (eds.): Osteoporosis: Genetics, Prevention and Treatment. 1998. ISBN: 0-7923-8366-4.
4. B.-Å. Bengtsson (ed.): Growth Hormone. 1999. ISBN: 0-7923-8478-4
5. C. Wang (ed.): Male Reproductive Function. 1999. ISBN 0-7923-8520-9
6. B. Rapoport and S.M. McLachlan (eds.): Graves' Disease: Pathogenesis and Treatment. 2000. ISBN: 0-7923-7790-7.
7. W. W. de Herder (ed.): Functional and Morphological Imaging of the Endocrine System. 2000. ISBN 0-7923-7923-9

FUNCTIONAL AND MORPHOLOGICAL IMAGING OF THE ENDOCRINE SYSTEM

edited by

Wouter W. de Herder M.D.

University Hospital Rotterdam
Rotterdam, The Netherlands

SPRINGER SCIENCE+BUSINESS MEDIA, LLC

Library of Congress Cataloging-in-Publication Data

Functional and morphological imaging of the endocrine system / edited by Wouter W. de Herder.
p. ; cm. – (Endocrine updates; 7)
Includes bibliographical references and index.
ISBN 978-1-4613-6950-9 ISBN 978-1-4615-4341-1 (eBook)
DOI 10.1007/978-1-4615-4341-1
1. Endocrine glands—Imaging. 2. Endocrine glands—Diseases—Diagnosis. 3. Endocrine glands—Tumors—Imaging. I. Herder Wouter W. de II. Series.
[DNLM: 1. Endocrine Diseases—radionuclide imaging. 2. Endocrine Diseases—ultrasonography. 3. Endocrine Glands—pathology. WK 140 F9787 2000]
RC655.5 .F86 2000
616.4'0754—dc21

00-057820

Originally published by Kluwer Academic Publishers, New York in 2000
Softcover reprint of the hardcover 1st edition 2000

Printed on acid-free paper.

CONTENTS

Adrenal

LIST OF CONTRIBUTORS

Anna Ali, M.D., Università di Torino, Turin, Italy.

Alberto Angeli, M.D., Università di Torino, Turin, Italy.

Emmanuelle Barrali, M.D., Centre Hospitalier Universitaire de Besançon, Besançon, France.

Jean-François Bonneville, M.D., Centre Hospitalier Universitaire de Besançon, Besançon, France.

Fabrice Bonneville, M.D., Centre Hospitalier Universitaire de Besançon, Besançon, France.

Françoise Cattin, M.D., Centre Hospitalier Universitaire de Besançon, Besançon, France.

Wouter W. de Herder, M.D., University Hospital Rotterdam, Rotterdam, the Netherlands.

Diego Ferone, M.D., "Federico II" University, Naples, Italy.

Brian Gorman, M.B., B.Ch., F.R.C.R., M.B.A., Mayo Medical School, Rochester, USA.

Milton D. Gross, M.D., University of Michigan, Ann Arbor, USA.

Ad R. Hermus, M.D., University Hospital Nijmegen, Nijmegen, the Netherlands.

Melanie P. Hiorns, M.R.C.P., F.R.C.R., St Bartholomew's Hospital, London, United Kingdom.

Dyde A. Huysmans, M.D., Catharina Hospital, Eindhoven, the Netherlands.

Guy Jacquet, M.D., Centre Hospitalier Universitaire de Besançon, Besançon, France.

Eric P. Krenning, M.D., University Hospital Rotterdam, Rotterdam, the Netherlands.

Gabriel P. Krestin, M.D., University Hospital Rotterdam, Rotterdam, the Netherlands.

Dik J. Kwekkeboom, M.D., University Hospital Rotterdam, Rotterdam, the Netherlands.

Steven W.J. Lamberts, M.D., University Hospital Rotterdam, Rotterdam, the Netherlands.

Mark E. Molitch, M.D., Northwestern University Medical School, Chicago, USA.

Giangiacomo Osella. M.D., Università di Torino, Turin, Italy.

Herman Pieterman, M.D., University Hospital Rotterdam, Rotterdam, the Netherlands.

Carl C. Reading, M.D., Mayo Medical School, Rochester, USA.

Rodney H. Reznek, F.R.C.P., F.R.C.R., St Bartholomew's Hospital, London, United Kingdom.

Brahm Shapiro, M.B., CH.B., Ph.D., University of Michigan, Ann Arbor, USA.

Paul Shreve, M.D., University of Michigan, Ann Arbor, USA.

Barry I. Shulkin, M.D., University of Michigan, Ann Arbor, USA.

Hervé L.J. Tanghe, M.D., University Hospital Rotterdam, Rotterdam, the Netherlands.

Massimo Terzolo, M.D., Università di Torino, Turin, Italy.

Lukas C. van Dijk, M.D., University Hospital Rotterdam, Rotterdam, the Netherlands.

Wilmar M. Wiersinga, M.D., Academic Medical Center, University of Amsterdam, Amsterdam, the Netherlands.

PREFACE

In 1895, Wilhelm Conrad Röntgen (re)discovered a variant of electromagnetic radiation, which he called X-rays. The clinical application of X-rays caused a dramatic change in medicine, starting with the creation of the new field of radiology. Approximately fifty years later, radiopharmaceuticals had become available for the diagnosis and treatment of various disorders. The disciplines of radiology and nuclear medicine are still expanding because of new discoveries, and advancements and improvements in techniques and instruments.
Our purpose of this issue of Endocrine Updates is to provide comprehensive but concise insights in modern imaging techniques and protocols for the diagnosis and treatment of a variety of endocrine disorders. For this purpose we have chosen to distinguish between "morphological imaging" and "functional imaging".
We fortunately acknowledge and appreciate the high quality of the contributions by eminent scientists and clinicians.

Wouter W. de Herder, M.D.
University Hospital Rotterdam,
Rotterdam, the Netherlands

PITUITARY

1

MAGNETIC RESONANCE IMAGING OF THE PITUITARY AREA: PATHOLOGIC ASPECTS

Jean-François Bonneville, M.D.
Fabrice Bonneville, M.D.
Emmanuelle Barrali, M.D.
Guy Jacquet, M.D.
Françoise Cattin, M.D.
University Centre HospitalierUniversitaire de Besançon
Besançon France

INTRODUCTION

Pituitary adenomas are the most common pathological lesions in the sellar region. Since the introduction of magnetic resonance imaging (MRI), these tumors are easier to diagnose and monitor. Imaging plays a decisive role for the diagnosis of hormone-producing pituitary adenomas. For example, the therapeutic approach in acromegaly or Cushing's disease is directly influenced by the results of pituitary MRI. Other lesions located in the sellar region, such as craniopharyngiomas, meningiomas, gliomas of the optic chiasm, germinomas and aneurysms of the circle of Willis are usually discovered because of visual defects, headaches, hypopituitarism, or diabetes insipidus, among other symptoms.

In this chapter, we will discuss MRI of pituitary microadenomas, picoadenomas and macroadenomas. We will also discuss the differential diagnosis of lesions in the hypothalamic-pituitary region and analyze the imaging results of these lesions.

Pituitary adenomas

MRI replaces practically all the previously used techniques for morphological investigation of pituitary adenomas. In addition to MRI, standard skull X-rays and CT-scans may still be needed for the demonstration of bony malformations, anatomical variants or calcifications (7,16,22,47).

We will first describe the MR aspect of pituitary adenomas according to size, sex, age, endocrine activity and some specific conditions.

MRI aspects according to size

Historically, pituitary adenomas are divided into two categories: pituitary microadenomas, which have a diameter smaller than 10 mm and pituitary macroadenomas, which have a diameter larger than 10 mm. We will also refer to picoadenomas, which have a diameter less than 3 mm, because these tumors may produce additional diagnostic problems.

Pituitary microadenomas and picoadenomas

Pituitary micro- and picoadenomas are almost uniformly localized within the sella. Therefore, these tumors rarely cause visual defects. However, exceptionally when the sella turcica is small or flat, a 10-mrn pituitary adenoma may be located very close to the optic chiasm. Usually, endocrine dysfunction is the first presenting symptom of these pituitary micro- and picoadenomas, but they may also be incidentally discovered. Changes of the bony sellar floor are more difficult to distinguish with MRI than with CT scanning. Depressions, slopes, and angulations of the sellar floor may be visualized with MRI, but cortical thinning cannot be visualized with MRI (10,25,41).

Pituitary microadenomas produce altered MR signals in the anterior pituitary (Figures 1-4). On the more heavily T1-weighted spin-echo images, pituitary microadenomas are usually demonstrated as rounded or oval, sometimes flattened or triangular intrasellar lesions, with loss of signal intensity when compared to the uninvolved anterior pituitary gland. In coronal sections of T2-weighted MR images, the signal intensity of pituitary adenomas typically resembles that of the temporal cortex of the brain, while the signal intensity of the normal anterior pituitary gland is very close to that of temporal white matter. However, in approximately one fourth of the cases the more heavily T1-weighted signal of the pituitary adenoma is very similar to that of the uninvolved pituitary gland and additional studies are necessary. Pituitary microadenomas can also cause high signal intensity on T1-weighted images, which is probably due to complete or partial hemorrhagic transformation of the adenoma. This is a frequent occurring phenomenon in prolactinomas.

On the more heavily T2-weighted, fast spin-echo MR images, the aspect of pituitary microadenomas varies, particularly with the type of endocrine activity. The diagnosis of microadenomas is easy when they demonstrate high intensity on T2-weighted images, although this signal may only be produced by a part of the adenoma. An increased intensity on T2-weighted images is found in more than 80% of microprolactinomas. However, hypersignals on T2-weighted images should not be confused with the lateral pituitary veins. Conversely, less clear isosignals or hyposignals on T2-weighted images can be found in two-thirds of all growth hormone-secreting microadenomas. Fast spin-echo T2-weighted images are particularly helpful for the identification of pituitary picoadenomas, for which T1-weighted images and even gadolinium-enhanced sequences are sometimes negative.

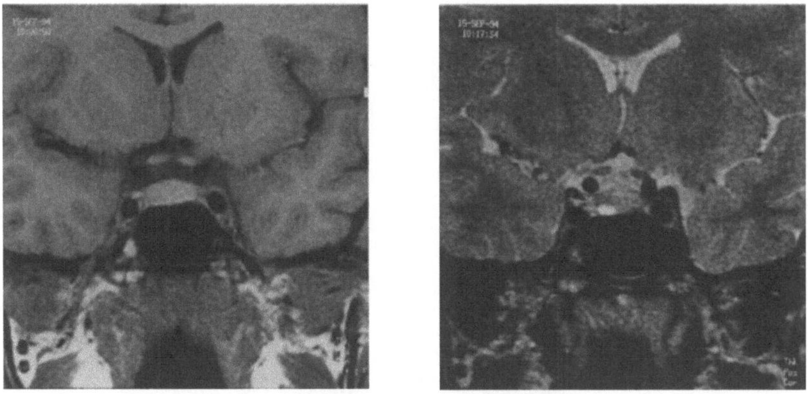

Figure 1. 18-year-old woman with oligomenorrhea and slight hyperprolactinemia.
Left: Coronal spin-echo T1-weighted image. Right: Turbo T2-weighted image.
A microadenoma is nearly invisible on the T1-weighted image, but hyperintense at the right side of the pituitary on the T2-weighted image.

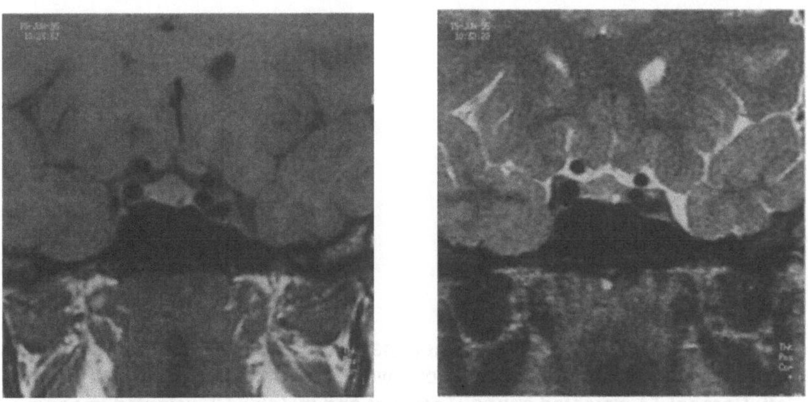

Figure 2. 24-year-old woman with oligomenorrhea and slight hyperprolactinemia.
Left: coronal spin-echo T1-weighted image. Right: Turbo T2-weighted image.
A picoadenoma with a diameter less than 2 mm is perfectly defined both on the T1-weighted image as a hypointense lesion and on the T2-weighted image as a hyperintense lesion.
The very convex aspect of the upper margins of the pituitary gland is an anatomic variant

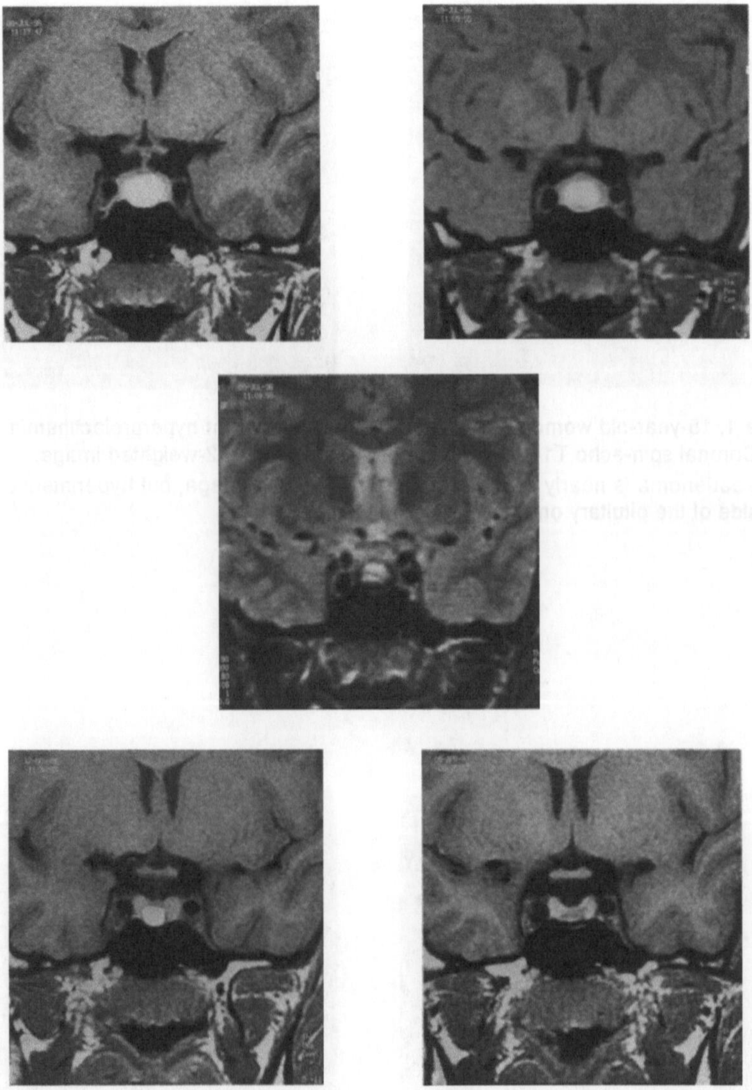

Figure 3. 17 -year-old girl with amenorrhea, galactorrhea, initially moderately increased serum prolactin levels and recent onset of severe headaches.
Top left: Coronal T1-weighted image. Top right and middle: T2-weighted images.
On the T1-weighted image a hypersignal fills the sellar fossa. Also depression of the sellar floor is shown. The signal is identical at the first echo on T2. At the second echo, there is a more heterogeneous aspect together with a hypointense margin.
4 months after the start of bromocriptine treatment.
Bottom left: Collapse of the lesion, which remains hemorrhagic with a thin peripheral hypointense margin. The upper margin of the pituitary has shrunk.
10 months after the onset of bromocriptine treatment.
Bottom right: The adenoma is no longer hemorrhagic, but appears as a hypointense triangular lesion.

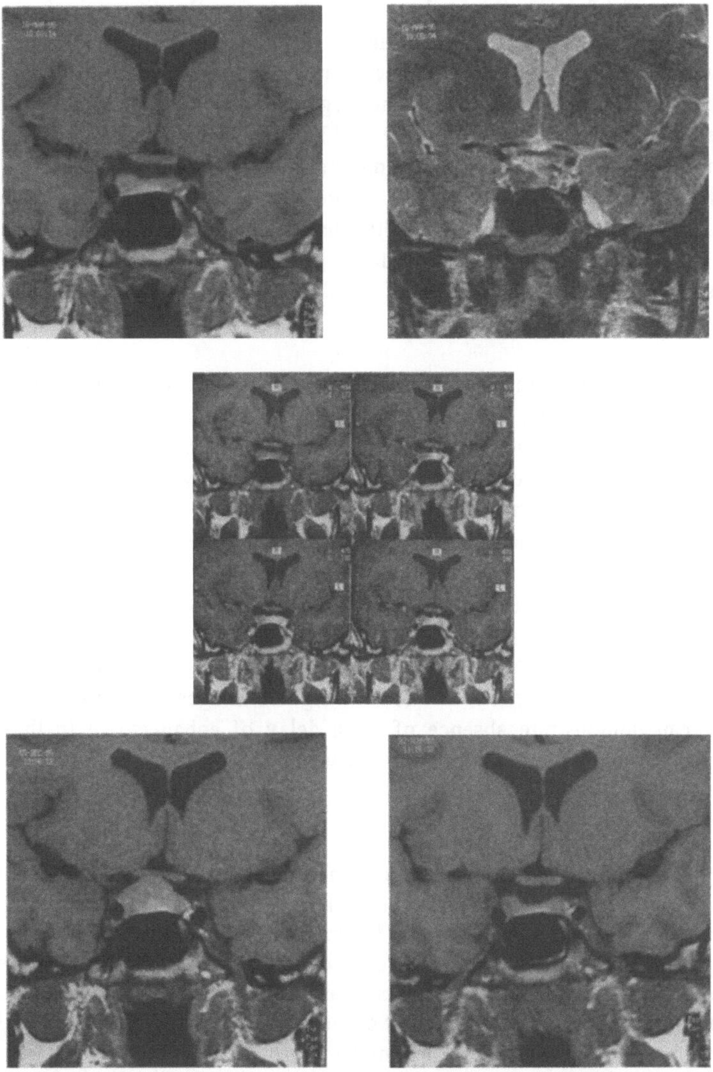

Figure 4. 38-year-old woman with amenorrhea and hyperprolactinemia.
Top left: coronal spin-echo T1-weighted image Top right: turbo spin-echo T2-weighted image. Middle: dynamic imaging after injection of gadolinium.
The pituitary adenoma, which is located at the right side of the pituitary, has identical signal intensity as the normal pituitary. It is shown as a local bulging of the upper margins of the pituitary. On the T2-weighted image, the adenoma appears hypointense. Dynamic imaging shows distinct enhancement of the sellar contents. Subsequently, pregnancy occurred with bromocriptine treatment.
Bottom left: at the 7th pregnancy month a marked increase of the adenoma volume with slight deformation of the optic chiasm is shown. Note the multiple disseminated small hemorrhages in the adenoma.
2 years later with bromocriptine therapy
Bottom right: almost total normalization of the pituitary gland.

When the T1- and fast T2-weighted images both confirm the diagnosis (for example a low intensity T1-weighted signal and a high intensity T2-weighted signal), gadolinium enhancement is not necessary. This is commonly the case in prolactinomas. On the contrary, when the diagnosis has not been formally established, enhanced imaging is mandatory (8,9,29,31,33,34,43). A half-dose of gadolinium, i.e. 0.05 mmol/kg body weight (BW), or sometimes even less (e.g. 0.03 mmol/kg BW), is injected intravenously and T1-weighted spin-echo coronal images are made. These images show a relative signal void of the adenoma, which may be surrounded by the intense enhancement of the normal pituitary gland in the following situations: 1) the tumor is extremely small, 2) the dose of gadolinium is too high, or 3) the visualization window is too large.

Additional techniques can also be used. Delayed sequences, 30 to 40 minutes after injection of the contrast agent can sometimes demonstrate enhancement of the adenoma. A good correlation has been found between the hypersignal of the adenoma on fast T2-weighted images and late enhancement. Usually, these lesions are weak at surgery. However adenomas, which are hypointense on T2-weighted images show absence of late enhancement and generally are solid at surgery and active hormone secreting. Dynamic imaging can be used routinely for the diagnosis of ACTH-secreting microadenomas (3,17,23,24). Complementary dynamic imaging can also be used in those cases when clinical signs strongly point to the presence of a pituitary adenoma, but first MR images have not been convincing enough (e.g. an isointense pituitary microadenoma on T1- and/or T2-weighted images). In these cases, dynamic imaging can demonstrate absence of, or a delay of enhancement in the pituitary adenoma as compared to the normal pituitary gland.

Pituitary macroadenomas (27,45)

Pituitary macroadenomas are intrasellar masses extending out of the sellar region, usually upwards into the optochiasmatic cistern or even higher, thereby compressing the third ventricle and sometimes the foramen of Monro. The tumor mass can also extend downwards into the sphenoid sinus, or laterally towards the cavernous sinus. What is expected of MRI differs for pituitary microadenomas and macroadenomas. When an intrasellar mass extending out of the sella is detected, the origin of the tumor (pituitary or extra-pituitary), its extension in relation to the various surrounding anatomical structures, its structure (firm, cystic, necrotic or hemorrhagic) and its enhancement should be determined. What is expected of MRI, therefore, is not so much a confirmation of the diagnosis, but rather assessment of the extension of the tumor and its differential diagnosis (Figures 5-7).

Pituitary macroadenomas are located central, usually in a remodeled sella turcica. MR imaging may show this remodeled and enlarged sella, with parts of the dorsum sellae missing. If additional morphological details are needed, a CT scan of the sellar region, or a standard skull X-ray may provide more information, particularly on changes in the sellar cortex. However, this may only occasionally be necessary. Macroadenomas with suprasellar extension often contain multiple cysts. Sometimes, one or more extensions into the optochiasmatic cistern can be clearly identified. Their spontaneous signal varies, but they usually appear brighter on T1-weighted spin-echo images than pituitary microadenomas. Macroadenomas are often inhomogeneous; particularly on fast T2-weighted images, with disseminated areas of hypersignal corresponding to cystic or necrotic parts of the adenoma. The adenomatous tissue usually enhances slightly after injection of gadolinium. However, the aim of enhanced imaging is to visualize normal non-pathologic pituitary tissue. This is usually shown as a strongly enhanced pseudocapsula usually located unilaterally, either above, or behind the adenoma and rarely below or in front of it. The coronal sections of enhanced T1-weighted images generally show a unilateral layer of normal pituitary tissue located between the adenoma and the contents of the cavernous sinus. This provides crucial information to the neurosurgeon. The hyperintense posterior lobe is usually modified. It appears either flattened or displaced and is well recognized on axial sections. Also an ectopic location of anti-diuretic hormone (ADH) secretion can be located in the pituitary stalk, which is compressed by the superior margins of the macroadenoma (Figure 8) (15). The pituitary stalk is tilted laterally. The positions of the optic chiasm and the pituitary macroadenoma are best studied on coronal sections, rather than on sagittal images. The optic chiasm may be difficult to identify when there is extensive suprasellar extension of the adenoma. In these cases, fast spin T2-weighted coronal sections could be helpful, as the optic chiasm appears clearly hypointense using this technique.

After gadolinium injection, a discrete meningeal enhancement is usually observed near the area where the meninges are in contact with the adenoma and particularly at the anterior part of the posterior cranial fossa, sometimes along a dural tail. This has previously been described in connection with meningiomas of the sellar area as well as with hypophysitis. In our experience, enhancement of the dura mater has no specificity whatsoever.

MR aspects according to sex and age

Prolactin-secreting microadenomas are common in young women. Some may remain dormant over a very long period. They usually do not develop after menopause. Prolactin-secreting adenomas usually have reached the macroadenoma phase when they are discovered in males. This is partly due to the fact that specific clinical signs are less manifest or are only recognized late in the curse of the disease, and partly because their development is probably different in men than in women. Cavernous sinus involvement of these prolactin-secreting macroadenomas is not exceptional.

Pituitary adenomas in children are rare but potentially very active tumors. Prolactin-secreting adenomas can be responsible for delayed puberty, while ACTH-secreting adenomas cause Cushing's disease.

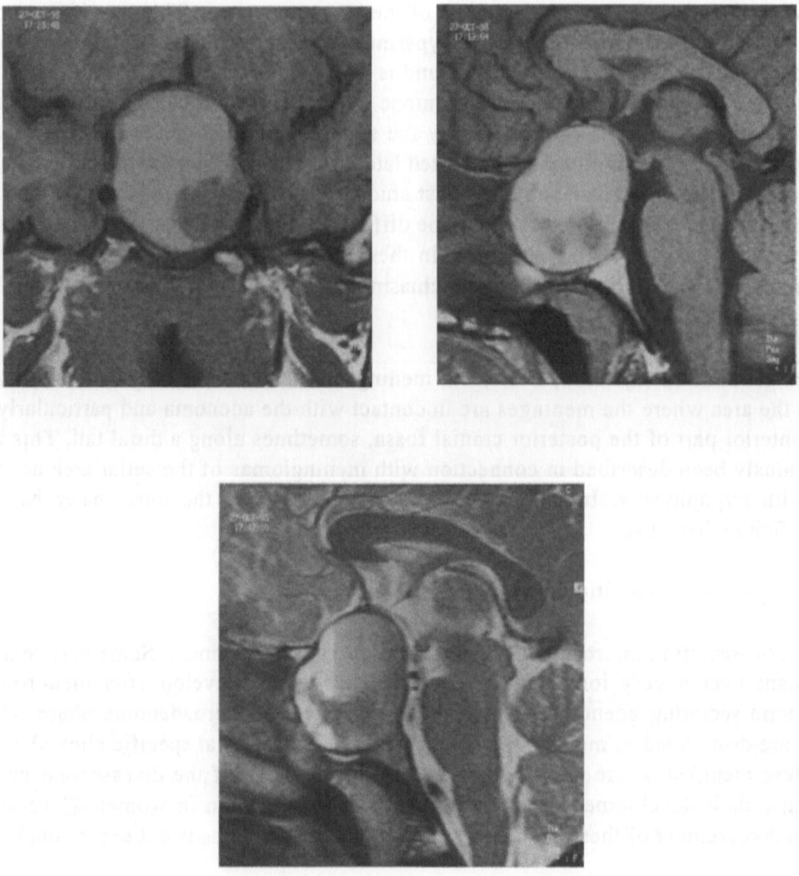

Figure 5. 19-year-old man with loss of visual acuity and visual field defects and severe hyperprolactinemia.

Top left: coronal spin-echo T1-weighted image. Top right: sagittal spin-echo T1-weighted image. Large pituitary adenoma with intra- and suprasellar extension, mainly hyperintense on the T1-weighted image with a left inferolateral fleshy part isointense compared to the temporal cortex. This hemorrhagic pituitary adenoma also elevates the optic chiasm. Bottom: On the T2-weighted turbo image a fluid level corresponding to sedimentation of different derivatives of blood degradation is shown

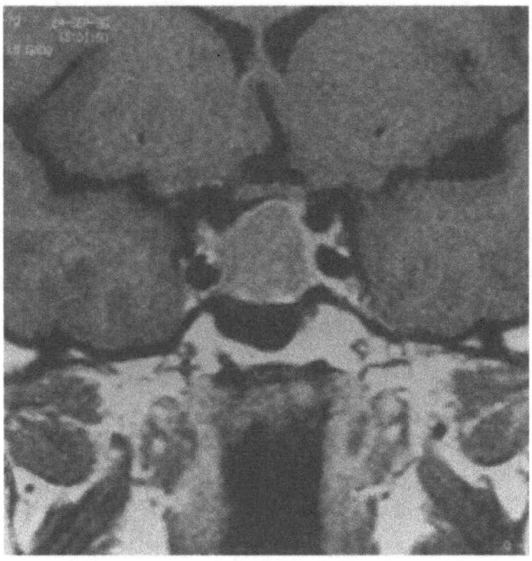

Figure 6. 25-year-old man with bilateral gynecomastia, slight impairment of the visual fields and severe hyperprolactinemia.
Coronal spin-echo T1-weighted image after intravenous injection of gadolinium showing a macroadenoma with suprasellar extension coming into close contact with the optic chiasm. At the left side, located between the adenomatous tissue and the cavernous sinus, and at the upper margin of the tumor, compressed normal pituitary tissue shows enhancement after gadolinium injection.

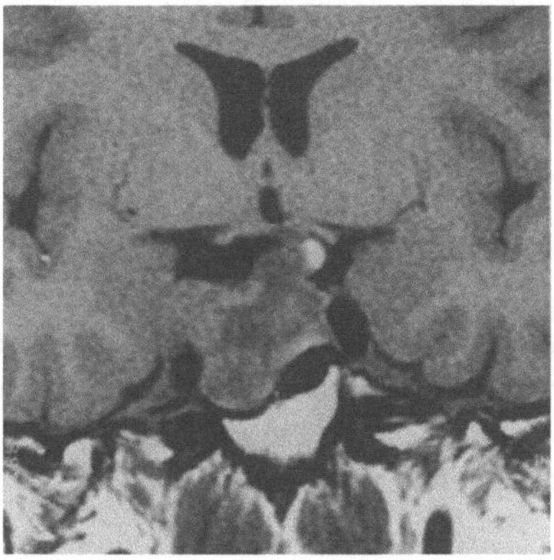

Figure 7. 21-year-old man with severe hyperprolactinemia.
Coronal spin-echo T1-weighted image showing a hypointense adenoma with intra- and suprasellar extension and elevation of the optic chiasm. There is accumulation of anti-diuretic hormone in an ectopic position at the base of the pituitary stalk. Invasion of the cavernous sinus is suspected at the right side, because of bulging of the lateral wall of the cavernous sinus at this side.

MR aspects according to hormonal secretion

Prolactinomas are usually discovered at the stage of microadenomas in women owing to distinctive clinical signs like amenorrhea, galactorrhea and hyperprolactinemia (30,37). They appear generally hypointense on T1-weighted images and 80% appear hyperintense on T2-weighted images. However, only part of the adenoma may give this hypersignal. Usually, there is a good correlation between the level of prolactin secretion and the size of the adenoma. However, prolactinomas, which appear hypointense on T2-weighted images, are generally more actively secreting than hyperintense tumors. Medical treatment with dopamine agonists generally decreases the size of the prolactinoma drastically. As a result, the radiological diagnosis becomes more difficult or even impossible in some of these medically treated patients (46). Therefore, pituitary MRI studies are strongly recommended before instituting medical treatment for prolactinomas.

When follow-up MRI studies are performed in the course of dopamine agonist therapy, peculiar scar tissue may be seen, which is characteristic for the former presence of a pituitary adenoma. This usually gives very local remodeling of the pituitary gland, forming a V at its superior aspect (Figure 5).

While prolactinomas and GH-secreting microadenomas are usually located laterally in the sella turcica, ACTH-secreting microadenomas (2,6,12,13,14,36) are generally smaller and often located along the median plane. Because of the poor prognosis and the good results of surgery for Cushing's disease, sequences and MR investigations should be repeated in these patients.

Growth hormone (GH)-secreting adenomas (28) have the unique characteristic of producing a hyposignal on T2-weighted images in 2/3 of cases. Spontaneous infarction or necrosis of GH-secreting adenomas is not exceptional. Some patients with acromegaly who were detected late in the course of the disease present with an enlarged, partial empty sella lined with adenomatous tissue, which is difficult to analyze. Medical treatment with somatostatin analogs decreases the size of the adenoma on average by 35% and normalizes serum IGF-I levels in 50% of cases.

Macroadenomas can be nonfunctioning, but also prolactin-secreting, gonadotropin-secreting and GH-secreting. The greater their size, the more heterogeneous they appear, as areas of cystic necrosis result from poor tumoral blood supply. Gonadotropin-secreting adenomas are often solid and have a strong tendency to recur.

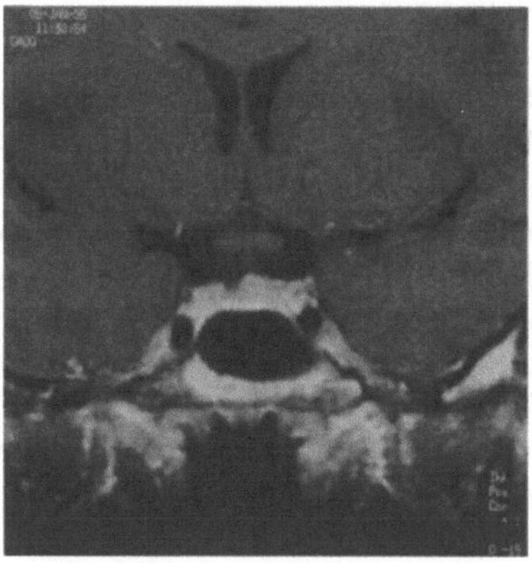

Figure 8. Microprolactinoma treated with bromocriptine. Coronal spin-echo T1-weighted image after injection of gadolinium showing localized depression of the upper margin of the pituitary.

Particular aspects

Hemorrhagic pituitary adenomas

Complete or partial hemorrhage occurs in 20% of pituitary adenomas. This is usually occult (Figures 3, 4 and 6). Pituitary apoplexy, usually presenting with headaches, meningism, cranial nerve paralysis and hypopituitarism is generally caused by massive hemorrhage of a pituitary macroadenoma. However, less abundant hemorrhages occur more frequently. Bromocriptine is claimed to be responsible for intratumoral hemorrhages in prolactinomas, although these have also been identified on MR images before institution of this therapy. Recurrent hemorrhages can cause repeated headaches. Intratumoral hemorrhages can be demonstrated by spontaneous hypersignals on Tl-weighted images. A fluid level can sometimes be seen within these hemorrhages. This is due to sedimented blood cell membranes and hemoglobin residues (deoxyhemoglobin, methemoglobin). Although there is no blood-brain barrier within the pituitary parenchyma, small linear or curved hyposignals can sometimes be found after intratumoral hemorrhage. These are caused by hemosiderin deposits (5,26,35,48).

Pituitary adenomas and pregnancy

The normal pituitary increases in height during pregnancy at a rate of 0.08 mm per week, implying a total increase of almost 3 mm during the whole pregnancy period. Pituitary adenomas also increase in volume during pregnancy (Figure 4). The normal pituitary has a longer Tl signal in pregnant women. Especially, increase of prolactinoma volume can be found after interruption of dopamine-agonist therapy in pregnancy. In pregnant prolactinoma patients, visual acuity and visual fields should be regularly checked and a follow-up MRI can be considered in specific situations (11,18,19,32)

Involvement of the cavernous sinus

Involvement of the cavernous sinus significantly affects the prognosis of pituitary adenomas. However, compression and infiltration of the cavernous sinus are difficult to differentiate (Figures 8, 9). Complete encircling of the intra-cavernous carotid artery by the tumor is the best sign of cavernous sinus involvement. Cavernous sinus involvement can particularly be ruled out when a strip of normal pituitary tissue can be identified between the tumor and the cavernous sinus. Large pituitary adenomas can apply pressure onto the cavernous sinus and cause convex deviation of its external wan without signs of infiltration. In case of massive infiltration, the cavernous sinus' intensity is identical to that of the intrasellar tumor on T1-weighted images, before and after gadolinium injection, as well as on T2-weighted images (1,4,21,38,39).

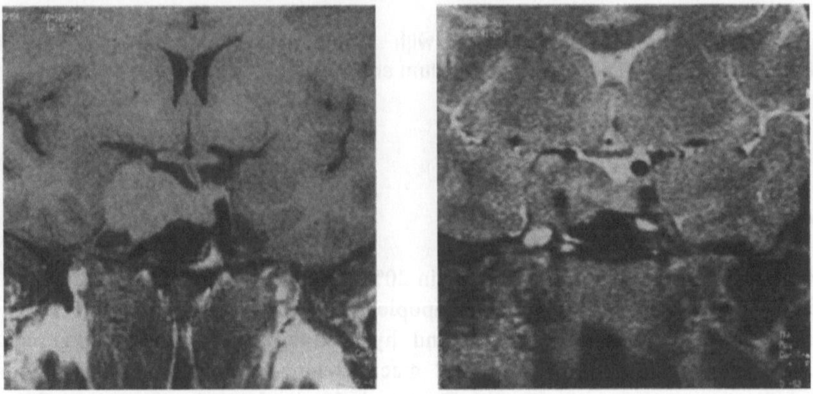

Figure 9. 40-year-old woman with active acromegaly.
Left: coronal spin-echo T1-weighted image Right: T2-weighted image
Pituitary adenoma with right intrasellar and mainly intracavernous extension. The right intracavernous internal carotid artery is completely encased by tumor tissue shown as an abnormal signal on the T1- and T2-weighted images. Note the convexity of the external limit of the cavernous sinus. The pituitary stalk is deviated to the tumor-contralateral side

Aspects after surgery

After transsphenoidal resection of a pituitary adenoma, the surgical cavity is often filled with packing material. These materials usually absorb blood and other secretory fluids. The presence of packing material, secretions and perhaps of periadenomatous adherences usually keeps the surgical cavity from collapsing in the days to weeks following surgery. Blood, secretions and packing material are slowly resorbed over the following 2 to 3 months (Figure 10). Still some fragments of blood-impregnated material can be found in the surgical cavity at this time. If the sellar diaphragm was torn at surgery, fat or muscle implants are usually inserted to prevent formation of a cerebrospinal fluid (CSF) fistula. However, their resorption takes much longer. Implanted fat slowly involutes and may produce a hypersignal on T1-weighted images up to 2 to 3 years after surgery

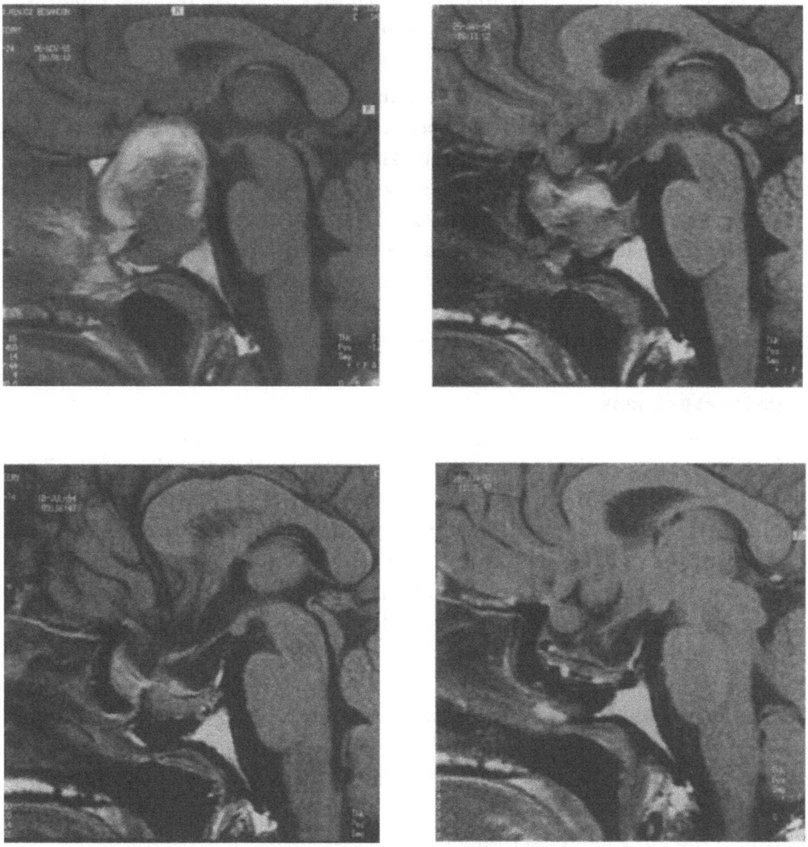

Figure 10. The same patient as in Figure 6.
Top left: sagittal T1-weighted image, 7 days after pituitary surgery
The upper rims of the lesion have not yet collapsed and the optic chiasm remains elevated. The surgical cavity has a heterogeneous aspect. Filling material has been implanted in the sellar fossa and muscle has been implanted in the sphenoid sinus because of a dural tear. The sellar floor has been restored with a part of the vomer. Apart from the material implanted by the surgeon, the surgical cavity is filled with blood and secretions.
Top right: sagittal T1-weighted image, 3 months after surgery.
The suprasellar component has collapsed. The optic chiasm is no longer compressed. Some blood remains visible as hyperintense material. The sella turcica is still filled with heterogeneous material.
Bottom left: sagittal T1-weighted image, 9 months after surgery.
The height of the intrasellar contents has further decreased.
Bottom right: Follow up MRI at 2 and a half years postoperatively, showing intrasellar expansion of the subarachnoid spaces and herniation of the rectus gyrus at the front part of the sella turcica. The sellar contents remain heterogeneous. The hypointense linear elements correspond to the restored sellar floor.

A postoperative follow-up MRI, 2 or 3 months after surgery is very useful to monitor further development of an adenoma remnant. An early MRI made 48 hours after surgery, checks for potential complications and may visualize residual tumor, usually appearing as a mass of identical intensity as the adenoma before surgery and commonly occupying a peripheral part of the space previously occupied by the complete adenoma. These early investigations also prove very helpful for the interpretation of follow-up MR studies. At this early stage the remaining normal pituitary tissue can be well characterized. This usually has an asymmetrical form, and at the base of the deviated hypophyseal stalk, a hypersignal caused by ectopic location of ADH secretion is frequently observed. The follow-up MRI at 2 or 3 months is essential to check for potential recurrence, which usually appears as a rounded or convex mass that is isointense with the initial tumor (40,42,44).

Other hypothalamic-pituitary pathologies

Craniopharyngiomas

Craniopharyngiomas arise from epithelial remnants of Rathke's pouch. They are almost invariably located in the optochiasmatic cistern. Frequently they extend into the sella. More than 50% of all craniopharyngiomas are first diagnosed in children, their peak incidence being between the ages of 5 and 10 years. A second peak can be found in adults aged 40 to 60 years. Both, their shape and size varies. Two categories of craniopharyngiomas can be distinguished: adamantinomatous and squamopapillary craniopharyngiomas (54,92).

Adamantinomatous craniopharyngiomas

Adamantinomatous craniopharyngiomas are classically described as suprasellar masses in pediatric patients and usually in boys. These are the most frequent occurring type of craniopharyngiomas. They present with symptoms of increased intracranial pressure, growth failure, visual disturbances and diabetes insipidus, but precocious puberty never occurs. Adamantinornatous craniopharyngiomas are polycyclical and typically contain cystic, calcified, and parenchymal parts (64,69,85,87,104). Cysts have been found in 90% of cases. These cysts contain cholesterol, triglycerids, methemoglobin, proteins and squamous epithelial cells. The signal intensity of cysts is mainly influenced by the protein content, usually being greater than or equal to 90 g/l and by the presence of unbound methemoglobin. However, cholesterol and triglycerids concentrations have little effect on the MR signal (51). A hypersignal on Tl-weighted images eliciting "motor oil" content is frequently found. Clear cysts and hypointense on Tl-weighted images. They can present as either hypo- or hyperintense signals on T2-weighted images. The parenchymal part of the craniopharyngioma and the walls of the cyst enhance with. Sometimes a complete or incomplete calcified ring can be found. Calcifications can be found in 90% of cases. CT may better demonstrate these. Although adamantinomatous craniopharyngiomas are usually encapsulated, they can extend anteriorly towards the optic chiasm, upward towards the third ventricle and especially posteriorly behind the optic chiasm. MRI plays an important role for assessment of tumor extension and for planning of the surgical access route. In 9-59% of cases, adamantinomatous craniopharyngiomas recur up to 30 years after first surgery. Their treatment consists of surgical resection and/or radiotherapy. The overall long-term prognosis is good. Patients usually require pituitary hormonal replacement therapy.

Squamopapillary craniopharyngiomas

Squamopapillary craniopharyngiomas generally affect young adults. Their aspect is that of a rounded mass which can either be solid or both solid and cystic. They rarely have calcifications and frequently are located within the third ventricle. These tumors appear hypointense on Tl-weighted images and more or less hyperintense on T2-weighted images. They show particularly intense gadolinium-enhancement, although this is mostly not homogeneous, because of necrotic areas. This type of tumor is encapsulated, and can be easily cleaved. Squamopapillary craniopharyngiomas show less frequent recurrences than adamantinomatous craniopharyngiomas.

Rathke's cleft cysts

Symptomatic forms of Rathke's cleft cysts are less common than craniopharyngiomas. They can be diagnosed at any age. Their origin is identical to that of craniopharyngiomas. They arise from squamous epithelial remnants of Rathke's pouch, but their walls only have a single layer of epithelium. Typically, the cysts contain mucous fluid. Less frequently, serous fluid or cellular remnants are found. They are rarely calcified. Most of these cysts are small and asymptomatic and they are usually incidentally discovered on a MRI. They can also show spontaneous involution. CT densities and MR signals of Rathke's cleft cysts reflect the cyst's chemical composition (53,75,79,83,91,98,106) (Figures 11, 12).

Mucous cysts appear hyperintense on both Tl- and T2-weighted images. Axial sections on Tl-weighted images are essential to differentiate cysts from the posterior pituitary. Using MRI, Rathke's cleft cysts may be difficult to distinguish from a hemorrhagic microadenoma and differentiation from cystic craniopharyngiomas is almost impossible. In these cases, only careful histological examination of the cyst walls can lead to an accurate diagnosis.

Cysts containing serous fluid are isointense to CSF while cysts containing cellular remnants resemble solid tumors. Rathke's cleft cysts generally do not enhance with gadolinium but a thin margin of enhancement may appear. Symptomatic cysts are either treated with drainage or surgical resection (74,99). They usually are non-invasive and do not recur often, thereby contrasting with the local aggressive behavior of craniopharyngiomas

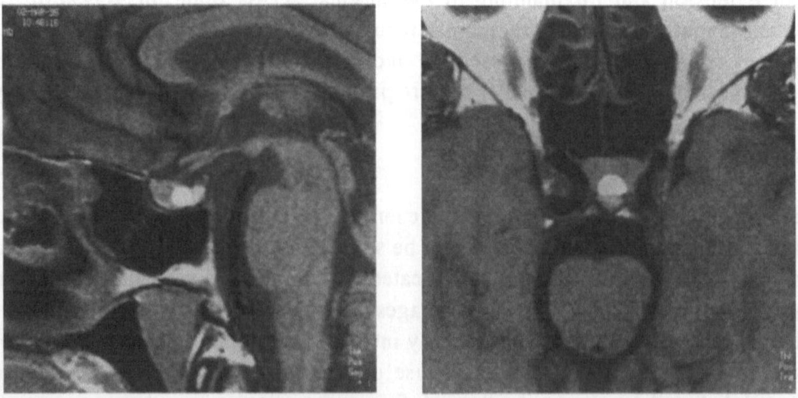

Figure 11. 41-year-old-woman with oligomenorrhea and slight hyperprolactinemia. Left: sagittal. Right: axial T1-weighted spin-echo images.
A round hyperintense intrasellar lesion is demonstrated in the midline, just in front of the posterior lobe. These findings are highly suggestive of a Rathke's cleft cyst.

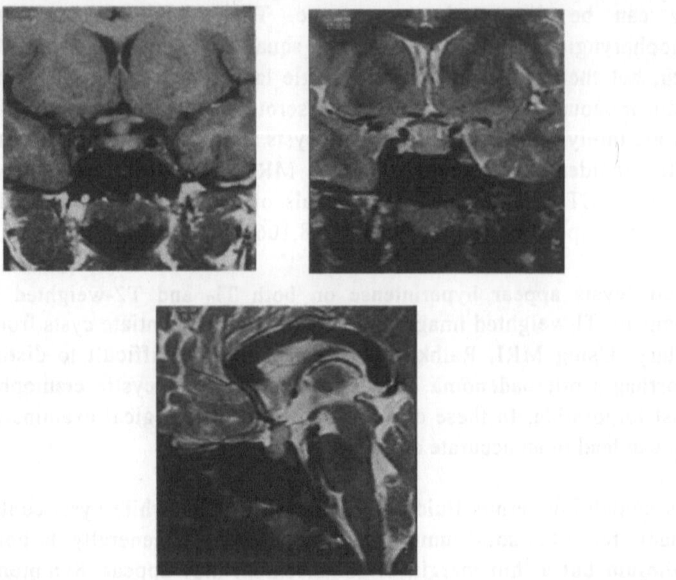

Figure 12. 13-year-old-girl. A supra- and intrasellar lesion was demonstrated, 4 years earlier, on a MRI performed for headaches, obesity and polyphagia. There was no endocrine dysfunction.
Follow-up MRI demonstrated a progressive increase in the size of the lesion.
Top left: coronal T1-weighted spin-echo image. Top right: coronal T2-weighted turbo spin-echo image. Bottom: sagittal T2-weighted turbo spin-echo image.
A hyperintense lesion is shown posteriorly in the sellar fossa with suprasellar extension reaching the inferior aspect of the optic chiasm. Tentative diagnoses were craniopharyngioma or Rathke's cleft cyst. At surgery a Rathke's cleft cyst with mucoid content was found.

Meningiomas

Approximately 10% of all meningiomas are located in the sella turcica. They can be located on the tuberculum sellae, the anterior clinoid process, the lesser wing of the sphenoid, the greater wing of the sphenoid, or the cavernous sinus (58). Meningiomas of the planum sphenoidale or the optic sulcus can extend backwards into the optochiasmatic cistern or downwards into the sella. Meningiomas are slow-growing tumors. Typical symptoms are visual field defects, ophthalmoplegia or exophthalmia. Meningiomas appear isointense with white matter on T1-weighted images and only rarely hypointense. On T2-weighted images, 50% of all meningiomas appears isointense, while 40% appears hyperintense. Such signal characteristics stress the need for indirect signs, such as mass effect, peri-lesional edema, hyperostosis and the visualization of CSF trapped between the tumor and the brain parenchyma. The tumor is best delineated after gadolinium injection. Its enhancement is intense and homogeneous, and the neighboring dura mater often appears thickened (Figure 13). Such changes in the dura mater, and more specifically the classically described dural tail, were long considered pathognomonic of meningiomas. Recently, however, dural tails have also been described in association with certain inflammatory diseases of the pituitary gland like lymphocytic adenohypophysitis and even with pituitary macroadenomas. Dynamic imaging may prove helpful for identifying normal pituitary tissue below the tumor, especially with large meningiomas of the jugum sphenoidale and of the optic sulcus that extend backwards and cover the sella turcica (101). Large meningiomas of the cavernous sinus often extend into the sella and displace the normal pituitary gland laterally and upwards. A second intention CT investigation can demonstrate bony changes and intratumoral calcifications, which, in certain cases, become conclusive arguments in favor of the diagnosis.

Chiasmatic and hypothalamic gliomas

Chiasmatic and hypothalamic gliomas are diagnosed within the first 10 years of life in 75% of cases. When chiasmatic gliomas are voluminous, they are often difficult to distinguish from hypothalamic gliomas, although they definitely are separate entities.

Chiasmatic gliomas

While sporadic cases do exist, chiasmatic gliomas are most often seen in relation with neurofibromatosis type I or von Recklinghausen's disease. Clinical signs are local skin pigmentations (café-au-lait spots) and visual complaints rather than endocrine dysfunctions. The tumor is isointense relative to the cerebral parenchyma on T1-weighted images and discretely hyperintense on T2-weighted images (Figure 14). The enhancement is variable. Characteristic signs are involvement of the optic nerves and lack of cystic components (55).

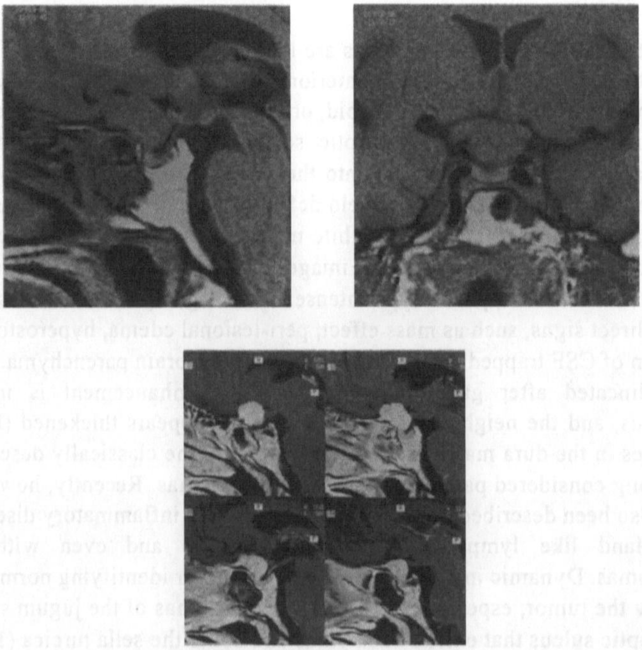

Figure 13. 49-year-old-man with recent loss of bilateral visual fields. Top left: sagittal T1-weighted spin-echo MR image. Top right: coronal T1-weighted spin-echo MR image. Bottom: sagittal T1-weighted spin-echo MR image after gadolinium injection.
A pre-sellar lesion inserted on the optic sulcus, enhancing markedly after gadolinium with thickening of the dura of the optic sulcus and planum sphenoidale is shown. The pituitary gland appears normal. These findings are pathognomonic for a pre-sellar meningioma.

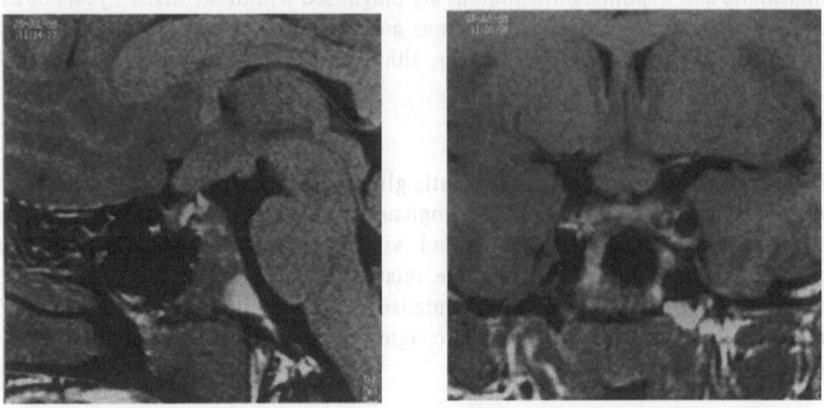

Figure 14. 13-year-old boy with neurofibromatosis type I and visual loss.
Left: sagittal T1-weighted spin-echo image. Right: coronal T1-weighted spin-echo image.
Images show thickening of the optic chiasm, but no involvement of the optic nerves.

Hypothalamic Gliomas

Hypothalamic gliomas arise from the floor of the third ventricle and are of ten presenting with diencephalic cachexia or Russel's syndrome. MR images feature identical signals as in chiasmatic gliomas, but cysts are more common (86).

Germinomas

Germinomas originate from germinal cells. They represent 0.5 to 2% of primitive cerebral tumors. Approximately 20% of germinomas are located within the sellar area. Other locations include the pineal region and the posterior aspect of the third ventricle. Suprasellar germinomas are either metastatic pineal tumors or primitive tumors, as bifocal occurrence has been reported. Germinomas affect children and young adults, aged 5 to 25, with a male predominance for pineal tumors. They often present with diabetes insipidus, which is indicative for involvement of the floor and walls of the third ventricle. Other clinical signs include visual field defects, optic nerve atrophy and increased intracranial pressure secondary to hydrocephalus, anterior pituitary deficiency, and diplopia. The diagnosis can be confirmed by analyzing CSF for the presence of tumor cells and by elevated levels of β-HCG in the blood or CSF. The aspect of germinomas is that of a mass in the optochiasmatic cistern, in the midline, centered on the pituitary stalk or located immediately behind it (66,99). Their MRI signal is homogeneous, which is a major difference with craniopharyngiomas, discretely hypointense on T1- and hyperintense on T2-weighted images. Intratumoral cysts are rare. The posterior pituitary does not produce a hypersignal on Tl-weighted images when diabetes insipidus is present. It is important to remember that clinical signs sometimes precede imaging features by several years and, therefore, that it is essential to continue monitoring children with diabetes insipidus with initial normal MRI studies.

Lymphocytic adenohypophysitis

Lymphocytic adenohypophysitis is an inflammatory process associated with lymphocytic infiltration of the pituitary gland. It usually occurs during pregnancy or in the post-natal period and presents with partial or complete hypopituitarism in association with visual field defects (71,88). Lymphocytic adenohypophysitis may also exclusively involve the posterior lobe and pituitary stalk. Granulomatous hypophysitis is a rare disorder, in which there are no lymphoid follicles but nodules of histiocytes and giant multinucleated cells at pathology.

Imaging can contribute to the diagnosis. The sella turcica often undergoes little modification in lymphocytic adenohypophysitis, whereas it appears deformed, enlarged and eroded in pituitary macroadenomas. Tl-weighted images of lymphocytic adenohypophysitis show a relatively hypointense signal, while the hypersignal demonstrated by the posterior lobe usually is unaltered. Most importantly, enhancement of the mass is both more intense and larger as compared with pituitary macroadenomas (Figure 15). Enhancement of the dura mater usually occurs, but is non-specific (50,78,88,94).

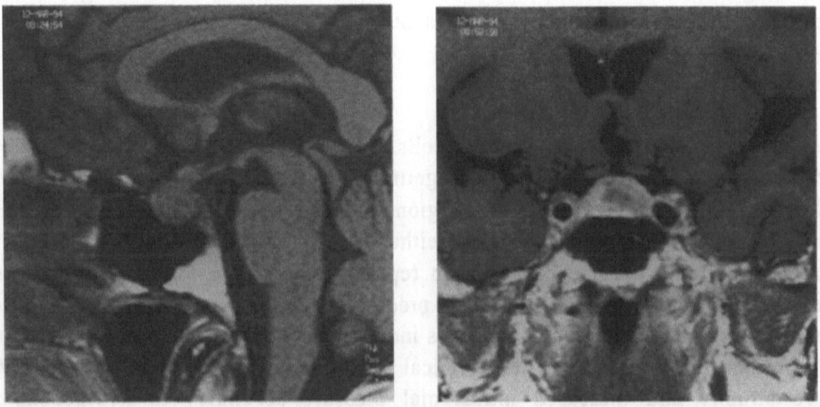

Figure 15. 7O-year-old woman presenting with hypopituitarism and an inflammatory syndrome.
Left: sagittal T1-weighted spin-echo image. Right: coronal T1-weighted spin-echo image after gadolinium.
Images show upward bulging of the pituitary gland and loss of the posterior lobe hypersignal. There is heterogeneous enhancement of the gland after gadolinium injection. Therapy with glucocorticoids resulted in shrinkage of the enlarged pituitary gland (not shown). The most likely diagnosis was: lymphocytic adenohypophysitis

Pituitary Metastases

Pituitary metastases account for about l% of sellar masses. They have been found both in the pituitary stalk and the posterior lobe. In decreasing order of frequency, breast, lung, stomach, and uterus cancer in females and lung, prostate, bladder, stomach and pancreas cancer in males may metastasize to the pituitary. In more than half the case in females, the primary cancer is breast cancer. Although pituitary metastases can be asymptomatic, they often present with diabetes insipidus caused by interruption of the hypothalamic-pituitary tract. The prognosis of a patient with a pituitary or pituitary stalk metastasis is poor, as it reflects diffuse dissemination of cancer. Most pituitary metastases are located intra- and suprasellar. Metastases with exclusively intrasellar localization have occasionally been found. The Tl-weighted MR image of a metastasis is isointense relative to the cerebral parenchyma and moderately hyperintense on T2-weighted images. Gadolinium enhancement varies (95).

Hamartomas of the tuber cinereum

Ectopic masses of normal nervous tissue, so-called "hamartomas" have a characteristic location in the interpeduncular cistern, behind the optic chiasm and pituitary stalk, and in front of the basilar artery. They present almost uniformly in early puberty in association with gelastic episodes. Hamartomas are well-delineated oval, sessile or pedunculated masses on the tuber cinereum. They display identical MR signals as brain parenchyma, but may demonstrate a discrete hypersignal on T2-weighted images. They do not enhance with gadolinium (57,59,62,67). These lesions are stable and non-progressive. The only differential diagnosis is hypothalamic glioma, especially when the lesion is hyperintense on T2-weighted images.

Empty sella syndrome

Empty sella is the result of a dehiscent sellar diaphragm due to intrasellar extension of the subarachnoid spaces. Consequently, the pituitary gland is pressed against the floor and the dorsum of the sella turcica. Primitive empty sella is caused by sellar diaphragm deficiency. This should be distinguished from secondary empty sella, which is caused by necrosis of the pituitary gland during the post-partum period as in Sheehan's syndrome, after medical shrinkage of the tumor, or after surgical removal of a pituitary tumor. Empty sella is often an accidental discovery in menopausal multiparous women. Classical symptoms are headaches, obesity, endocrine dysfunction (hyperprolactinemia, anterior pituitary deficiency), rhinorrhea, and campimetrical deficit. The MR diagnosis is usually easy as the intrasellar liquid content is well demonstrated on Tl- and T2-weighted images. Artifacts due to liquid flow on fast Spin-echo T2-weighted images can create mass images within the optochiasmatic cistern leading to an erroneous interpretation and the false diagnosis of empty sella. Sagittal sections are preferred, as they visualize the entire pituitary stalk in its usual median position. The sellar fossa may appear enlarged and the pituitary gland is thin and pressed against the sellar floor. Ptosis of the optic chiasm may be observed. The pituitary stalk must be identified within the optochiasmatic cistern in order to exclude an intrasellar cyst. An asymmetrical sella along with a deviated pituitary stalk is strongly suggestive of secondary empty sella. The posterior pituitary may be less frequently visualized in association with empty sella.

Central diabetes insipidus

Central diabetes insipidus is a fluid balance disorder characterized by production of excessive amounts of very dilute urine. Nephrogenic diabetes insipidus is the result of a congenital or acquired defect in the renal tubules, whereas central diabetes insipidus is due to the inappropriate secretion of ADH secondary to a hypothalamic-pituitary disorder. Cranial trauma or surgery in the pituitary area is responsible for approximately 50% of cases of central diabetes insipidus, while 25% is idiopathic. Other causes of diabetes insipidus include sellar tumors (like metastases and Christmas), hypothalamic tumors (like germinomas and hypothalamic gliomas) and granulomas (like histiocytosis X, sarcoidosis or tuberculosis) (15). Also a rare form of congenital central diabetes insipidus has been reported. In almost all cases of central diabetes insipidus, the Tl hypersignal of the posterior lobe is absent (56,65,81,97,102). Although the clinical presentation of patients with primary polydipsia overlaps that of diabetes insipidus, the posterior lobe remains hyperintense on T1-weighted images in primary polydipsia.

Traumatic rupture of the pituitary stalk

In traumatic rupture of the pituitary stalk, MR images fail to visualize the hypophyseal stalk and an ectopic neurohypophysis can be demonstrated if the rupture occurred below the middle third of the pituitary stalk (68).

Histiocytosis X, Langerhans cell histiocytosis or eosinophilic granuloma

Histiocytosis X, also called Langerhans cell histiocytosis or eosinophilic granuloma is characterized by the pathologic proliferation of histiocytes. The benign unifocal form usually presents with a solitary lytic bone lesion without involvement of the hypothalamic-pituitary axis. In contrast, the much more aggressive multifocal form which mainly occurs in children presents as a classic triad of diabetes insipidus, exophthalmia, and lytic bone lesions (Hand-Schüller-Christian disease). In these cases, granulomas can be demonstrated in the hypothalamus and pituitary stalk (Figure 16). MRI can demonstrate thickening of the pituitary stalk together with an enhanced hypothalamus (80,90,103).

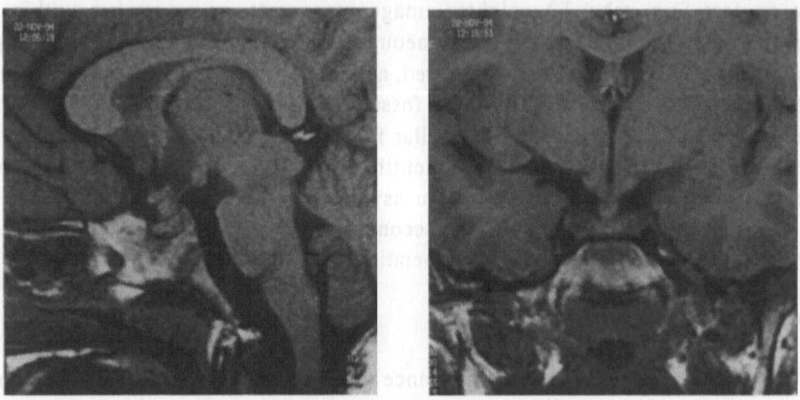

Figure 16. 6-year-old girl with polyuria and polydipsia for 3 months. A radiograph of the left hand showed a lytic phalange lesion (not shown).
Left: sagittal T1-weighted spin-echo image. Right: coronal T1-weighted spin-echo image. Images show absence of the posterior lobe hypersignal and thickening of the pituitary stalk suggestive of granuloma, likely histiocytosis X.

Sarcoidosis

Sarcoidosis is a chronic granulomatous disease involving several organs, but showing particular preference for the lungs and mediastinal lymph nodes. Five per cent of patients affected by pulmonary sarcoidosis develop central disorders including cranial nerve disorders and/or hypothalamic-pituitary dysfunction like diabetes insipidus or anterior pituitary deficiencies. MRI can show a thickened pituitary stalk, absence of the posterior lobe hypersignal, a hypothalamic mass, or leptomeningitis of the skull base (61,70,93,96).

Non-tumoral pediatric hypopituitarism

OH deficiency in children results in growth retardation, dentition defects and bone maturation defects. This disorder affects twice as many boys as girls. In almost half the cases, there is a history of perinatal trauma, anoxia, hypoxia, or breech presentation. Pituitary imaging is normal in 60% of cases. In the remaining 40%, a hypoplastic or aplastic anterior pituitary lobe may be demonstrated. However, it should be remembered that demonstration of an isolated hypoplastic anterior pituitary lobe has poor diagnostic value. A correlation between the size of the anterior pituitary and OH deficiency has not been demonstrated. MR may also show a hypoplastic or aplastic pituitary stalk, which is either isolated or associated with an ectopic posterior pituitary. The ectopic posterior pituitary can be demonstrated as a rounded hyperintense signal hanging from the median eminence on Tl-weighted images (48,49,52,73,76,82,84,89) (Figure 17). Non-tumoral pediatric hypopituitarism may be associated with other midline malformations, like total or partial agenesis of the corpus callosum and septal agenesis or hypoplasia (De Morsier's septooptic pituitary dysplasia).

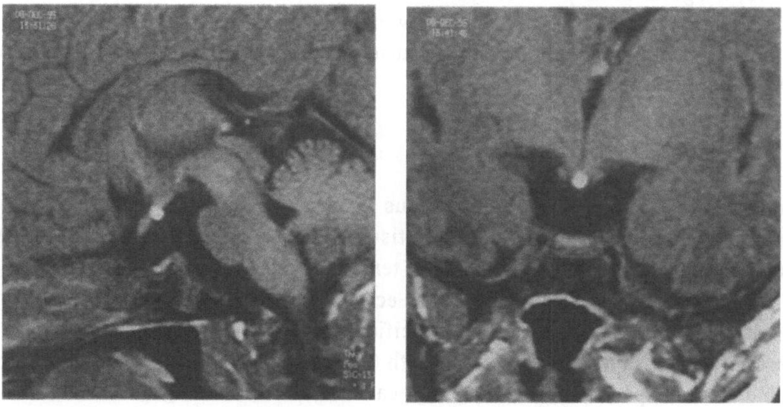

Figure 17. 3-week-old newborn with GH deficiency.
Left: sagittal T1-weighted spin-echo MR image. Right: coronal T1-weighted spin-echo MR image.
Images show hypoplasia of the anterior pituitary lobe (maximal height: 1,5 mm). The hypersignal on the T1-weighted sequence of the anterior lobe is physiological in the newborn. The pituitary stalk is absent. An ectopic posterior lobe is located at the level of the median eminence.

Rare intra- and suprasellar lesions

Pituitary abscesses

Infection can spread via the hematogenic dissemination or from an adjacent infection focus in the cavernous sinus or sphenoid bone. Generally, there is an underlying pituitary lesion such as a pituitary adenoma, craniopharyngioma, or Rathke's cleft cyst. MRI of a pituitary abscess shows a rounded mass in the pituitary region. Its center produces a hyposignal on Tl-weighted images and gadolinium-enhancement delineates a peripheral margins.

Choristomas

Choristomas also called granular cell tumors or Abrikossof's tumors are primitive pituitary tumors. Small choristomas are often discovered at autopsy. Small choristomas are asymptomatic, but they can cause diabetes insipidus when they grow. Their aspect is that of an intrasellar mass located either posteriorly or in the infundibulum (60). They may become a surgical hazard because they are highly vascularized.

Epidermoid cysts

Epidermoid cysts are usually epithelial cysts containing squamous cells and keratin debris. They may be located within the optochiasmatic cistern. They most commonly are diagnosed in adults between the age of 40 and 60 years. MR images show a lobulated, irregular mass producing a signal very similar to that of CSF, but often a slight hypersignal on both T1- and T2-weighted images (100,105). They can be distinguished from arachnoid cysts because of their hyperdensity on the proton density-weighted images.

Dermoid cysts

Dermoid cysts have a less homogenous aspect on T1-weighted images than epidermoid cysts, since they include fatty tissue. This produces a marked hypersignal on the upper part of the image, which is of ten classified as an artifact due to chemical shift. The differential diagnosis is an ectopic posterior lobe, but the clinical presentation is completely different. Calcifications are often recognized. These are better identified with MR imaging than with CT scans. Dermoid cysts can rupture into the subarachnoid space and, subsequently, cause chemical meningitis.

Arachnoid cysts

Approximately 10% of arachnoid cysts are located within the optochiasmatic cistern. Their signal is identical to that of CSF in every sequence and a mass effect on the third ventricle can be shown (63,107). MR imaging of the CSF flow may prove helpful, as it will demonstrate stagnated fluid within the cyst. Most arachnoid cysts present in children with hydrocephalus. In older patients with no hydrocephalus, presenting symptoms include epileptic seizures, hypopituitarism, or signs caused by the compression of adjacent nervous structures.

Pathologies of the cavernous sinus

Meningiomas of the cavernous sinus

Meningiomas of the cavernous sinus generally present with oculomotor nerve palsies with an unpredictable course (like spontaneous remission, or deterioration during pregnancy) and/or exophthalmia. Pituitary dysfunction may also occur, depending on involvement of the sella. Bone changes are limited to signs of chronic increased pressure. Unlike meningiomas of the sphenoid lesser wing or jugum, hyperostosis and calcification are rare. The aspect is that of a mass in the cavernous sinus with a convex lateral wall and Gasser's ganglion can often not be identified. The tumor is homogenous, isointense relative to white matter on Tl-weighted images and either iso- or hypointense on T2-weighted images or rarely slightly hyperintense. Enhancement with gadolinium appears intense and homogeneous, and becomes more pronounced if dynamic imaging is used. The dura mater of both the lateral wall of the cavernous sinus and the free edge "of the tentorium are thickened. Posterior tumoral extension along the free border of the tentorium accounts for the non-specific "dural tail" aspect that can also appear in other tumoral pathologies such as metastases and lymphomas. The intracavernous part of the internal carotid artery is often encased in the tumor, which causes its lumen to become smaller (77).

Aneurysms

A variety of aneurysms may occur in the sellar area. The main variants are aneurysms of the intracavernous and supraclinoid parts of the internal carotid artery, of the anterior and posterior communicating arteries, and of the tip of the basilar artery. Aneurysms are well-delineated lesions with flow void on both Tl- and T2-weighted images. Their diagnosis may be difficult if the aneurysm is partially or completely thrombosed. In that case a lamellar hypersignal on Tl-weighted images will be found. Finally it is not unusual to visualize a hypointense ring of hemosiderin on T2-weighted images. MR Angiography should be considered for confirming the diagnosis.

Metastases

The most common primary cancers are breast and lung carcinomas. The MR images of these metastases show iso- or hypointense masses within the cavernous sinus on Tl-weighted images and hyperintense signals on T2-weighted images. Their enhancement with gadolinium is intense.

Rare tumors in the cavernous sinus

Neurinomas

Neurinomas of the trigeminal (Vth) nerve originate from Schwann cells of the sensitive root at its retrogasserian part. These neurinomas typically develop in a hourglass pattern around the petrosal apex. They usually present with neuralgia of the Vth nerve. MRI shows a well-delineated, rounded or lobulated mass that is iso- or hypointense on T1- and hyperintense on T2-weighted images. They enhance intensely with gadolinium (108).

Lymphomas

The cavernous sinus may be unilaterally or bilaterally infiltrated by lymphoma tissue, resulting in widening. Lymphomas show intense enhancement with gadolinium.

Epidermoid cysts

Epidermoid cysts may either have their primary localization in the cavernous sinus, or are extensions of cysts located on the petrosal apex. Because of their heterogeneity, these lesions produce a hyposignal on Tl-weighted images and a hypersignal on T2-weighted images. They do not enhance with gadolinium.

Cavernous hemangiomas

Hemangiomas are either iso-, or hypointense on Tl- and hyperintense on T2-weighted images. They appear homogenous and enhance intensely with gadolinium. The surrounding dura mater does not appear thickened (72). The differential diagnosis with meningiomas may be very difficult.

References

1. Ahmadi J, North CM, Segall HD, Zee CS, Weiss MH. Cavernous sinus invasion by pituitary adenomas. AJR Am J Roentgenol 1986;10:193
2. Barrou Z. Magnetic resonance imaging in Cushing disease. Prediction of surgical results Presse Med 1997;26:7.
3. Bonneville JF, Cattin F, Gorczyca W, Hardy J. Pituitary micro-adenomas: Early enhancement with dynamic CT -implications of arterial blood supply and potential importance. Radiology 1993;187:857.
4. Brami F, Roux FX, Leriche B, Kalamarides M. Invasion du sinus caverneux par les adénomes hypophysaires: mythe ou réalité. Journées françaises de radiologie. Paris, 17-23 Oct. 1995.
5. Brismon MH. Symptoms of pituitary apoplexy rapidly reversed with bromocriptine. J Neurosurg 1996;85:1153.
6. Colombo N, Loli P, Vignati F, Scialfa G. MR of corticotropin-secreting pituitary microadenomas. AJNR 1994;15:1591.
7. Davis PC, Hoffman JC Jr, Spencer T, et al. MR Imaging of pituitary adenoma: CT, clinical and surgical correlation. AJNR 1987;8:107.
8. Davis PC, Hoffman JC Jr, Malko JA, et al. Gadolinium-DTPA and MR imaging of pituitary adenoma: a preliminary report. AJNR 1987;8:817.
9. Davis PC, Gokhale KA, Josep GJ. Pituitary adenoma: correlation of half dose gadolinium enhanced MRI with surgical findings in 26 patients. Radiology 1991;180:779.
10. Davis PC, Hoffman JC Jr, Spencer T, Tindall GT, Braun IF.MR Imaging of pituitary adenoma: CT, clinical, and surgical correlation. AIR Am J Roentgenol 1987;195:797.
11. Dietemann JL, Portha C, Cattin F, Mollet E, Bonneville JF. CT Follow-up of microprolactinomas during bromocriptine-induced pregnancy. Neuroradiology 1983;25:133.
12. Doppman JL, Frank JA, Dwyer AJ, et al. Gadolinium DTPA enhanced MR imaging of ACTH-secreting microadenomas of the pituitary gland. J Comput Assist Tomogr 1988;12:728.
13. Dwyer AD, Frank JA, Doppman JL, et al. Pituitary adenomas in patients with Cushing disease: initial experience with Gd-DTPA-enhanced MR imaging. Radiology 1987:163:421.
14. El Gammal T, Brooks BS, Hoffman WH.MR imaging of the ectopic bright signal of posterior pituitary regeneration. AJNR 1989;10:323.
15. Elster AD. Modem imaging of pituitary. Radiology 1993;187:1.
16. Finelli DA, Kaufman B. Varied microcirculation of pituitary adenomas at rapid, dynamic contrast-enhanced MR imaging. Radiology 1993;189:205.
17. Genzell C, Wang CF. Outcome of pregnancy in women with pituitary adenoma. Fertil Steril 1979:31:363.
18. Goluboff LG, Ezrin C. Effect of pregnancy on the somatotroph and the prolactin cell of the human adenohypophysis. J Clin Endocrinol Metab 1969;29:1533.
19. Reschke K. Hyperthyroidism in TSH-producing hypophyseal adenoma. Dtsch Med Wochenschr 1997;122:150.
20. Knosp E, Kitz K, Steiner E, Matula CR. Pituitary adenomas with parasellar invasion Acta Neurochir 1991;53:65.
21. Kucharczyk W, Davis DO, Kelly WM, Sze G, Norman D, Newton TH. Pituitary adenomas: high-resolution MR imaging at 1.5 T. Radiology 1986;161:761.
22. Kucharczyk W, Bishop JE, Plewes DB, et al. Dynamic MR imaging of pituitary microadenomas with FSE T1-weighted shared view MRI. SMRM Annual Meeting 1993. New York.

23. Kucharczyk W, Bishop JE, Plewes DB, Keller MA, George s. Detection of pituitary microadenomas: comparison of dynamic keyhole fast spin-echo, unenhanced, and conventional contrast-enhanced MR imaging. AJNR 1994;163:671.
24. Kulkarni MV, Lee KF , McArdle CB, Yeakley JW, Haar FL. 1.5- T MR imaging of pituitary microadenomas: technical considerations and CT correlation. AJNR 1988;9:5.
25. Kyle CA, Laster RA, Burton EM, Sanford RA. Subacute pituitary apoplexy: MR and CT appearance. J Comput Assist Tomogr 1990;14:40.
26. Lundin P, Bergström K, Nyman R, Lundberg PO, Muhr C. Macroprolactinomas: serial MR imaging in long term bromocriptine therapy. AJNR 1992;13:1279.
27. Lundin P, Long-term octreotide therapy in growth hormone-secreting pituitary adenomas: evaluation with serial MR AJNR 1997;18:765.
28. Macpherson P, Hadley DM, Teasdale E, Teasdale G. Pituitary microadenomas: does gadolinium enhance their demonstration? Neuroradiology 1989;31:293.
29. Merran S. Prolactin Pituitary microadenoma. Presse Med 1997:26:395.
30. Miki Y, Matsuo M, Nishizawa S, et al. Pituitary adenomas and normal pituitary tissue: enhancement patterns on gadopentetate-enhanced MR images. Radiology 1990;177:35.
31. Molitch ME, Pregnancy and the hyperprolactinemic women. N Engl J Med 1985;312:1364.
32. Nakamura T, Schorner W, Bittner RC, et al. Value of paramagnetic contrast agent gadolinium-DTPA in the diagnosis of pituitary adenomas. Neuroradiology 1988:30:951.
33. Newton DR, Dillon WP, Norman D, Newton TH, Wilson CB. Gd-DTPA-enhanced MR imaging of pituitary adenomas. AJNR 1989;10:949.
34. Ostrov SG, Quencer RM, Hoffman JC, Davis PC, Hasso AN, David NJ. Hemorrhage within pituitary adenomas: how often associated with pituitary apoplexy syndrome? AJNR 1989;10:503.
35. Peck WW, Dillon WP, Norman D, Newton TH, Wilson CB. High-resolution MR imaging of microadenomas at 1.5 T: experience with Cushing disease. AJNR 1988;9:1085.
36. Pojunas KW, Daniels DL, Williams AL, Haughton VM. MR imaging of prolactin-secreting microadenomas. AJNR 1986;7:209.
37. Scotti G, Vu CV, Dillon WP, et al. MR imaging of cavernous sinus involvement by pituitary adenomas. AJNR 1988;9:657.
38. Scotti G, Yu CY, Dillon WP, et al. MRI of cavernous sinus invasion by pituitary adenomas. AJR Am J Roentgenol 1988;151:799.
39. Scotti G, Anzalone N, Triulzi F, Pieralli C, Parazzini C, Bozzi M. MR evaluation of post-surgical changed in transsphenoidal surgery for pituitary adenomas. Rivista di Neuroradiol 1991;4:57.
40. Stadnik T, Stevenaert A, Beckers A, Luypaert R, Buisseret T, Osteaux M. Pituitary microadenornas: diagnosis with two-and three -dimensional MR imaging at 1.5 T before and after injection of gadolinium. Radiology 1990;176:419.
41. Steiner E, Knosp E, Herold CJ, et al. Pituitary adenomas: findings of postoperative MR imaging. Radiology 1992;185:521.
42. Steiner E, Imhof H, Knosp E. Gd-DTPA-enhanced high-resolution MR imaging of pituitary adenomas. RadioGraphics 1989;9:587.
43. Teng MMH, Huang C, Chang T. The pituitary mass after transsphenoidal hypophysectomy. AJNR 1988;9:23.
44. Van de Straete S. Aggressive pituitary macroadenoma: CT and MR appearances. J Belge Radiol 1996;76:255.
45. Weissbuch SS. Explanation and implications of MR signal changes within pituitary adenomas after bromocriptine therapy. AJNR 1986;7:214.
46. Wolpert SM. The radiology of pituitary adenomas. Semin Roentgenol 1984;19:53.

47. Youssem DM, Arrington JA, Zinreich SJ, Kumar Al, Bryan RN. Pituitary adenomas: possible role of bromocriptine in intratumoral hemorrhage. Radiology 1989;170:239.
48. Abrahams JJ, Trefelner E, Boulware SD. Idiopathic growth hormone deficiency: MR findings in 35 patients. AJR Am J Roentgenol 1991;156:599.
49. Adamsbaum C, Houang M, Andre C, Richard I, Ginisty D, Chaussain JL, G Kalifa. Imagerie par résonance magnétique des hypopituitarismes non tumoraux de l'enfant. Rev Im Med 1993;5:251.
50. Ahmadi J, Meyers G, Segall HD, Sharma OP, Hinton DR. Lymphocytic adenohypophysitis: contrast-enhanced MR imaging in five cases. Radiology 1995;195:30.
51. Ahmadi J, Destian S, Apuzzo MLJ, Segall HD, Zee CS. Cystic fluid in craniopharyngiomas: MR imaging and quantitative analysis. Radiology 1992; 182:783.
52. Argyropoulou M, Perignon F, Brauner R, Brunelle F. Magnetic resonance imaging in the diagnosis of growth hormone deficiency. J Pediatr 1992;120:886.
53. Asari S, Ito T, Tsuchida S, Tsutsui T. MR appearance and cyst content of Rathke cleft cysts. J Comp Assist Tomogr 1990;14:532.
54. Atlas SW. The sella turcica and parasellar region. Kucharczyk W, Montanera WJ, Becker LE in: Magnetic Resonance Imaging of the Brain and Spine. 2nd ed. Philadelphia, Pa: Lippincott-Raven 1996.
55. Bognanno IR, Edwards MK, Lee TA, et al. Cranial MR imaging in neurofibromatosis. AJNR 1988;9:461
56. Bourlière B, Kalifa G, Chausain JL, Demange P, Sellier N. IRM et diabète insipide. Valeur de l'hypersignal de la région sellaire. Rev lm Med 1990;2:373.
57. Boyko OB, Curnes JT, Oakes WJ, Burger PC. Hamartomas of the tuber cinereum: CT MR and pathologic findings. AJNR 1991;12:309.
58. Bradac B, Riva A, Schoiner W, Stura G. Cavernous sinus meningiomas: an MRI study. Neuroradiology 1987;29:578.
59. Burton EM, Ball WS, Crane K, Dolan LM. Hamartomas of tuber cinereum: comparison of MR and CT findings in 4 cases. AJNR 1989;10:497.
60. Cone L, Srinivasan M, Romanul FCA. Granular cell tumor (choristoma) of the neurohypophysis: two cases and a review of the literature. AJNR 1990;11:403.
61. Cooper SD, Brady MB, Williams JP , et al. Neurosarcoidosis: evaluation using CT and MRI. J Comput Assist Tomogr 1988;12:96.
62. Diebler C. Ponsot G. Hamartomas of the tuber cinereum. Neuroradiology 1983;25:93.
63. Dietemann JL, Schultz A, Zollner G, Sanoussi S, Maitrot D, Buchheit F. lntrasellar arachnoid cysts: computed tomography and MRI. A propos de 2 cas. J Neuroradiol 1997:24:168.
64. Freeman MP, Kessler RM, Allen JH, Price AC. Craniopharyngioma CT and MR imaging in nine cases. J Comput Assist Tomogr 1987;11:810.
65. Fujisawa I, Nishimura K, Asato R, et al. Posterior lobe of the pituitary in diabetes insipidus: MR findings. J Comput Assist Tomogr 1987;11:221.
66. Fujisawa I, Asato R, Okumura R, et al. Magnetic resonance imaging of neurohypophyseal germinomas. Cancer 1991;68:1009.
67. Hahn Fl, Leibrock LG, Huseman CA, Makos MM. The MR appearance of hypothalamic hamartoma. Neuroradiology 1988;30:65.
68. Halimi P, Sigal R, Doyon D, et al. Post-traumatic diabetes insipidus: MR demonstration of pituitary stalk rupture. J Comput Assist Tomogr 1988;12:135.
69. Harwood-Nash DC. Neuroimaging of childhood craniopharyngioma. Pediatr Neurosurg 1994;21(suppl 1):2.
70. Hayes WS, Sherman JL, Stem BJ, Citrin CM, Pulaski PD. MR and CT evaluation of intracranial sarcoidosis. AJR Am J Roentgenol 987;149:1043.

71. Higuchi M, Arita N, Mori S, et al. Pituitary granuloma and chronic inflammation of hypophysis: clinical and immunohistochemical studies. Acta Neurochir 1993;121:152.
72. Katayama Y, Tsubokova T, Miyazaki S, Yoshida K, Himi K. Magnetic resonance imaging of cavernous sinus cavernous hemangiomas. Neuroradiology 1991;33:118.
73. Kelly WM, Kucharczyk W, Kucharczyk J, Kjos B, Peck WW, Norman M, Newton TH Posterior pituitary ectopia: an MR feature of pituitary dwarfism. AJNR 1988;9:453.
74. Kleinschmidt-DeMasters BK, Lillehei KO, Stears JC. The pathologic, surgical, and MR spectrum of Rathke cleft cysts. Surg Neurol 1995;44:19.
75. Kucharczyk W, Peck WW, Kelly WM, Norman D, Newton TH. Rathke cleft cysts: CT, MR imaging and pathologic features. Radiology 1987;165:491.
76. Kuroiwa T, Okabe Y, Hasuo K, Yasumori K, Mizushima A, Masuda K. MR imaging of pituitary dwarfism. AJNR 1991;12:161.
77. Lanzino G, Hirsch WL, Pomonis S, Sen CN, Sekhar LN. Cavernous sinus tumors: neuroradiologic and neurosurgical considerations on 150 operated cases. Neurosurg Sci 1992;36:183.
78. Levine SN, Benzel EC, Fowler MR, Shroyer JV, Mirfakhraee Mo Lymphocytic hypophysitis: clinical, radiological and magnetic resonance imaging characterization. Neurosurgery 1988;22:937.
79. Maggio WW, Cail WS, Brookman IR, Persing JA, Jane JA. Rathke's cleft cyst: computed tomographic and magnetic resonance imaging appearances. Neurosurgery 1987;21:60.
80. Maghnie M, Arico M, Villa A, et al. MR of the hypothalamic pituitary axis in Langerhans cell histiocytosis. AJNR 1992;13:1365.
81. Maghnie M, Genovese E, Bernasconi S, Binda S, Arico M. Persistent high MR signal of the posterior pituitary gland in central diabetes insipidus. AJNR 1997;18:1749.
82. Mizushima K, Masuda K. MR imaging of pituitary dwarfism. AJNR 1991;12:161
83. Nemoto Y, Inoue Y, Fukuda T, et al. MR appearance of Rathke's cleft cysts. Neuroradiology 1988;30:155.
84. Pellini C, Dinatale B, De Angelis R, Bressani N, Scotti G, Triulzi F, Chiumello G. Growth hormone deficiency in children: role of magnetic resonance imaging in assessing aetiopathogenesis and prognosis in idiopathic hypopituitarism. Eur J Pediatr 1990;149:536.
85. Pigeau I, Sigal R, Halimi P, Comoy J, Doyon D. MRI features of craniopharyngiomas at 1.5 tesla: a series of 13 cases. J Neuroradiol 1988;15:276.
86. Poussaint TY, Barnes PD, Nichols K, Anthony DC, Cohen L, Tarbell NJ, Goumnerova L. Diencephalic syndrome: clinical features and imaging findings. AJNR 1997:18:1499.
87. Pusey E, Kortman KB, Flannigan BD, Tsuruda J, Bradley WO. MR of craniopharyngiomas: tumor delineation and characterization. AJNR 1987;8:439.
88. Quencer RM. Lymphocytic adenohypophysitis: autoimmune disorder of the pituitary gland. AJNR 1980;1:343.
89. Root W. Magnetic resonance imaging in hypopituitarism. J Clin Endocrinol Metab 1991;72:10.
90. Rosenfield NS, Abrahams J, Komp D. Brain MR in patients with Langerhans cell histiocytosis: findings and enhancement with Gd-DTPA. Pediatr Radial 1990;20:433.
91. Ross DA, Norman D, Wilson CB. Radiologic characteristics and results of surgical management of Rathke's cleft cysts in 43 patients. Neurosurgery 1992;30:173.
92. Sartoretti-Schefer S, Wichmann W, Aguzzi A, Valavanis A. MR differentiation of adamantinous and squamous-papillary craniopharyngiomas. AJNR 1997;18:77.
93. Sato N, Sze G, Kim JH. Cystic pituitary mass in neurosarcoidosis. AJNR 1997;18:1182
94. Sato N, Sze G, Endo K. Hypophysitis: endocrinologic and dynamic MR findings. AJNR 1998;19:439.

95. Schubiger O, Haller D. Metastases to the pituitary-hypothalamic axis. Neuroradiology 1992;34:131.
96. Seltzer S, Mark AS, Atlas SW. CNS sarcoidosis: evaluation with contrast-enhanced MR imaging. AJNR 1991;12:1227.
97. Silva MB, Carlier R, Parlier-Cuau C, Schaison G, Doyon D. Imagerie normale et pathologique de la tige pituitaire. J Radiol 1993;74;355.
98. Sumida M, Uozumi T, Mukada K, Arita K, Kurisu K, Eguchi K. Rathke cleft cysts: correlation of enhanced MR and surgical findings. AJNR 1994;15:525.
99. Takeuchi J, Handa H, Nagata I. Suprasellar germinoma. J Neurosurg 1978;49:41
100. Tampieri D, Melanson D, Ethier R. MR imaging of epidermoid cysts. AJNR 1989;10:351.
101. Taylor SL, Barakos JA, Harsh GR, Wilson CB. Magnetic resonance imaging of tuberculum sellae meningiomas: preventing preoperative misdiagnosis as pituitary adenoma. Neurosurg 1992;31:621.
102. Tien R, Kucharczyk J, Kucharczyk W. MR imaging of the brain in patients with diabetes insipidus. AJNR 1991;12:533.
103. Tien RD, Newton TH, Mc Dermott MW, Dillon WP, Kucharczyk W. Thickened pituitary stalk on MR images in patients with diabetes insipidus and Langerhans cell histiocytosis. AJNR 1990;11:703.
104. Tsuda M, Takahashi S, Higano S, Kurihara N, Ikeda H, Sakamoto K. CT and MR imaging of craniopharyngioma. Eur Radiol 1997;7:464.
105. Vion-Dury J, Vincentelli F, Jiddane M, et al. MR imaging of epidermoid cysts. Neuroradiology 1987;29:333.
106. Voelker JL, Campbell RL, Muller J. Clinical, radiographic and pathologic features of symptomatic Rathke's cleft's cysts. J Neurosurg 1991;74:535.
107. Wiener SN, Pearlstein AE, Eiber A. MR imaging of intracranial arachnoid cysts. J Comput Assist Tomogr 1987;11:236.
108. Yuh W TC, Wright DC, Barlan Tl, et al. MR imaging of primitive tumor of trigeminal nerve and Meckel's cave. AJNR 1988;9:665.

2

BILATERAL SIMULTANEOUS INFERIOR PETROSAL SINUS SAMPLING (BSIPSS)

Wouter W. de Herder, M.D.
Steven W.J. Lamberts, M.D.
Hervé L.J. Tanghe, M.D.
Herman Pieterman, M.D.
University Hospital Rotterdam
Rotterdam, the Netherlands

INTRODUCTION – Cushing's syndrome

Traditionally, spontaneous Cushing's syndrome is divided into corticotropin (ACTH)-dependent and ACTH-independent. In the first category are Cushing's disease, accounting for approximately 75% of Cushing's syndrome, ectopic ACTH secretion and the rare ectopic CRF syndrome (1). ACTH-producing pituitary tumors are usually relatively small as compared to other pituitary adenomas. The mean size of these adenomas is 5-6 mm, but tumors as small as 1-2 mm have been documented (2). Transsphenoidal microsurgery is the primary treatment for patients with Cushing' s disease (3). In the past, the differential diagnosis of ACTH-dependent Cushing's syndrome using the available diagnostic endocrine tests was sometimes very difficult (4).

In 1977, Corrigan and co-workers first introduced the technique of venous sampling of the pituitary venous effluent for the differential diagnosis of ACTH-dependent Cushing's syndrome (5). Since that time, the technique and procedure of bilateral simultaneous inferior petrosal sinus sampling (BSIPSS) for ACTH measurements has been further refined. In many referral centers, BSIPSS has become an established diagnostic procedure in patients with ACTH-dependent Cushing's syndrome. It is an invasive technique requiring a skilled and experienced team (6). Since BSIPSS cannot differentiate between normal individuals or patients with Cushing's disease, confirmation of ACTH-dependent hypercortisolism is first required.

Drainage of venous blood from each half of the anterior pituitary gland tends to remain lateralized as it successively flows through multiple small tributaries via the cavernous sinuses into the inferior petrosal sinuses (6). Sometimes, mixing of venous blood from the two sites of the anterior pituitary gland may occur (7). Because of its proximity to the anterior pituitary, inferior petrosal sinus ACTH levels are higher than in the peripheral blood.

Petrosal sinus sampling - Cushing's syndrome

Since about 86% of the ACTH-secreting microadenomas are located laterally in the pituitary (8) a dominant and non-dominant drainage of pituitary ACTH-rich blood to the inferior petrosal sinuses will ensue. Therefore, unilateral sampling may miss a central source and simultaneous bilateral inferior petrosal sampling is essential (9,10). A significant gradient between the inferior petrosal sinus and peripheral plasma ACTH levels is indicative of Cushing's disease. In most recent studies, a inferior petrosal sinus to peripheral plasma ACTH gradient greater than or equal to 2.0 at baseline has been considered diagnostic of Cushing's disease (11-14). However, episodical tumoral ACTH secretion can possibly result in a basal gradient less than 2 (15,16). The sensitivity of the test can be increased by continuing the sampling procedure during 15-20 min. after the administration of a 100 μg bolus (or 1 μg/kg body weight (BW)) of ovine corticotropin-releasing hormone (CRH), or recombinant human CRH bolus in a peripheral vein. In most studies, a inferior petrosal sinus to peripheral plasma ACTH gradient greater than or equal to 3.0 in post-CRH samples has been considered diagnostic of Cushing's disease (11-13,15,17-26,72)(Figure 1). In case CRH is not available, pretreatment with desmopressin (10 μg i.v. bolus) (14), naloxone (125 μg/kg BW i.v. bolus) (27), or metyrapone (6 x 750 mg p.o.) (28) has been successfully used to enhance the inferior petrosal sinus to peripheral gradient.

Presently, more than 30 publications have evaluated the role of BSIPSS in the diagnostic approach to patients with ACTH-dependent Cushing's syndrome and contain information on more than 600 successful samplings. Among these is one of the largest and most referred to series from the National Institutes of Health (USA) in 246 patients with Cushing's disease and 20 with ectopic ACTH secretion. Applying the criteria of a post-CRH inferior petrosal sinus to peripheral ACTH gradient greater than or equal to 3.0, the sensitivity and specificity of BSIPSS in this series equaled 100 and 100%, respectively. However, 32 patients were excluded from analysis, since the authors were unable to formally classify them. Obviously, inclusion of these patients would have influenced the very favorable outcome of this study (11). The mean sensitivity and specificity of BSIPSS in the published series is still very high and equals 96% and 100%, respectively. False negative results have been described in 4% (13,20,21,29-33), whereas false positive results have been obtained in a patient with combined ectopic ACTH and CRH secretion (34).

Anatomical variants in the size and number of venous anastomoses, or technical problems may preclude successful simultaneous sampling from both inferior petrosal sinuses in some patients (6,7,13,73). Patients can experience slight discomfort in the ear caused by periostal stretching in the jugular fossa during the final phase of catheter positioning (35). The most common complication of BSIPSS is groin hematoma (6). Rarely, serious complications like pulmonary embolism (36) and brain stem ischemia occur (37-39). Therefore, heparinisation of patients is generally recommended (37).

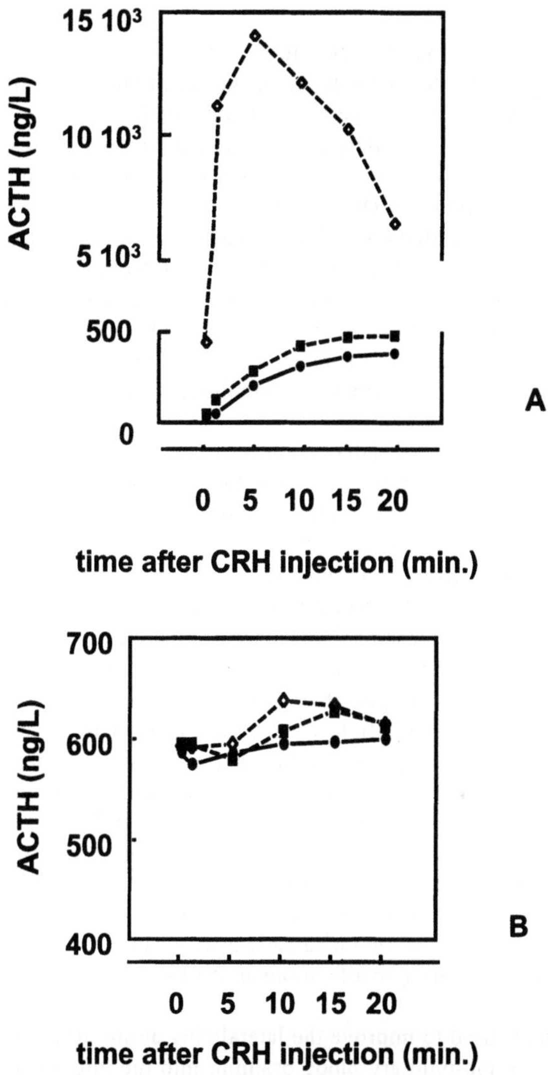

Figure 1. Simultaneous sampling for corticotrophin (ACTH) determinations of the left (◊) and right (■) inferior petrosal sinus and a femoral vein (●), before and after CRH (1 µg/kg i.v.). A: Cushing's disease caused by a 7-mm. corticotroph adenoma located at the left side of the pituitary gland. Note the presence of a significant gradient between the ipsilateral (left) inferior petrosal sinus and the contralateral sinus or the peripheral vein pointing to a pituitary origin of ACTH secretion, presumably located at the left side of the pituitary gland. B: Cushing's syndrome caused by ectopic secretion of ACTH by an 8-mm. bronchial carcinoid. Note the absence of a gradient between the left and right inferior petrosal sinus, or between both petrosal sinus and the peripheral vein pointing to a non-pituitary source of ACTH production.

Mean sensitivities of computer tomography and MRI (with the use of gadolinium contrast-enhancement) for the localization of ACTH-producing pituitary adenomas is about 47% and more than 70%, respectively. However, false positive localization may occur, because MRI detects pituitary microadenomas in 10% of healthy individuals. As already mentioned earlier, about 86% of the ACTH-secreting microadenomas are located laterally in the pituitary (8). In Cushing's disease, the usefulness of BSIPSS for the intrapituitary lateralization of microadenomas is subject to controversy. A generally accepted cut-off lateralization limit for the intersinus ACTH gradient (ISG) of 1.4 has been shown to be consistent with the ipsilateral lateralization of a microadenoma in 68% to 85% of the patients (11-13,20,72). Adjunctive CRH stimulation in order to further dissociate ACTH levels on the ipsi- versus contra-lateral side does not seem to improve this diagnostic accuracy.

An erroneous or unequivocal lateralization of the pituitary lesion by a falsely lateralized ISG has been reported in 18% to 41% of cases (13,22,40,41). Also, reversal of the ISG may occur after administration of CRH (12,13,42). Mamelak and coworkers have demonstrated asymmetrical venous drainage in as many as 39% of patients with Cushing's disease and this may explain some of the false lateralisations with BSIPSS (43). Misleading lateralization results have also been found in patients previously operated upon, presumably because of postoperative rearrangement in the venous drainage (44). On the other hand, a significant ISG may be absent because of a central localization of the responsible corticotroph tumor, or in case of diffuse corticotroph hyperplasia, or multiple corticotroph adenomas. As already mentioned earlier, BSIPSS has only diagnostic value in the differential diagnosis of ACTH-dependent Cushing's syndrome. Interestingly, some healthy normal individuals with normal petrosal sinus anatomy also show unilateral ACTH gradients (45,46). In contrast to patients with Cushing's disease, this is not the result from cortisol excess suppressing normal corticotrophs and causing Crooke's hyalinization. However, in patients with ACTH-dependent Cushing's syndrome, reduction or normalization of serum cortisol by cortisol-lowering medications may cause recovery of non-tumorous corticotrophs thereby resulting in alterations in the ISG.

Several groups have tried to improve the lateralizing ability of BSIPSS by correcting for the influence of non-pituitary blood draining into the inferior petrosal sinus. For this purpose, the ACTH concentrations were corrected for the levels of other anterior pituitary hormones, like growth hormone (GH), prolactin (PRL), gonadotropins and their alpha subunit and thyrotropin (TSH) (29,31,44,47-50). However, in a significant number of examinations, these hormone levels also showed a inferior petrosal sinus to peripheral gradient, which was closely associated with the ACTH gradient. This gradient could be due to either co-secretion of these hormones by the adenoma, or by a paracrine effect of the tumor on adjacent pituitary tissue (51).

We advocate MRI with Gd-DTPA contrast enhancement as the first-line approach for localization of pituitary adenomas in Cushing's disease. BSIPSS should be reserved for the assessment of patients with Cushing's disease with a normal or equivocal pituitary MRI (13,72). Ideally, bilateral petrosal sinus sampling should guide the neurosurgeon's initial examination of the pituitary gland in search for small lesions. The question is whether exploration should indeed start at the side ipsilateral to the ACTH gradient and whether ipsilateral hemihypophysectomy should be performed in case a microadenoma cannot be visualized at operation, because in about half of the cases the tumor may be at the contralateral side (72).

Cavernous sinus sampling–Cushing's syndrome

Teramoto and co-workers have validated the technique of simultaneous super-selective sampling from both cavernous sinuses. According to these authors, only basal ACTH sampling would be sufficient and adjunctive CRH stimulation would not be needed (52). Others have also used this technique (53-55,74). Although cavernous sinus to peripheral ACTH gradients are generally higher than those for the inferior petrosal sinus, this technique generally does not have more accuracy than BSIPSS for the differential diagnosis of ACTH-dependent Cushing's syndrome (56,74). However, bilateral simultaneous cavernous sinus sampling for ACTH measurements before and after CRH stimulation may be more accurate than BSIPSS for predicting intrapituitary tumor localization (74). The major disadvantages of bilateral cavernous sinus sampling, however, are the significantly added expense of the catheters and, possibly, the increased risk of cavernous sinus thrombosis (56).

Jugular venous sampling–Cushing's syndrome

Initial studies have shown that sampling from both jugular bulbs without adjunctive CRH stimulation was not sufficiently sensitive for the differential diagnosis of ACTH-dependent Cushing's syndrome (5,17,57,58). Recently, Doppman and coworkers have reassessed the clinical usefulness of the technique of bilateral jugular vein sampling (59). To obtain maximal sensitivity with this technique, CRH-stimulation is essential. This technique is a much easier and simpler procedure than BSIPSS. There are, however, several disadvantages of bilateral jugular vein sampling. First, it has a lower sensitivity than BSIPSS (80% in this series) when using the same cut-off limits for the jugular vein to peripheral plasma ACTH gradient as for the inferior petrosal sinus gradient (59). Second, BSIPSS is still recommended for confirmation in patients who do not show diagnostic jugular vein to peripheral plasma ACTH gradients (59).

Petrosal sinus sampling–other pituitary disorders

BSIPSS with the use of hypothalamic-releasing factors has successfully lateralised a TSH- producing adenoma in a patient with central hyperthyroidism and GH-producing adenoma in a patient with acromegaly. In both patients high-resolution CT did not show the presence of an adenoma, whereas MRI was normal in the patient with acromegaly (60). In additional patients with acromegaly and no demonstrable tumor on pituitary CT or MRI, a inferior petrosal sinus to peripheral gradient for GH both before and after GH-releasing hormone (GHRH) was shown. However, lateralization of the adenomas in the pituitary on the basis of the intersinus gradient for GH was not reliable (61,62).

Petrosal sinus sampling-experimental studies

Bilateral inferior petrosal sinus sampling has been used for the experimental study of pituitary levels and dynamics of a number of other hormones and peptides, mostly in patients with Cushing's disease, like: atrial natriuretic peptide (63), CRH (64), AVP (vasopressin) (65-68), alpha-melanocyte-stimulating hormone (69), tumor necrosis factor alpha (70) and beta-endorphin (71).

General conclusions

BSIPSS is the most sensitive diagnostic technique for the differential diagnosis of ACTH-dependent Cushing'' syndrome. It's usefulness for the intrapituitary lateralization of corticotroph adenomas is still a matter of controversy. Sampling at levels more proximal or distal does not add extra advantages. The clinical usefulness in other pituitary tumor syndromes seems more limited.

References

1. Orth DN. Cushing's syndrome. N Engl J Med. 1995;332:791.
2. Kaye TB, Crapo L. The Cushing syndrome: an update on diagnostic tests. Ann Intern Med 1990;112:434.
3. Aron DC, Findling JW, Tyrrell JB. Cushing's disease. Endocrinol Metab Clin North Am 1987;16:705.
4. Aron DC, Raff H, Findling JW. Effectiveness versus efficacy: the limited value in clinical practice of high dose dexamethasone suppression testing in the differential diagnosis of adrenocorticotropin-dependent Cushing's syndrome. J Clin Endocrinol Metab 1997;82:1780.
5. Corrigan DF, Schaaf M, Whaley RA, Czerwinski CL, Earll JM. Selective venous sampling to differentiate ectopic ACTH secretion from pituitary Cushing's syndrome. N Engl J Med 1977;296:861.
6. Miller DL, Doppman JL. Petrosal sinus sampling: technique and rationale. Radiology 1991;178:37.
7. Doppman JL, Krudy AG, Girton ME, Oldfield EH. Basilar venous plexus of the posterior fossa: a potential source of error in petrosal sinus sampling. Radiology 1985;155:375.
8. Mampalam TJ, Tyrrell JB, Wilson CB. Transsphenoidal microsurgery for Cushing disease. A report of 216 cases. Ann Intern Med 1988;109:487.
9. Manni A, Latshaw RF, Page R, Santen RJ. Simultaneous bilateral venous sampling for adrenocorticotropin in pituitary-dependent Cushing's disease: evidence for lateralization of pituitary venous drainage. J Clin Endocrinol Metab 1983;57:1070.
10. Oldfield EH, Chrousos GP, Schulte HM, et al. Preoperative lateralization of ACTH-secreting pituitary microadenomas by bilateral and simultaneous inferior petrosal venous sinus sampling. N Engl J Med 1985;312:100.
11. Oldfield EH, Doppman JL, Nieman LK, et al. Petrosal sinus sampling with and without corticotropin-releasing hormone for the differential diagnosis of Cushing's syndrome. N Engl J Med 1991;325:897.
12. Landolt AM, Schubiger O, Maurer R, Girard J. The value of inferior petrosal sinus sampling in diagnosis and treatment of Cushing's disease. Clin Endocrinol 1994;40:485.
13. de Herder WW, Uitterlinden P, Pieterman H, et al. Pituitary tumour localization in patients with Cushing's disease by magnetic resonance imaging. Is there a place for petrosal sinus sampling? Clin Endocrinol 1994;40:87.
14. Booth GL, Redelmeier DA, Grosman H, Kovacs K, Smyth HS, Ezzat S. Improved diagnostic accuracy of inferior petrosal sinus sampling over imaging for localizing pituitary pathology in patients with Cushing's disease. J Clin Endocrinol Metab 1998;83:2291.
15. Cuneo R, Ross D, MacFarlane M, Espiner E, Donald RA. Sequential inferior petrosal venous sampling for Cushing's disease. N Engl J Med 1985;313:582
16. Yamamoto Y, Davis DH, Nippoldt TB, Young WFJ, Huston J, Parisi JE. False-positive inferior petrosal sinus sampling in the diagnosis of Cushing's disease. Report of two cases. J Neurosurg 1995;83:1087.
17. Findling JW, Aron DC, Tyrrell JB, et al. Selective venous sampling for ACTH in Cushing's syndrome: differentiation between Cushing disease and the ectopic ACTH syndrome. Ann Intern Med 1981;94:647.
18. Hauffa BP, Stolecke H, Schulte HM. Cushing disease: successful preoperative lateralization of an ACTH- producing pituitary microadenoma by simultaneous bilateral inferior petrosal venous sinus sampling with corticotropin-releasing hormone

stimulation. Eur J Pediatr 1986;145:559.

19. Landolt AM, Valavanis A, Girard J, Eberle AN. Corticotrophin-releasing factor-test used with bilateral, simultaneous inferior petrosal sinus blood-sampling for the diagnosis of pituitary- dependent Cushing's disease. Clin Endocrinol 1986;25:687.
20. Snow RB, Patterson RHJ, Horwith M, Saint LL, Fraser RA. Usefulness of preoperative inferior petrosal vein sampling in Cushing's disease. Surg Neurol 1988;29:17.
21. McCance DR, McIlrath E, McNeill A, et al. Bilateral inferior petrosal sinus sampling as a routine procedure in ACTH-dependent Cushing's syndrome. Clin Endocrinol 1989;30:157.
22. Boolell M, Gilford E, Arnott R, McNeill P, Cummins J, Alford F. An overview of bilateral synchronous inferior petrosal sinus sampling (BSIPSS) in the pre-operative assessment of Cushing's disease. Aust N Z J Med 1990;20:765.
23. Findling JW, Kehoe ME, Shaker JL, Raff H. Routine inferior petrosal sinus sampling in the differential diagnosis of adrenocorticotropin (ACTH)-dependent Cushing's syndrome: early recognition of the occult ectopic ACTH syndrome. J Clin Endocrinol Metab 1991;73:408.
24. Tabarin A, Greselle JF, San-Galli F, et al. Usefulness of the corticotropin-releasing hormone test during bilateral inferior petrosal sinus sampling for the diagnosis of Cushing's disease. J Clin Endocrinol Metab 1991;73:53.
25. Colao A, Merola B, Tripodi FS, et al. Simultaneous and bilateral inferior petrosal sinus sampling for the diagnosis of Cushing's syndrome: comparison of multihormonal assay, baseline multiple sampling and ACTH-releasing hormone test. Horm Res 1993;40:209.
26. Strack TR, Schild HH, Bohl J, Beyer J, Schrezemeir J, Kahaly G. Selective bilateral blood sampling from the inferior petrosal sinus in Cushing's disease: effects of corticotropin-releasing factor and thyrotropin-releasing hormone on pituitary secretion. Cardiovasc Intervent Radiol 1993;16:287.
27. Torpy DJ, Jackson RV, Grice JE, Hockings GI, Strakosch CR, Topliss DJ. Naloxone stimulation of ACTH secretion during petrosal sinus sampling in Cushing's syndrome. Clin Exp Pharmacol Physiol 1993;20:299.
28. Cuneo RC, Lee W, Harper J, et al. Metyrapone pre-treated inferior petrosal sinus sampling in the differential diagnosis of ACTH-dependent Cushing's syndrome. Clin Endocrinol 1997;46:607.
29. Crock PA, Pestell RG, Calenti AJ, et al. Multiple pituitary hormone gradients from inferior petrosal sinus sampling in Cushing's disease. Acta Endocrinol (Copenh) 1988;119:75.
30. Boscaro M, Rampazzo A, Paoletta A, et al. Selective venous sampling in the differential diagnosis of ACTH- dependent Cushing's syndrome. Neuroendocrinology 1992;55:264.
31. McNally PG, Bolia A, Absalom SR, Falconer-Smith J, Howlett TA. Preliminary observations using endocrine markers of pituitary venous dilution during bilateral simultaneous inferior petrosal sinus catheterisation in Cushing's syndrome: is combined CRF and TRH stimulation of value? Clin Endocrinol 1993;39:681.
32. Lopez J, Barcelo B, Lucas T, et al. Petrosal sinus sampling for diagnosis of Cushing's disease: evidence of false negative results. Clin Endocrinol 1996;45:147.
33. Heppner C, Becker K, Saeger W, et al. Occult eutopic Cushing's syndrome--failure of simultaneous bilateral petrosal sinus sampling to diagnose pituitary-dependent Cushing's syndrome. Eur J Endocrinol 1997;137:74.
34. Young J, Deneux C, Grino M, Oliver C, Chanson P, Schaison G. Pitfall of petrosal sinus sampling in a Cushing's syndrome secondary to ectopic adrenocorticotropin-corticotropin releasing hormone (ACTH-CRH) secretion. J Clin Endocrinol Metab 1998;83:305.
35. Schild H, Strack T, Gunther R, et al. Selektive Blutentnahme aus dem Sinus petrosus inferior mit digitaler Subtraktionsangiographie. Fortschr Rontgenstr 1986;144:627.

36. Diez JJ, Iglesias P. Pulmonary thromboembolism after inferior petrosal sinus sampling in Cushing's syndrome. Clin Endocrinol 1997;46:777
37. Miller DL, Doppman JL, Peterman SB, Nieman LK, Oldfield EH, Chang R. Neurologic complications of petrosal sinus sampling. Radiology 1992;185:143.
38. Seyer H, Honegger J, Schott W, et al. Raymond's syndrome following petrosal sinus sampling. Acta Neurochir (Wien) 1994;131:157.
39. Sturrock ND, Jeffcoate WJ. A neurological complication of inferior petrosal sinus sampling during investigation for Cushing's disease: a case report. J Neurol Neurosurg Psychiatry 1997;62:527.
40. McCance DR, McIlrath E, McNeill A, et al. Bilateral inferior petrosal sinus sampling as a routine procedure in ACTH-dependent Cushing's syndrome. Clin Endocrinol 1989;30:157.
41. Tabarin A, Greselle JF, San-Galli F, et al. Usefulness of the corticotropin-releasing hormone test during bilateral inferior petrosal sinus sampling for the diagnosis of Cushing's disease. J Clin Endocrinol Metab 1991;73:53.
42. Miller DL, Doppman JL, Nieman LK, et al. Petrosal sinus sampling: discordant lateralization of ACTH-secreting pituitary microadenomas before and after stimulation with corticotropin- releasing hormone. Radiology 1990;176:429.
43. Mamelak AN, Dowd CF, Tyrrell JB, McDonald JF, Wilson CB. Venous angiography is needed to interpret inferior petrosal sinus and cavernous sinus sampling data for lateralizing adrenocorticotropin- secreting adenomas. J Clin Endocrinol Metab 1996;81:475.
44. Vignati F, Berselli ME, Scialfa G, Boccardi E, Loli P. Bilateral and simultaneous venous sampling of inferior petrosal sinuses for ACTH and PRL determination: preoperative localization of ACTH- secreting microadenomas. J Endocrinol Invest 1989;12:235.
45. Yanovski JA, Cutler GBJ, Doppman JL, et al. The limited ability of inferior petrosal sinus sampling with corticotropin-releasing hormone to distinguish Cushing's disease from pseudo-Cushing states or normal physiology. J Clin Endocrinol Metab 1993;77:503.
46. Kalogeras KT, Nieman LK, Friedman TC, et al. Inferior petrosal sinus sampling in healthy subjects reveals a unilateral corticotropin-releasing hormone-induced arginine vasopressin release associated with ipsilateral adrenocorticotropin secretion. J Clin Invest 1996;97:2045.
47. Tanaka K, Shimizu N, Nagata M, Seki T, Nagai J. Identification of source of excessive ACTH production by improved selective venous sampling: simultaneous assay of PRL as a pituitary marker. Endocrinol Jpn 1984;31:195.
48. Schulte HM, Allolio B, Gunther RW, et al. Selective bilateral and simultaneous catheterization of the inferior petrosal sinus: CRF stimulates prolactin secretion from ACTH-producing microadenomas in Cushing's disease. Clin Endocrinol 1988;28:289.
49. Zovickian J, Oldfield EH, Doppman JL, Cutler GBJ, Loriaux DL. Usefulness of inferior petrosal sinus venous endocrine markers in Cushing's disease. J Neurosurg 1988;68:205.
50. Vignati F, Berselli ME, Boccardi E, Branca V, Loli P. Stimulatory effect of oCRH on alpha-subunit secretion during petrosal sinus sampling in patients with Cushing's disease. Horm Metab Res 1992;24:524.
51. Tabarin A, Corcuff JB, Rashedi M, et al. Multihormonal response to corticotropin-releasing hormone in inferior petrosal sinus blood of one patient with Cushing's disease: comparison with *in vitro* secretion of the tumoral corticotropes. Acta Endocrinol (Copenh) 1992;127:284.
52. Teramoto A, Nemoto S, Takakura K, Sasaki Y, Machida T. Selective venous sampling directly from cavernous sinus in Cushing's syndrome. J Clin Endocrinol Metab 1993;76:637.

53. Aoki S, Okubo T, Sasaki Y, et al. Direct cavernous sinus sampling. Radiat Med 1993;11:196.
54. Vandorpe RA, Fox AJ, Pelz DM, Lee DH. Direct sampling of the cavernous sinus in Cushing's disease. Can Assoc Radiol J 1994;45:234.
55. Oliverio PJ, Monsein LH, Wand GS, Debrun GM. Bilateral simultaneous cavernous sinus sampling using corticotropin- releasing hormone in the evaluation of Cushing disease. Am J Neuroradiol 1996;17:1669.
56. Doppman JL, Nieman LK, Chang R, et al. Selective venous sampling from the cavernous sinuses is not a more reliable technique than sampling from the inferior petrosal sinuses in Cushing's syndrome. J Clin Endocrinol Metab 1995;80:2485.
57. Anonymous. Jugular-vein sampling of ACTH. N Engl J Med 1977;297:730.
58. Drury PL, Ratter S, Tomlin S, et al. Experience with selective venous sampling in diagnosis of ACTH- dependent Cushing's syndrome. Br Med J (Clin Res Ed) 1982;284:9.
59. Doppman JL, Oldfield EH, Nieman LK. Bilateral sampling of the internal jugular vein to distinguish between mechanisms of adrenocorticotropic hormone-dependent Cushing syndrome. Ann Intern Med 1998;128:33.
60. Frank SJ, Gesundheit N, Doppman JL, et al. Preoperative lateralization of pituitary microadenomas by petrosal sinus sampling: utility in two patients with non-ACTH-secreting tumors. Am J Med 1989;87:679.
61. Crock PA, Gilford EJ, Henderson JK, et al. Inferior petrosal sinus sampling in acromegaly. Aust N Z J Med 1989;19:244.
62. Doppman JL, Miller DL, Patronas NJ, et al. The diagnosis of acromegaly: value of inferior petrosal sinus sampling. Am J Roentgenol 1990;154:1075.
63. Colao A, Pivonello R, Ferone D, et al. Plasma atrial natriuretic factor levels in the inferior petrosal sinus blood of patients with Cushing's disease before and after corticotropin- releasing hormone administration. J Endocrinol Invest 1998;21:257.
64. Yanovski JA, Nieman LK, Doppman JL, et al. Plasma levels of corticotropin-releasing hormone in the inferior petrosal sinuses of healthy volunteers, patients with Cushing's syndrome, and patients with pseudo-Cushing states. J Clin Endocrinol Metab 1998;83:1485.
65. Nussey SS, Page SR, Peterson DB, et al. Corticotrophin releasing hormone (CRH1-41) stimulates the secretion of adrenocorticotrophin, vasopressin and oxytocin but not adrenocorticotrophin precursors: evidence from petrosal sinus sampling in man. Clin Endocrinol 1991;34:51.
66. Colao A, Ferone D, Di Sarno A, et al. Vasopressin levels in Cushing's disease: inferior petrosal sinus assay, response to corticotrophin-releasing hormone and comparison with patients without Cushing's disease. Clin Endocrinol 1996;45:157.
67. Friedman TC, Yanovski JA, Nieman LK, et al. Inferior petrosal sinus arginine vasopressin concentrations in normal volunteers and patients with Cushing's disease. J Clin Endocrinol Metab 1996;81:3068.
68. Yanovski JA, Friedman TC, Nieman LK, et al. Inferior petrosal sinus AVP in patients with Cushing's syndrome. Clin Endocrinol 1997;47:199.
69. Colao A, Merola B, Cataldi M, et al. Alpha-melanocyte-stimulating hormone is present in the inferior petrosal sinuses in patients with Cushing's disease. Neuroendocrinology 1993;58:227.
70. Merola B, Longobardi S, Colao A, et al. Tumor necrosis factor-alpha increases after corticotropin-releasing hormone administration in Cushing's disease. In vivo and in vitro studies. Neuroendocrinology 1996;64:393.
71. Colao A, Merola B, Spaziante R, et al. Adrenocorticotropic hormone and beta-endorphin concentrations in the inferior petrosal sinuses in Cushing's disease and other pituitary diseases. J Endocrinol Invest 1992;15:807.

72. Kaltsas GA, Giannulis MG, Newell-Price JDC, et al. A critical analysis of the value of simultaneous inferior petrosal sinus sampling in Cushing's disease and the occult ectopic adrenocorticotropin syndrome. J Clin Endocrinol Metab 1999;84:487.
73. Doppman JL, Chang R, Oldfield EH, Chrousos G, Stratakis CA, Nieman LK. The hypoplastic inferior petrosal sinus: a potential source of false-negative results in petrosal sampling for Cushing's disease. J Clin Endocrinol Metab 1999;84:533.
74. Graham KE, Samuels MH, Nesbit GM, et al. Cavernous sinus sampling is highly accurate in distinguishing Cushing's disease from the ectopic adrenocorticotropin syndrome and in predicting intrapituitary tumor location. J Clin Endocrinol Metab 1999;84:1602.

3
SCINTIGRAPHY OF PITUITARY TUMORS

Wouter W. de Herder, M.D.
Diego Ferone, M.D.
Dik J. Kwekkeboom, M.D.
Steven W.J. Lamberts, M.D.
University Hospital Rotterdam
Rotterdam, the Netherlands
"Federico II" University
Naples, Italy

INTRODUCTION

Several neoplastic and non-neoplastic lesions may arise within the sellar and parasellar regions (Table 1). Among these, pituitary adenomas are the most common. Almost all pituitary tumors are benign, although they may display signs of local invasion or show histological evidence of malignancy. However, generally these tumors can be designated malignant only when distant metastases are present. Adenomas with a diameter less than 10 mm are classified as microadenomas, whereas those greater than 10 mm are considered macroadenomas. Pituitary adenomas are subclassified into clinically functioning - according to the hormone secreted - and clinically non-functioning. Among the hormone products secreted are prolactin (PRL), growth hormone (GH), adrenocorticotropic hormone (ACTH), thyroid stimulating hormone (TSH), gonadotropins (LH and FSH), glycoprotein hormone subunits (SU) or mixtures of these products. The majority of the so-called clinically functioning pituitary macroadenomas either secrete inappropriate amounts of pituitary hormones, or inactive hormonal fragments. The differential diagnosis of pituitary tumors is currently based on clinical, endocrinological and radiological characteristics. Active hormone-secreting pituitary adenomas are easily diagnosed because of signs and symptoms related to hormonal hypersecretion. Clinically non-functioning adenomas generally do not produce specific hormonal syndromes, but often hypopituitarism results from insufficient secretion of anterior pituitary hormones. The differential diagnosis of these tumors is mainly achieved using neuroradiological studies. However, even with the use of modern imaging techniques the differential diagnosis still may be difficult in some cases. The recent development of improved imaging techniques in nuclear medicine may allow further biochemical and functional characterization of these tumors, thus providing useful additional information about the characteristics of the sellar mass.

Table 1. Lesions arising within the sellar and parasellar regions.

NEOPLASTIC LESIONS	NON-NEOPLASTIC LESIONS
Pituitary adenomas	**Granulomas and inflammatory lesions**
PRL-secreting	tuberculosis
GH-secreting	sarcoidosis
ACTH-secreting	giant cell granuloma
TSH-secreting	abscess (bacterial and fungal)
gonadotropin-secreting	lymphocytic hypophysitis
glycoprotein hormone subunit-secreting	lymphocytic infundibulohypophysitis
plurihormonal-secreting	histiocytosis X (eosinophilic granuloma)
null cell (oncocytoma)	echinococcal cyst
nonsecreting	
Other benign lesions	**Miscellaneous**
meningioma	vascular aneurysms
enchondroma	arachnoid cyst
gangliocytoma	sphenoidal mucocele
hypothalamic hamartoma	empty sella syndrome
myoblastoma	
Germ cell tumors	
germinoma	
dermoid cyst	
teratoma	
dysgerminoma	
Cell rest tumor	
craniopharyngioma	
Rathke's cleft cyst	
chordoma	
cholesteatoma	
lipoma	
colloid cyst	
Gliomas	
optic glioma	
oligodendroglioma	
ependymoma	
astrocytoma	
microglioma	
infudibuloma	
Metastatic tumors	

Dopamine D2 receptor analogs and long-acting somatostatin analogs have been increasingly used as medical therapy of patients with prolactinomas, GH-secreting and TSH-secreting pituitary tumors. The potential use of these drugs in other clinically functioning and non-functioning pituitary tumors is not yet established.

However, the presence of large numbers and/or the high affinity of dopamine D2 and/or somatostatin receptors on the diverse subtypes of pituitary adenomas, enables their visualization with radionuclide-coupled receptor analogs.

Dopamine D2 receptor imaging

Pituitary PRL secretion is under the tonic inhibitory control of dopamine secreted from the hypothalamus through stimulation of dopamine D2 receptors on the lactotrope cells. Dopamine D2 receptors have been identified in the majority of prolactinomas and in a considerable number of growth hormone secreting, and gonadotropin-secreting, or clinically nonfunctioning pituitary adenomas (NFPAs) (1-4). The presence of high numbers of high affinity D2 receptors on prolactinomas is the pharmacological basis for therapy with dopamine receptor agonist drugs, like the ergot-derived substances bromocriptine, pergolide and cabergoline and the nonergot dopamine agonist quinagolide (4). In these tumors, dopamine D2 receptor agonists successfully control the pathological tumoral secretion and may also cause significant tumor reduction (5). In bromocriptine-resistant prolactinomas D2 receptor density is markedly reduced as compared to dopamine agonist-sensitive prolactinomas (6). Kwekkeboom and coworkers have shown that treatment with quinagolide of patients with NFPAs can result in a reduction of tumor size in some patients (7). However, dopamine agonist-sensitive and -resistant NFPAs are clinically indistinguishable.

Muhr and coworkers and Bergström and coworkers have performed positron emission tomography (PET) studies using ^{11}C-labeled raclopride and N-methylspiperone for *in vivo* measurement of D2 receptors in prolactinomas and GH-secreting pituitary adenomas (8,9). They have demonstrated higher dopamine receptor binding in patients responsive to dopamine agonists than in therapy-resistant patients. Lucignani and coworkers have studied 16 patients with tumors in the sellar and parasellar regions using PET (10). These authors have determined the uptake of [^{18}F]fluoro-ethyl-spiperone for the differential diagnosis and clinical management of patients harboring these lesions. The uptake of [^{18}F]fluoro-ethyl-spiperone was significantly higher in clinically nonfunctioning pituitary adenomas than in meningiomas or craniopharyngiomas. It was concluded that this technique can be useful, particularly in those cases in which conventional radiological methods fail to make a certain diagnosis.

Imaging of the dopaminergic systems using single photon emission tomography (SPET) has also become feasible, due to the recent development of iodinated neuroligands and advancements in SPET technology. Both the widespread availability and the lower operating costs of SPET, as compared with PET suggest that SPET imaging of neurotransmitter systems may become a more important clinical tool. D2-receptor imaging in pituitary adenomas is feasible with SPET using ^{123}I-S-(-)-N-[(1-ethyl-2-pyrrolidinyl)methyl]-2-hydroxy-3-iodo-6-methoxybenzamide (^{123}I-IBZM) and ^{123}I-(S)-N-[(1-ethyl-2-pyrrolidinyl) methyl]-5-iodo-2, 3-dimethoxybenzamide (^{123}I-epidepride). At present, ^{123}I-IBZM is the most widely used SPET radiopharmaceutical for demonstrating the presence of D2 receptors. A number of studies have shown that SPET with ^{123}I-IBZM of the pituitary region was positive in dopamine agonist-sensitive PRL-secreting and clinically nonfunctioning macroadenomas. However, it was negative in dopamine-resistant PRL- and GH-secreting macroadenomas and dopamine agonist-sensitive microprolactinomas (11-15). Most physicians treating patients with PRL-secreting adenomas will generally "blindly" start dopaminergic therapy first, as resistance of these tumors to dopamine agonists is rare. Furthermore, the sensitivity of ^{123}I-IBZM SPET is probably too low to visualize adenomas with a diameter < 10 mm (13,14). In the study by de Herder and coworkers, significant uptake of the radioligand in the pituitary region was observed in 5 out of 19 patients (26%) with NFPA. In 2 out of 3 scan-positive NFPA patients that were treated with quinagolide, shrinkage of the pituitary tumors was observed, although one of these tumors was also treated with octreotide, as this tumor showed an increased pituitary uptake of ^{111}In-pentetreotide (13,14). Treatment with quinagolide resulted in stabilization of tumor growth in the other scan-positive patient (13,14). In the study by Ferone and coworkers, significant uptake of the radioligand in the pituitary region was observed in 3 out of 6 patients with NFPA. In 2 out of 3 scan-positive NFPA patients that were treated with quinagolide, shrinkage of the pituitary tumors was observed. ^{123}I-IBZM SPET is not sensitive enough to visualize dopamine D2 receptors on GH-secreting pituitary tumors (13-15). In a patient with a metastatic malignant macroprolactinoma, ^{123}I-IBZM SPET failed to visualize the primary tumor, whereas the uptake in a metastasis was lower than that observed for the striatum. A partial response of this metastatic tumor to dopamine D2 receptor agonists could be demonstrated *in vivo* and *in vitro* (16). In another patient with a mixed TSH/α-SU/PRL-secreting pituitary macroadenoma, SPET with ^{123}I-IBZM and [^{111}In-DTPA-d-Phe^{0}]-octreotide (^{111}In-pentetreotide, OctreoScan^{111}) both visualized the tumor (see also later). An acute *in vivo* response of the tumor to the somatostatin analog octreotide and the dopamine D2 receptor agonist bromocriptine could be demonstrated. However, long-term combined treatment did not result in tumor regression, or a decrease in circulating hormone levels. Thus, the demonstration of receptors *in vivo* in these patients did not predict the outcome of medical therapy with these two receptor agonists (17). Therefore, the sensitivity of ^{123}I-IBZM SPET for imaging pituitary adenomas is also rather poor, which is presumably the result of the relatively low target-to-background ratio of ^{123}I-IBZM binding (11,12,14,15). Consequently, investigators have been actively seeking SPET radiopharmaceuticals for the D2 receptor with greater receptor affinity.

Recent studies have demonstrated that the substituted benzamide derivative, epidepride, is a high affinity, low lipophilicity ligand (Kd = 20-30 pM and log k_w = 2.05), which generally provides high target-to-background uptake and hence high image quality (18-20). For comparison, the Kd of IBZM is in the range of 0.3-1.2 nM (21-23). It has been demonstrated that ^{123}I-epidepride is superior to ^{123}I-IBZM for studying striatal dopamine D2 receptors (24). Pirker and coworkers have shown that SPET and ^{123}I-epidepride provides high quality images of dopamine D2 receptor-positive pituitary adenomas (25). de Herder and coworkers have compared ^{123}I-epidepride and ^{123}I-IBZM SPET for *in vivo* imaging of dopamine receptors in NFPAs and dopamine agonist-sensitive macroprolactinomas (26). In parallel with studies demonstrating a much greater relative striatal uptake of ^{123}I-epidepride than of ^{123}I-IBZM, they have also observed a much higher uptake of ^{123}I-epidepride in NFPAs and macroprolactinomas than of ^{123}I-IBZM. All 4 macroprolactinomas showed specific binding of ^{123}I-epidepride within the area of the macroadenoma, but specific binding of ^{123}I-IBZM was only demonstrated in one of these tumors. Specific binding of ^{123}I-epidepride was shown in 60% of NFPA (n = 15), but specific binding of ^{123}I-IBZM was only shown in 40%. Therefore, ^{123}I-epidepride is superior to ^{123}I-IBZM for the visualization of D2 receptor on pituitary macroadenomas (Figures 1 - 2).

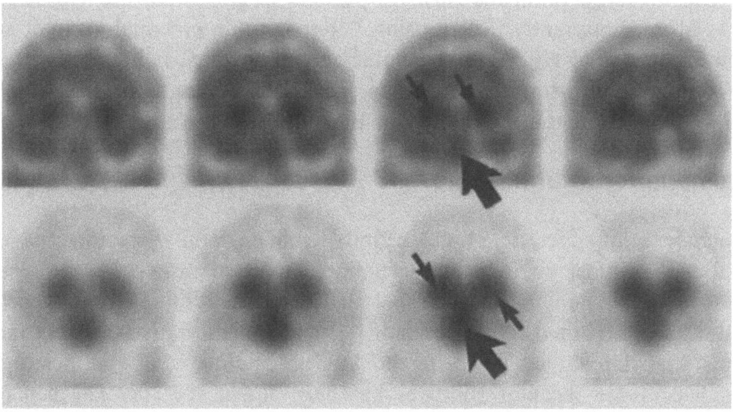

Figure 1. Coronal SPET images in a patient with a clinically nonfunctioning pituitary macroadenoma. Top panel: ^{123}I-IBZM. Note the relatively high background radioactivity, high uptake in the basal ganglia (thin arrows) and low uptake in the pituitary tumor (large arrow). Bottom panel: ^{123}I-epidepride. Note the low background radioactivity, high uptake in the basal ganglia (thin arrows) and pituitary tumor (large arrow).

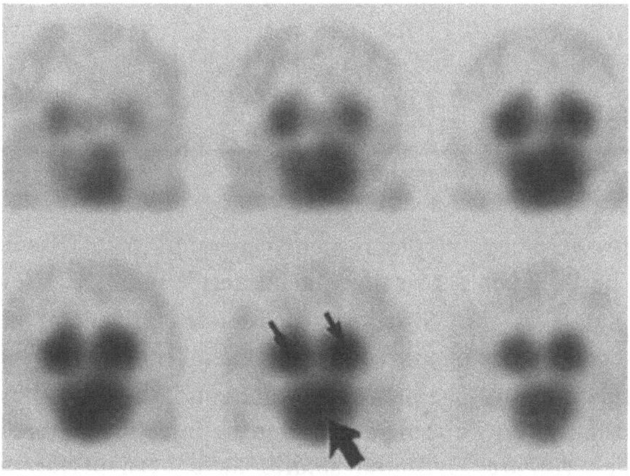

Figure 2. Coronal (left panel) ^{123}I-epidepride SPET images in a patient with a very large clinically nonfunctioning pituitary macroadenoma. Note the low background radioactivity, high uptake in the basal ganglia (thin arrows) and very high uptake in the pituitary tumor (large arrow).

Discrimination of NFPAs from other pathologies in the sellar region is generally not difficult when modern MRI protocols are applied. Clinically functioning and non-functioning pituitary adenomas may present with hyperprolactinemia as a secondary phenomenon. The specificity of D2 receptor SPET for the differentiation of prolactinomas from these tumors will probably be low, because dopamine D2 receptors have also been demonstrated on clinically non-functioning tumors (2). However, D2 receptor SPET might be of additional discriminatory merit in case of problems in the differential diagnosis: a positive SPET would point to a pituitary adenoma. More importantly, SPET using ^{123}I-epidepride potentially might serve to predict the response of NFPAs to dopamine agonist therapy. In patients with NFPA, *in vivo* scintigraphy with ^{123}I-epidepride may then be used for the selection of patients, who may potentially benefit from dopaminergic therapy.

Somatostatin receptor imaging

High numbers of specific, high affinity somatostatin receptors have been demonstrated on most neuroendocrine tumors. Six somatostatin receptor subtypes have been cloned in human tissues (Table 2). They differ with regard to their binding of natural somatostatin-14, somatostatin-28 and somatostatin analogs, including octreotide and lanreotide. In different human pituitary tumors, heterogeneous expression of these receptor subtypes has been found (27-30). The somatostatin analogs octreotide and lanreotide bind with high affinity to sst_2, sst_3 and sst_5.

Table 2. Characteristics of the six cloned human somatostatin receptors subtypes.

	sst_1	sst_{2A}	sst_{2B}	sst_3	sst_4	sst_5
Amino acids	391	369	356	418	388	363
M.W. (kDa)	42.6	41.3	39.9	45.7	41.9	39.1
mRNA (kb)	4.8	8.5	2.5	5.0	4.0	4.0
G protein coupling	Yes	yes	n.d.	yes	yes	yes
Chromosomal Localization	14q13	17q24	17q24	22q13.1	20p11.2	16p13.3

n.d. = not determined, M.W. = molecular weight

In patients with acromegaly, the responsiveness of the GH-secreting tumors to octreotide can be tested in a so-called "acute test": serum GH levels are measured after an acute single dose of 50-100 μg octreotide. GH and/or insulin-like growth factor-I (IGF-I) can also be measured in a so-called "chronic test" after 1-3 months of 300 μg octreotide therapy. The presence of octreotide-binding sites on GH-secreting tumors allows their *in vivo* visualization after the injection of a radionuclide-labeled octreotide analog (Figure 3). Initial studies have been performed with ^{123}I-^{3}Tyr-octreotide. This radioligand does not visualize the normal pituitary. Therefore, pituitary uptake of radioactivity after ^{123}I-^{3}Tyr-octreotide always points to the presence of a somatostatin-receptor positive pathologic process. A good correlation has been demonstrated between scan positivity for ^{123}I-^{3}Tyr-octreotide and the *in vitro* receptor positivity, or the *in vivo* GH response in the acute octreotide test (31,32). Nowadays, ^{111}In-pentetreotide is almost exclusively used as radiopharmaceutical for the visualization of receptors for octreotide and ^{123}I-^{3}Tyr-octreotide has been abandoned both for practical and financial reasons. In contrast to ^{123}I-^{3}Tyr-octreotide, the non-pathologic anterior pituitary gland also takes up ^{111}In-pentetreotide. Therefore, most studies have been using either a visual scoring system, or cut off values have been determined for an uptake index calculated from the uptake of radioactivity in the pituitary region of interest (ROI) divided by the uptake in a fixed background ROI. Conflicting results, especially in clinically nonfunctioning pituitary adenomas, may be caused by differences in subjective evaluation of these images. A fixed ROI method without background correction might also be a reliable approach for measuring pituitary uptake of ^{111}In-pentetreotide and may allow for separation of somatostatin receptor-positive tumors from the normal pituitary (33,34).

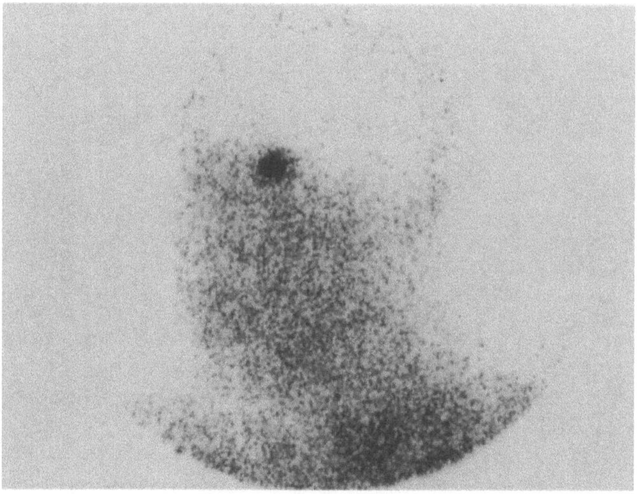

Figure 3. ^{111}In-pentetreotide images in a patient with active acromegaly caused by a somatotroph pituitary macroadenoma.

Several studies in patients with acromegaly have shown a close association between the increased ^{111}In-pentetreotide uptake in the pituitary tumor and the inhibition of the excessive GH secretion in the acute octreotide test (35-37) or the chronic octreotide test (38,39). However, others could not reproduce these findings (40-43). A close association between the increased ^{111}In-pentetreotide uptake in TSH-secreting pituitary adenomas and inhibition of the excessive TSH secretion in an acute octreotide test has also been shown (44). Somatostatin receptor scintigraphy (SRS) was negative a limited number of patients with microprolactinomas and ACTH-secreting pituitary microadenomas (43). SRS was positive in patients with infiltrating macroprolactinomas and invasive ACTH-secreting macroadenomas (43).

Until now, the *in vivo* effects of somatostatin analogs on NFPAs to are very difficult to predict. Various studies have demonstrated positive effects of this therapy on tumor size, visual field disturbances, or excessive secretion of tumor products (45-47). Like in acromegaly, some studies in NFPAs have shown a correlation between pituitary uptake of ^{111}In-pentetreotide and the inhibition of tumor growth, or excessive hormonal secretion (like FSH, LH or glycoprotein hormone subunits in some patients), or the improvement in visual field defects by somatostatin analog therapy (35,45). Generally, negative SRS predicted failure of somatostatin analogs to produce any kind of response in NFPAs in these studies (35). However, other studies could also not show any correlation between SRS-positivity and tumor response in NFPAs (40,41). The absence of a therapeutic effect of somatostatin analogs in these patients might result from a defect in the coupling-transduction process of somatostatin receptors in the tumor (48) (Figure 4).

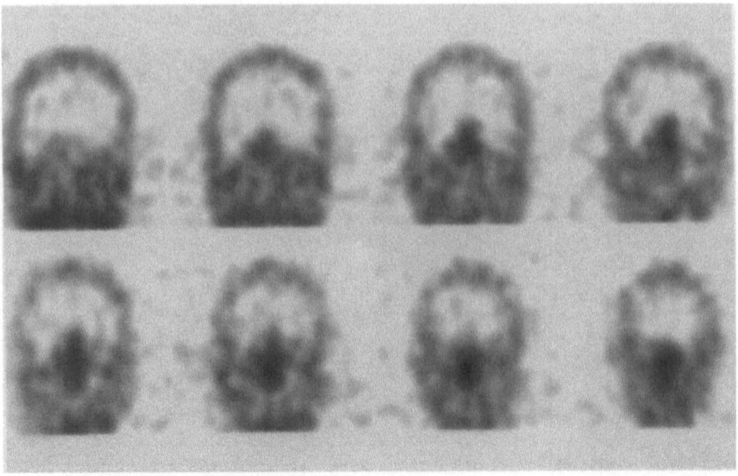

Figure 4. Coronal ^{111}In-pentetreotide SPET image in a patient with a clinically nonfunctioning pituitary macroadenoma (the same patient as in Figure 1). Note the high uptake in the pituitary tumor (arrow).

A large variety of lesions in and around the pituitary region express somatostatin receptors and, therefore, can be visualized by SRS. The majority of meningiomas and class III and IV gliomas, some metastases from breast carcinomas and other adenocarcinomas, osteosarcomas, Hodgkin and non-Hodgkin lymphomas, abscesses and granulomatous lesions, angioleiomyomas, chordomas and haemangiopericytomas can be visualized by SRS. Class I and II gliomas, neurinomas, neurofibromas epidermoids, ependymomas plasmacytomas, craniopharyngiomas and other cystic lesions are generally negative on SRS. SRS allows post-surgical differentiation between scar tissue, radionecrosis and recurrent meningiomas. In some patients SRS may aid in the preoperative diagnosis and staging of skull base tumors, although it is not tumor-specific (49,50-52).

In the near future, ^{99m}Tc-labeled peptides may also become available for somatostatin receptor imaging of pituitary tumors (53). In a preliminary study, one of these new radiotracers has been used for imaging neuroendocrine tumors including pituitary adenomas (Figure 5) (54). It may also become feasible to label newer somatostatin analogs with other receptor binding characteristics than octreotide. The combined use of three-step immunoscintigraphy with an anti-chromogranin A monoclonal antibody and SRS may potentially further discriminate non-neuroendocrine masses of the pituitary region from non-functioning pituitary adenomas (55,56).

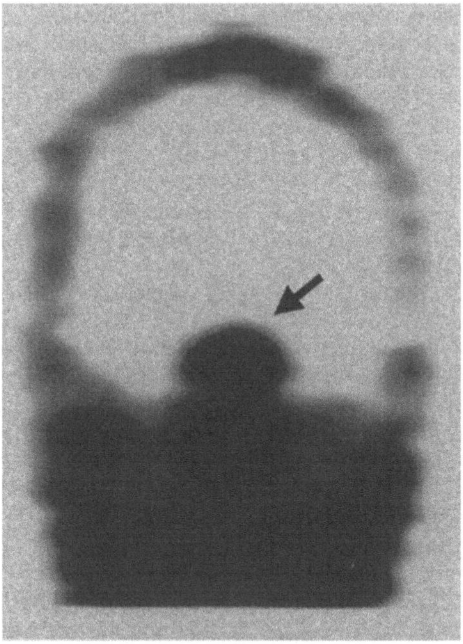

Figure 5. Coronal SPET image of the head in a patient with a TSH-secreting pituitary macroadenoma obtained 1 hr. after the injection of 10 mCi of ^{99m}Tc-P829 (Image kindly provided by Dr. S. Lastoria).

References

1. Serri O, Marchisio AM, Collu R, Hardy J, Somma M. Dopaminergic binding sites in human pituitary adenomas other than prolactinomas. Horm Res. 1984;19:97.
2. Bevan JS, Burke CW. Non-functioning pituitary adenomas do not regress during bromocriptine therapy but possess membrane-bound dopamine receptors which bind bromocriptine. Clin Endocrinol. 1986;25:561.
3. Koga M, Nakao H, Arao M, et al. Demonstration of specific dopamine receptors on human pituitary adenomas. Acta Endocrinol (Copenh). 1987;114:595.
4. Bevan JS, Webster J, Burke CW, Scanlon MF. Dopamine agonists and pituitary tumor shrinkage. Endocr Rev. 1992;13:220.
5. Vance ML, Thorner MO. Prolactinomas. Endocrinol Metab Clin North Am. 1987;16:731.
6. Pellegrini I, Rasolonjanahary R, Gunz G, et al. Resistance to bromocriptine in prolactinomas. J Clin Endocrinol Metab. 1989;69:500.
7. Kwekkeboom DJ, Lamberts SW. Long-term treatment with the dopamine agonist CV 205-502 of patients with a clinically non-functioning, gonadotroph, or alpha- subunit secreting pituitary adenoma. Clin Endocrinol. 1992;36:171.
8. Muhr C, Bergstrom M, Lundberg PO, et al. Dopamine receptors in pituitary adenomas: PET visualization with 11C-N-methylspiperone. J Comput Assist Tomogr. 1986;10:175.
9. Bergstrom M, Muhr C, Lundberg PO, Langstrom B. PET as a tool in the clinical evaluation of pituitary adenomas. J Nucl Med. 1991;32:610.
10. Lucignani G, Losa M, Moresco RM, et al. Differentiation of clinically non-functioning pituitary adenomas from meningiomas and craniopharyngiomas by positron emission tomography with [^{18}F]fluoro-ethyl-spiperone. Eur J Nucl Med. 1997;24:1149.
11. Pirker W, Brucke T, Riedl M, et al. Iodine-123-IBZM-SPECT: studies in 15 patients with pituitary tumors. J Neural Transm Gen Sect. 1994;97:235.
12. Scillitani A, Dicembrino F, Di Fazio P, et al. *In vivo* visualization of pituitary dopaminergic receptors by iodine-123 methoxybenzamide (IBZM) correlates with sensitivity to dopamine agonists in two patients with macroprolactinomas. J Clin Endocrinol Metab. 1995;80:2523.
13. de Herder WW, Lamberts SW. Imaging of pituitary tumours. Baill Clin Endocrinol Metab 1995;9:367.
14. de Herder WW, Reijs AE, Kwekkeboom DJ, et al. *In vivo* imaging of pituitary tumours using a radiolabelled dopamine D2 receptor radioligand. Clin Endocrinol. 1996;45:755.
15. Ferone D, Lastoria S, Colao A, et al. Correlation of scintigraphic results using ^{123}I-Methoxybenzamide with hormone levels and tumor size response to quinagolide in patients with pituitary adenomas. J Clin Endocrinol Metab. 1998;83:248.
16. Assies J, Verhoeff NP, Bosch DA, Hofland LJ. Intracranial dissemination of a macroprolactinoma. Clin Endocrinol. 1993;38:539.
17. Verhoeff NP, Bemelman FJ, Wiersinga WM, van Royen EA. Imaging of dopamine D2 and somatostatin receptors *in vivo* using single-photon emission tomography in a patient with a TSH/PRL- producing pituitary macroadenoma. Eur J Nucl Med. 1993;20:555.
18. Joyce JN, Janowsky A, Neve KA. Characterization and distribution of [^{125}I]epidepride binding to dopamine D2 receptors in basal ganglia and cortex of human brain. J Pharmacol Exp Ther. 1991;257:1253.
19. Kessler RM, Whetsell WO, Ansari MS, et al. Identification of extrastriatal dopamine D2 receptors in post mortem human brain with [^{125}I]epidepride. Brain Res. 1993;609:237.
20. Ichise M, Ballinger JR. SPECT imaging of dopamine receptors. J Nucl Med. 1996;37:1591.

21. Verhoeff NP, Bobeldijk M, Feenstra MG, et al. *In vitro* and *in vivo* D2-dopamine receptor binding with [^{123}I]S(-) iodobenzamide ([^{123}I]IBZM) in rat and human brain. Int J Rad Appl Instrum [B]. 1991;18:837.
22. Brucke T, Tsai YF, McLellan C, et al. *In vitro* binding properties and autoradiographic imaging of 3- iodobenzamide ([^{125}I]-IBZM): a potential imaging ligand for D-2 dopamine receptors in SPECT. Life Sci. 1988;42:2097.
23. de Paulis T, Janowsky A, Kessler RM, Clanton JA, Smith HE. (S)-N-[(1-ethyl-2-pyrrolidinyl)methyl]-5-[^{125}I]iodo- 2-methoxybenzamide hydrochloride, a new selective radioligand for dopamine D-2 receptors. J Med Chem. 1988;31:2027.
24. Leslie WD, Abrams DN, Greenberg CR, Hobson D. Comparison of iodine-123-epidepride and iodine-123-IBZM for dopamine D2 receptor imaging. J Nucl Med. 1996;37:1589.
25. Pirker W, Riedl M, Luger A, et al. Dopamine D2 receptor imaging in pituitary adenomas using iodine-123-epidepride and SPECT. J Nucl Med. 1996;37:1931.
26. de Herder WW, Reijs AM, de Swart J, et al. Comparison of iodine-123 epidepride and iodine-123 IBZM for dopamine D2 receptor imaging in clinically non-functioning pituitary macroadenomas and macroprolactinomas. Eur J Nucl Med. 1999;26:46.
27. Miller GM, Alexander JM, Bikkal HA, Katznelson L, Zervas NT, Klibanski A. Somatostatin receptor subtype gene expression in pituitary adenomas. J Clin Endocrinol Metab. 1995;80:1386.
28. Panetta R, Patel YC. Expression of mRNA for all five human somatostatin receptors (hSSTR1-5) in pituitary tumors. Life Sci. 1995;56:333.
29. Greenman Y, Melmed S. Expression of three somatostatin receptor subtypes in pituitary adenomas: evidence for preferential SSTR5 expression in the mammosomatotroph lineage. J Clin Endocrinol Metab. 1994;79:724.
30. Greenman Y, Melmed S. Heterogeneous expression of two somatostatin receptor subtypes in pituitary tumors. J Clin Endocrinol Metab. 1994;78:398.
31. Faglia G, Bazzoni N, Spada A, et al. *In vivo* detection of somatostatin receptors in patients with functionless pituitary adenomas by means of a radioiodinated analog of somatostatin ([^{123}I]SDZ 204-090). J Clin Endocrinol Metab. 1991;73:850.
32. Ur E, Mather SJ, Bomanji J, et al. Pituitary imaging using a labelled somatostatin analogue in acromegaly. Clin Endocrinol. 1992;36:147.
33. van Royen EA, Verhoeff NP, Meylaerts SA, Miedema AR. Indium-111-DTPA-octreotide uptake measured in normal and abnormal pituitary glands. J Nucl Med. 1996;37:1449.
34. Colao A, Lastoria S, Ferone D, et al. The pituitary uptake of ^{111}In-DTPA-D-Phe^{1}-octreotide in the normal pituitary and pituitary adenomas. J Endocrinol Invest. 1999;in press:
35. Broson-Chazot F, Houzard C, Ajzenberg C, et al. Somatostatin receptor imaging in somatotroph and non-functioning pituitary adenomas: correlation with hormonal and visual responses to octreotide. Clin Endocrinol. 1997;47:589.
36. Legovini P, De ME, Billeci D, Conti B, Zoli P, Conte N. ^{111}Indium-pentetreotide pituitary scintigraphy and hormonal responses to octreotide in acromegalic patients. J Endocrinol Invest. 1997;20:424.
37. Gorges R, Cordes U, Engelbach M, et al. Prediction of pharmacological effect of octreotide in acromegaly by means of ^{111}In-pentetreotide scintigraphy and calculation of a pituitary uptake index. Nuklearmedizin 1997;36:117.
38. Boni G, Ferdeghini M, Bellina CR, et al. [^{111}In-DTPA-D-Phe]-octreotide scintigraphy in functioning and non- functioning pituitary adenomas. Q J Nucl Med. 1995;39:90.
39. Colao A, Ferone D, Lastoria S, et al. Prediction of efficacy of octreotide therapy in patients with acromegaly. J Clin Endocrinol Metab. 1996;81:2356.

40. Plockinger U, Reichel M, Fett U, Saeger W, Quabbe HJ. Preoperative octreotide treatment of growth hormone-secreting and clinically nonfunctioning pituitary macroadenomas: effect on tumor volume and lack of correlation with immunohistochemistry and somatostatin receptor scintigraphy. J Clin Endocrinol Metab. 1994;79:1416.
41. Plockinger U, Bader M, Hopfenmuller W, Saeger W, Quabbe HJ. Results of somatostatin receptor scintigraphy do not predict pituitary tumor volume- and hormone-response to ocreotide therapy and do not correlate with tumor histology. Eur J Endocrinol. 1997;136:369.
42. Rieger A, Rainov NG, Elfrich C, et al. Somatostatin receptor scintigraphy in patients with pituitary adenoma. Neurosurg Rev. 1997;20:7.
43. de Herder WW, Kwekkeboom DJ, Reijs AE et al. Receptor scintigraphy with somatostatin analogues and dopamine antagonists of pituitary tumours. In: von Werder K, Fahlbusch R, eds. Pituitary adenomas. From basic research to diagnosis and therapy. Elsevier Science BV, 1996:93.
44. Losa M, Magnani P, Mortini P, et al. Indium-111 pentetreotide single-photon emission tomography in patients with TSH-secreting pituitary adenomas: correlation with the effect of a single administration of octreotide on serum TSH levels. Eur J Nucl Med. 1997;24:728.
45. de Bruin TW, Kwekkeboom DJ, van 't Verlaat JW, et al. Clinically nonfunctioning pituitary adenoma and octreotide response to long term high dose treatment, and studies *in vitro*. J Clin Endocrinol Metab. 1992;75:1310.
46. Warnet A. The role of octreotide (Sandostatin) in non-growth hormone-, non-thyroid-stimulating hormone-, and non-prolactin-secreting adenomas. Metabolism 1992;41:59.
47. Warnet A, Timsit J, Chanson P, et al. The effect of somatostatin analogue on chiasmal dysfunction from pituitary macroadenomas. J Neurosurg. 1989;71:687.
48. Oppizzi G, Cozzi R, Dallabonzana D, et al. Scintigraphic imaging of pituitary adenomas: an *in vivo* evaluation of somatostatin receptors. J Endocrinol Invest. 1998;21:512.
49. Luyken C, Hildebrandt G, Krisch B, Scheidhauer K, Klug N. Clinical relevance of somatostatin receptor scintigraphy in patients with skull base tumours. Acta Neurochir Suppl (Wien). 1996;65:102-4:102.
50. Maini CL, Sciuto R, Tofani A, et al. Somatostatin receptor imaging in CNS tumours using ^{111}In-octreotide. Nucl Med Commun. 1995;16:756.
51. Scheidhauer K, Hildebrandt G, Luyken C, Schomacker K, Klug N, Schicha H. Somatostatin receptor scintigraphy in brain tumors and pituitary tumors: first experiences. Horm Metab Res Suppl. 1993;27:59.
52. Schmidt M, Scheidhauer K, Luyken C, et al. Somatostatin receptor imaging in intracranial tumours. Eur J Nucl Med. 1998;25:675.
53. Pearson DA, Lister-James J, McBride WJ, et al. Somatostatin receptor-binding peptides labeled with technetium-99m: chemistry and initial biological studies. J Med Chem. 1996;39:1361.
54. Ferone D, Colao A, Lastoria S, et al. Somatostatin-receptor scintigraphy with ^{99m}Tc-labeled synthetic peptide P829 in neuroendocrine tumors. J Endocrinol Invest 1996;19:(Abstract)
55. Colombo P, Siccardi AG, Paganelli G, et al. Three-step immunoscintigraphy with anti-chromogranin A monoclonal antibody in tumours of the pituitary region. Eur J Endocrinol. 1996;135:216.
56. Magnani P, Paganelli G, Siccardi AG, et al. Combined use of ^{111}In-labeled pentetreotide and three-step immunoscintigraphy with antichromogranin A monoclonal antibody in the diagnosis of pituitary adenomas. Cell Biophys. 1994;24-25:307.

4
PITUITARY INCIDENTALOMAS

Mark E. Molitch, M.D.
Northwestern University Medical School
Chicago, IL 60611 USA

INTRODUCTION

The routine use of the high resolution methods of imaging of magnetic resonance imaging (MRI) and computed tomography (CT) for most central nervous system (CNS) diseases has created the dilemma for the clinician of the radiologist being able to detect asymptomatic masses in the pituitary, referred to as "pituitary incidentalomas" (5-7,14,21,38,45,48,60,66). It is the purpose of this chapter to provide information and guidelines for the evaluation of the patient incidentally found to have a mass lesion of the pituitary on a CT or MRI scan that has been performed for some other reason (Figure 1).

TYPES OF PITUITARY MASS LESIONS

A number of lesions may be present within the sella turcica (13,16,10,42,63) (See Table 1, Chapter 1). Certainly the most common lesion is the pituitary adenoma. Adenomas < 10 mm in diameter are designated microadenomas and those >10 mm in diameter are designated macroadenomas. Areas of invasion and extrasellar extension are important.

The most common tumor is a prolactin (PRL)-secreting tumor (prolactinoma) and the next most common is a clinically nonfunctioning tumor. The latter frequently secrete intact gonadotropins or their glycoprotein subunits (alpha and/or beta) *in vivo* or *in vitro*; technically, therefore, most are really gonadotroph adenomas (1). Rarely, clinically non-functioning tumors will be found to stain positively for adrenocorticotropic hormone (ACTH) or growth hormone (GH) but do not secrete these hormones in excess and such patients do not have Cushing's disease or acromegaly (1). The natural history of GH and ACTH-producing tumors that do not cause the classical symptoms of acromegaly and Cushing's disease is not known.

A number of other sellar lesions may mimic a pituitary adenoma (See Table 1, Chapter 1) and in many cases, the diagnosis can only be made histologically. There are some differentiating characteristics, however, for some types of lesions. Lymphocytic hypophysitis usually manifests in women in the peripartum period (46). Metastatic cancer frequently causes oculomotor palsies and diabetes insipidus - findings usually absent in pituitary adenomas (56). Artifacts mimicking pituitary lesions include beam-hardening effects with CT and susceptibility distortions with MRI (16).

AUTOPSY FINDINGS

Pituitary adenomas have been found at autopsy in 1.5 to 27 per cent of subjects not suspected of having pituitary disease while alive (4,6,9,10,15,25,28,30,34,39-41, 43,49,51,52,59,61,62) (Table 2).

Table 2. Frequency of Pituitary Adenomas Found at Autopsy

Study	Number Of Pituitaries Examined	Number of Adenomas Found	Freq. (%)	Number of Macro-adenomas	Stain for PRL (%)
Susman (61)	260	23	8.8	-	-
Costello (9)	1,000	225	22.5	0	-
Sommers (59)	400	26	6.5	0	-
McCormick& Halmi (34)	1,600	140	8.8	0	-
Kovacs et al (25)	152	20	13.2	2	53
Landolt (28)	100	13	13.0	0	-
Mosca et al (40)	100	24	24.0	0	23
Burrow et al (4)	120	32	26.7	0	41
Parent et al (43)	500	42	8.4	1	-
Muhr et al (41)	205	3	1.5	0	-
Schwezinger and Warzok (52)	5,100	485	9.5	0	-
Coulon et al (10)	100	10	10.0	0	60
Chambers et al (6)	100	14	14.0	0	-
Siqueira & Guembarovski (57)	450	39	8.7	0	-
El-Hamid et al (15)	486	97	20.0	0	48
Scheithauer et al (51)	251	41	16.3	0	66
Marin et al (30)	210	35	16.7	0	32
Mosca et al (39)	111	13	11.7	0	
Sano et al (49)	166	15	9.0	0	47
Teramoto et al (62)	1,000	51	5.1	0	30
TOTAL	12,411	1,408	11.3	3	

The average frequency of finding an adenoma for the 12,411 pituitaries in these studies was 11.3%. PRL immunohistochemistry was performed in 298 of these pituitaries with 46 per cent staining positively for PRL (4,10,15,25,28,30,49,62). There were no age or sex predilections for finding such tumors. In these postmortem studies all but three of the tumors were less than 10 mm in diameter (Table 2) and these three were less than 15 mm in diameter. The relative lack of macroadenomas in these studies suggests that growth from micro- to macroadenomas must be either exceedingly uncommon and/or that virtually all macroadenomas come to clinical attention and therefore are not included in autopsy findings. A recent paper that reported 3 macroadenomas at autopsy (2) highlights this fact.

As noted in Table 1, Chapter 1, not all sellar lesions are pituitary adenomas. Chambers et al (6) found that of 24 lesions > 3mm in diameter in 100 pituitaries, 11 were microadenomas, 6 were pars intermedia cysts, 4 were foci of metastatic tumor and 3 were pituitary infarcts. In addition there were 14 pars intermedia cysts and 3 pituitary microadenomas < 3 mm in diameter. Teramoto et al (62) found 61 lesions in 1000 pituitaries that were > 2 mm in diameter and of these, 18 were adenomas, 2 were focal hyperplasias, 37 were Rathke's cleft cysts, and 4 were hemorrhages.

CT and MRI SCANS IN NORMAL INDIVIDUALS

Three series have evaluated CT scans of the sellar area in normal subjects who were having such scans for reasons unrelated to possible pituitary disease. Chambers et al (6) found discrete areas of low density > 3 mm in diameter in 10 of 50 such subjects. In our study of 107 normal women, we found 7 who had focal hypodense areas and 5 who had focal high density regions > 3 mm in diameter (66). In a third study, Peyster et al. (45) found focal hypodense areas > 3 mm in diameter in only 8 of 216 subjects.

Two similar studies have been carried out using MRI. Chong et al (7) found focal pituitary gland hypodensities 2-5 mm (mean 3.9 mm) in 20 of 52 normal subjects with nonenhanced images using a 1.5-T scanner and 3 mm thick sections. With similar scans but with gadolinium-DTPA enhancement, Hall et al (21) found that in 100 normal volunteers focal areas of decreased intensity > 3mm in diameter compatible with the diagnosis of adenoma were found in 34, 10 and 2 volunteers, depending upon whether there was agreement on the diagnosis between 1, 2 or 3 independent reviewing neuroradiologists.

Sellar lesions > 10 mm in diameter have not been found in studies of consecutive normal individuals, similar to the very limited number found at autopsy. However, macroadenomas have been reported as incidental findings (5) and I have seen many such patients with large pituitary tumors found incidentally on scans done because of head trauma or other reasons (e.g. Figure 1). In the two series of patients reported with pituitary incidentalomas (14,48), 29 of 52 patients had macroadenomas.

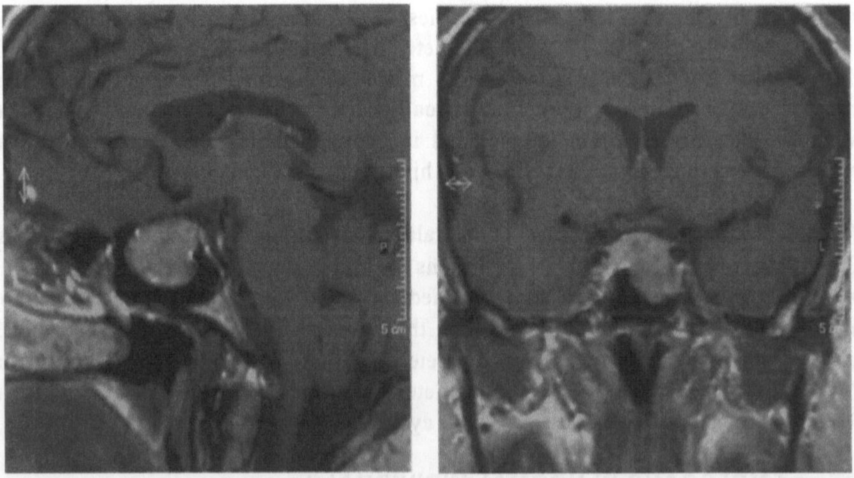

Figure 1. MRI scan *Left* sagittal view and *Right* coronal view, carried out to rule out lesions of internal auditory canals causing vertigo. This 53 year old man was eventually found to have a prolactin of 1596 ng/ml. His vertigo last 3 days and never returned. He denied sexual dysfunction and otherwise felt well. Additional testing revealed low Free T_4 and testosterone levels but normal cortisol levels. He is currently being treated with cabergoline.

DIAGNOSTIC EVALUATION

Endocrinologic Evaluation

As the most common lesion in the sella is a pituitary adenoma, it is reasonable to evaluate patients for hormone oversecretion, regardless of the size of the lesion seen. Many of the changes occurring with hormone oversecretion syndromes may be quite subtle and only slowly progressive and, therefore, screening for hormonal oversecretion is warranted even in patients with no clinical evidence of hormone oversecretion (Table 3). "Silent" somatotroph and corticotroph adenomas have been reported many times but it is not clear whether such patients with minimal clinical evidence of hormone oversecretion are free from the increased risk for the more subtle cardiovascular, bone, oncological, and possibly other adverse effects we usually associated with such tumors. Screening for hormone oversecretion in such patients has been questioned as to its cost-effectiveness but many of the premises used in these analyses were incorrect, i.e. they used assumptions based on the population at large rather than the published data on actual cases of incidental tumors (23). Evidence from these published series demonstrates that such screening is worthwhile, as 1 of the18 patients studied by Reincke et al (48) turned out to have a GH-secreting tumor and in another series in which tumor size was not specified 6/31 patients had prolactinomas and 1 had elevated GH levels (19).

Table 3. Screening Tests for Pituitary Hormone Oversecretion

Hormone	**Test**
GH	Elevated Insulin-like Growth Factor I (somatomedin C level) Failure to suppress GH levels to < 2 ng/ml with oral glucose load
ACTH	Elevated 24-hour urinary free cortisol level Failure to suppress cortisol levels to < 7 ng/ml (193 nmol/L with 1 mg of dexamethasone given orally 2300 - 2400h the previous night
PRL	Elevated basal levels, repeated at least once, Exclusion of other causes by history, physical examination, chemistry screening and thyroid function tests
Optional FSH/LH	Elevated basal levels of FSH, LH and alpha subunit
TSH	Elevated basal levels of T_4, T_3 resin uptake, T_3 with nonsuppressed or elevated levels of TSH

Prolactinomas are the most common of the hormone secreting tumors. In addition, there are a large number of medications and conditions that may cause hyperprolactinemia (36), so that the finding of hyperprolactinemia in a patient with a "tumor" on scan may be a false-positive finding (12). These conditions can generally be excluded on the basis of a careful history and physical examination, routine laboratory screening and checking of thyroid function (36). One important cause of hyperprolactinemia needs to be emphasized. Large pituitary lesions (nonsecreting adenomas, craniopharyngiomas, meningiomas etc.) can cause moderate hyperprolactinemia by interfering with stalk function and the transmission of PRL inhibitory factors (37). Rarely do PRL levels get above 200 ng/ml in this fashion, however (37).

For GH oversecretion, probably the best single screening test is the Insulin-like Growth Factor I (IGF-I) level, as basal GH levels fluctuate tremendously (35). If only GH measurements are available, then GH levels should be shown to suppress to < 2ng/ml after an oral glucose load (35). Measurement of IGF binding protein 3 (IGFBP3) adds little as an aid in diagnosing acromegaly (11). When any of these tests are positive, more detailed evaluation is necessary to establish the diagnosis definitively (35).

Although the 24 hour urinary free cortisol and overnight 1 mg dexamethasone suppression tests usually are considered to be equal in screening for Cushing's disease (47), in this circumstance of looking for very early hormone oversecretion, the latter test probably would have higher discriminatory value and generally is easier to perform accurately in clinical practice. Another alternative might be the measurement of a midnight salivary cortisol (47). When these screening tests are positive, more detailed testing will be necessary to establish the diagnosis definitively (47).

Gonadotroph adenomas can generally be evaluated on a screening basis by measuring basal FSH, LH and subunit levels (55); isolated FSH and LH subunit hypersecretion may be able to be evaluated in the future if radioimmunoassays become commercially available. The primary reason to establish this diagnosis is to use the abnormal hormone/subunit as a tumor marker whose change may indicate tumor growth or regression after surgery. The hormone oversecretion itself causes no ill effects and the only benefit of finding an elevation would be to help in establishing the diagnosis of a pituitary adenoma vs. a non-adenomatous lesion such as a craniopharyngioma.

Thyrotroph cell adenomas cause biochemical as well as clinical hyperthyroidism. The unusual feature in these patients is an inappropriately normal or even elevated, rather than depressed TSH level (55).

Microadenomas do not generally cause disruption of normal pituitary function. Of the 22 patients with suspected microadenomas evaluated in the series of Reincke et al (48) and Donovan and Corenblum (14), all had normal pituitary function. Larger lesions may cause varying degrees of hypopituitarism because of compression of the hypothalamus, the hypothalamic-pituitary stalk, or the pituitary itself. Of the 27 patients with suspected macroadenomas evaluated in the series of Reincke et al (48) and Donovan and Corenblum (14), 5 were found to have partial hypopituitarism. Patients with larger lesions should be evaluated for hypopituitarism, as hypopituitarism has been associated with increased mortality (3). The workup of hypopituitarism has been recently reviewed elsewhere (27).

Radiologic Evaluation

The index abnormality being discussed is an abnormality found during a scan. For lesions > 1 cm in diameter, the important differential resides between pituitary adenomas and other mass lesions. MRI may be done as a secondary procedure if a mass is first detected on CT scan, as MRI can reveal far more anatomic detail of the lesion itself and its relationship to surrounding structures (16,42,64). MRI can demonstrate the decreased signal of flowing blood and therefore can better determine the presence of aneurysms (13,16,42). Aneurysms and adenomas may coexist, however, and occasionally magnetic resonance arteriography may be necessary. The specific radiologic aspects of craniopharyngiomas, Rathke's cleft cysts, meningiomas, etc. vs. pituitary adenomas have been reviewed elsewhere (13,16,20,42,63). Because of the lack of specificity of many of the radiologic signs, however, in many cases the only sure way of diagnosing a lesion is by obtaining tissue.

In patients with lesions < 10 mm, there is a similar lack of specificity and artifacts may contribute to the confusion in establishing a diagnosis (16). Several studies have compared radiologic studies to operative findings. In three papers from the Montreal General Hospital that analyzed preoperative direct coronal CT scans for ACTH-, PRL-, and GH-secreting adenomas resected by Dr. Jules Hardy, Marcovitz et al calculated the following respective sensitivities - 63%, 91.9% and 81.2%, specificities - 62.5% 25%, and 100% and overall accuracies - 62.8%, 87.7%, and 81.2% (31-33).

Similarly poor sensitivity (30%) and accuracy (39%) of CT for Cushing's syndrome was reported from the NIH (50). Somewhat better data have been reported for MRI using 1.5 T systems, Peck et al (44) reporting a sensitivity of 71% and specificity of 87% for ACTH-secreting adenomas. Johnson et al (22) performed both CT and MRI on patients undergoing surgery and found that correct diagnoses of microadenomas were made in 8/14 cases with CT and in 12/14 cases with MRI. Specific features such as focal hypo- or hyperdense areas and deviation of the stalk are not specific for the presence of a pituitary adenoma or other lesions (38). In addition, it is important to avoid diagnosing a tumor simply on the basis of a slight increase in size of the pituitary, as the normal pituitary increases in size during the normal physiologic states of adolescence (17) and pregnancy (18) and is hyperintense during pregnancy (18). The increase in size during pregnancy continues into the first postpartum week with some pituitaries increasing to almost 12 mm in height; the pituitaries then rapidly return to normal size despite postpartum breast-feeding (18). Pituitary volume may also be seen to be homogeneously increased with depression (26).

RECOMMENDATIONS

The degree to which patients need evaluation needs to be balanced against such things as patient age and other associated illnesses in accord with standard clinical judgment. The primary two things to be considered are: (1) that this is a functioning pituitary adenoma for which specific treatment might be necessary to correct the hormonal hypersecretion and (2) that this is an adenoma or other lesion that potentially cause future problems for the patient because of enlargement (Figure 2). With respect to the first consideration, patients can be evaluated and screened for hormonal oversecretion as discussed above and treated appropriately.

If there is no evidence of hormone oversecretion, then follow-up will depend upon considerations of tumor growth. With respect to pituitary microadenomas, it is known that for prolactinomas, at least, the cumulative risk of significant tumor enlargement over 5 - 7 years is about 5-7 per cent (24,29,53,58,65). This low risk of significant enlargement is likely to be true for nonsecreting adenomas as well. The risks of significant enlargement of Rathke's cleft cysts, intrasellar craniopharyngiomas, etc. are unknown, but they also seem to enlarge slowly. There is one case report of a patient whose relatively large, probable craniopharyngioma did not enlarge over a 5 year period of observation (54) but there are no other series in which a substantial number of such patients have been followed without intervention. Therefore, a reasonable approach may be to repeat the scan at yearly intervals for two years and, if there is no evidence of growth of the lesion, subsequently lengthen the interval between scans. Because of the radiation exposure with CT (8), consideration should be given to performing the repeat scans with MRI. Surgery does not seem to be indicated for such nonsecreting lesions unless growth is demonstrated. In the series of patients evaluated by Reincke et al (48), 1 of 7 patients with suspected microadenomas showed evidence of tumor enlargement (5 to 9 mm) over an 8 year follow up period and one patient had a regression in tumor size from 8 to 4 mm. In the series of patients evaluated by Donovan and Corenblum (14), none of the 15 patients with suspected microadenomas showed evidence of tumor growth over a mean of 6.7 years of follow-up.

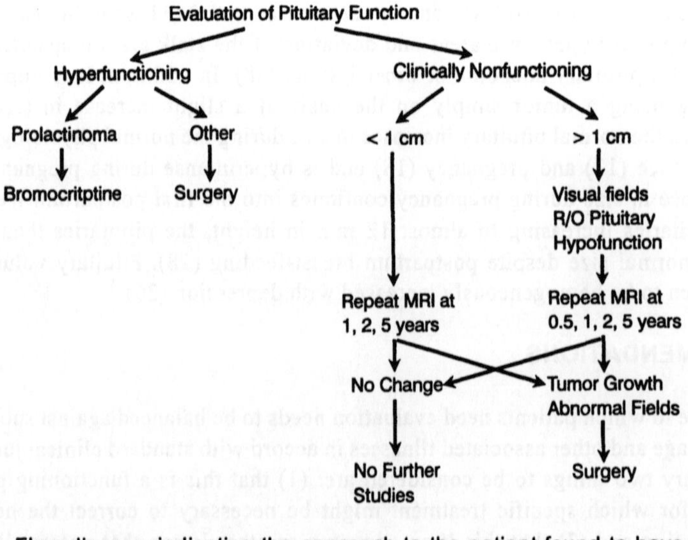

Figure 2. Flow diagram indicating the approach to the patient found to have a pituitary incidentaloma. The first step is to evaluate patients for pituitary hyperfunction and then treat those found to be hyperfunctioning. Of patients with tumors that are clinically non-functioning, those with macroadenomas are evaluated further for evidence of chiasmal compression and hypopituitarism. Scans are then repeated at progressively longer intervals to assess for enlargement of the tumors. (Reproduced from Molitch ME. Evaluation and treatment of the patient with a pituitary incidentaloma. J.Clin.Endocrinol.Metab 1995;80:3-6. Copyright, the Endocrine Society).

Lesions greater than 1 cm in diameter have already indicated a propensity for growth. A careful evaluation of the mass effects of these tumors is indicated, including evaluation of pituitary function and visual field examination. If a completely asymptomatic lesion is thought to be a pituitary adenoma on the basis of radiologic and clinical findings, then a decision could be made to simply repeat scans (MRI rather than CT to reduce irradiation, as above) on a yearly basis, surgery being deferred until there is evidence of tumor growth. As mentioned, however, the size of these lesions already indicates evidence of tumor growth and early surgery may be of benefit. About 10 - 15 per cent of nonsecreting adenomas respond to bromocriptine with tumor shrinkage and some may also respond to octreotide (55) so that a trial of medical therapy may be worthwhile in the completely asymptomatic patient. If no therapy is chosen initially, repeating scans at 6 and 12 months and then yearly to monitor for any increase in tumor size seems warranted. If there is no size change, the interval can subsequently be lengthened. Certainly, with any evidence of significant tumor growth, surgery should be performed.

In the series of Reincke et al (48), 4 of their 11 patients with incidentally found macroadenomas were operated upon initially because of visual field abnormalities in 2, chiasmal displacement in 1 and the demonstration of GH excess in 1. The other 7 patients were followed for 17 - 48 months. Two of these patients had increases in the size of their lesions from 22 to 25 mm and 14 to 20 mm in diameter over about 1.5 years. In the series of Donovan and Corenblum (14), 4 of their 16 patients with suspected macroadenomas experienced tumor enlargement over a mean follow-up period of 6.1 years, increase ranging from 2 to 5 mm. In 1 of these 4 the enlargement was associated with visual field impairment and he was found to have a craniopharyngioma at surgery. Another developed pituitary apoplexy following heparinization for coronary angiography, The other two patients continue to be followed with no further intervention or complications.

SUMMARY

Incidental pituitary masses are being found commonly during CT and MRI scans done for a variety of reasons. Screening for hormone oversecretion by these tumors appears to be warranted. For patients with lesions > 1cm, patients should also be screened for hypopituitarism.

In the absence of visual field abnormalities or hypothalamic /stalk compression, it may be appropriate to observe such patients carefully with repeated MRI scans. A limited amount of data suggests that significant tumor enlargement will occur in < 5% of patients with lesions < 1 cm in diameter. Significant growth occurs in just over one-quarter of lesions > 1 cm in diameter. Hemorrhage into such tumors is uncommon but anticoagulation may predispose to this complication. When there is no evidence of visual field deficits, an attempt at medical therapy with a dopamine agonist or octreotide is reasonable, realizing that only about 10% of such patients will respond with a decrease in tumor size. Alternatively, careful, periodic observation without intervention may determine that the lesion is not growing. Surgery is indicated if there is evidence of tumor enlargement, especially when such growth is accompanied by compression of the optic chiasm, cavernous sinus invasion or the development of pituitary hormone deficiencies.

References

1. Serri O, Marchisio AM, Collu R, Hardy J, Somma M. Dopaminergic binding sites in human pituitary adenomas other than prolactinomas. Horm Res. 1984;19:97.
2. Bevan JS, Burke CW. Non-functioning pituitary adenomas do not regress during bromocriptine therapy but possess membrane-bound dopamine receptors which bind bromocriptine. Clin Endocrinol. 1986;25:561.
3. Asa SL. The pathology of pituitary tumors. Endocrinol Metab Clin North Am. 1999;28:XX.
2. Auer RN, Alakija P, Sutherland GR. Asymptomatic large pituitary adenomas discovered at autopsy. Surg Neurol. 1996;46:28.
3. Bates AS, Van't Hoff W, Jones PJ, et al. The effect of hypopituitarism on life expectancy. J Clin Endocrinol Metab. 1996;81:1169.
4. Burrows GN, Wortzman G, Rewcastle NB, et al. Microadenomas of the pituitary and abnormal sellar tomograms in an unselected autopsy series. N Engl J Med. 1981;304:156.
5. Chacko AG, Chandy MJ. Incidental pituitary macroadenomas. Brit J Neurosurg. 1992;6:233.
6. Chambers EF, Turski PA, LaMasters D, et al. Regions of low density in the contrast-enhanced pituitary gland: normal and pathologic processes. Radiology 1982;44:109..
7. Chong BW, Kucharczyk AW, Singer W, et al. Pituitary gland MR: a comparative study of healthy volunteers and patients with microadenomas. Am J Neuroradiol 1994;15:675.
8. Conway BJ, McCrohan JL, Antonsen RG, et al. Average radiation dose in standard CT examinations of the head: results of the 1990 NEXT Survey. Radiology 1992;184:135.
9. Costello RT. Subclinical adenoma of the pituitary gland. Am J Pathol. 1936;12:205.
10. Coulon G, Fellmann D, Arbez-Gindre F, et al. Les adenome hypophysaires latents. Etude autopsique. Sem Hop Paris. 1983;59:2747.
11. de Herder WW, van der Lely AJ, Janssen JAMJL et al. IGFBP-3 is a poor parameter for assessment of clinical activity in acromegaly. Clin Endocrinol. 1995;43:501.
12. Dombrowski RC, Romeo JH, Aron DC. Verapamil-induced hyperprolactinemia complicated by a pituitary incidentaloma. Ann Pharmacother. 1995;29:999.
13. Donovan JL, Nesbit GM. Distinction of masses involving the sella and suprasellar space: Specificity of imaging features. Am J Roentgenol. 1996;167:597.
14. Donovan LE, Corenblum B. The natural history of the pituitary incidentaloma. Arch Intern Med. 1995;153:181.
15. El-Hamid MWA, Joplin GF, Lewis PD. Incidentally found small pituitary adenomas may have no effect on fertility. Acta Endocrinol. 1998;117:361.
16. Elster AD. Modern imaging of the pituitary. Radiology 1993;187:1.
17. Elster AD, Chen MYM, Williams DW III, et al. Pituitary gland: MR imaging of physiologic hypertrophy in adolescence. Radiology 1990;174:681.
18. Elster AD, Sanders TG, Vines FS, et al. Size and shape of the pituitary gland during pregnancy and post partum: measurement with MR imaging. Radiology 1991;181:531.
19. Feldkamp J, Becker A, Santen R, Seppel T, Schlaghecke R. Incidentalomas of the pituitary gland. Eur J Endocrinol. 1994;130(Suppl. 2):144.
20. Freda PU, Post KD. Differential diagnosis of sellar masses. Endocrinol Metab Clin North Am. 1999;28:XX.
21. Hall WA, Luciano MG, Doppman JL, et al. Pituitary magnetic resonance imaging in normal human volunteers: occult adenomas in the general population. Ann Intern Med. 1994;120:817.
22. Johnson MR, Hoare RD, Cox T, et al. The evaluation of patients with a suspected pituitary microadenoma: computed tomography compared to magnetic resonance imaging. Clin Endocrinol. 1992;36:335.

23. King JT Jr, Justice AC, Aron DC. Management of incidental pituitary microadenomas: a cost-effectiveness analysis. J Clin Endocrinol Metab. 1997;82:3625.
24. Koppelman MCS, Jaffe MJ, Rieth KG, et al. Hyperprolactinemia, amenorrhea, and galactorrhea. Ann Intern Med 1984;100:115.
25. Kovacs K, Ryan N, Horvath E. Pituitary adenomas in old age. J Gerontol. 1980;35:16.
26. Krishnan KRR, Doraiswamy PM, Lurie SN, et al. Pituitary size in depression. J Clin Endocrinol Metab. 1991;72:256.
27. Lamberts SW, de Herder WW, van der Lely AJ. Pituitary insufficiency. Lancet 1998;352:127.
28. Landolt AM. Biology of pituitary microadenomas. In: Faglia G, Giovanelli MA, MacLeod RM, eds. Pituitary Microadenomas. New York: Academic Press; 1980, p.107.
29. March CM, Kletzky OA, Davajan V, et al. Longitudinal evaluation of patients with untreated prolactin-secreting pituitary adenomas. Am J Obstet Gynecol. 1981;139:835.
30. Marin F, Kovacs KT, Scheithauer BW, et al. The pituitary gland in patients with breast carcinoma: a histologic and immunocytochemical study of 125 cases. Mayo Clin Proc.1992;67:949.
31. Marcovitz S, Wee R, Chan J, et al. The diagnostic accuracy of preoperative CT scanning in the evaluation of pituitary ACTH-secreting adenomas. Am J Radiol. 1987;149:803.
32. Marcovitz S, Wee R, Chan J, et al. Diagnostic accuracy of preoperative CT scanning of pituitary prolactinomas. Am J Neuroradiol. 1988;9:13.
33. Marcovitz S, Wee R, Chan J, et al. Diagnostic accuracy of preoperative CT scanning of pituitary somatotroph adenomas. Am J Neuroradiol. 1988;9:19.
34. McCormick WF, Halmi NS. Absence of chromophobe adenomas from a large series of pituitary tumors. Arch Pathol 1971;92:231.
35. Melmed S. Acromegaly. N Engl J Med.1990;322:966.
36. Molitch ME. Diagnosis and treatment of prolactinomas. Adv Intern Med 1999;44:117.
37. Molitch ME, Reichlin S. Hypothalamic hyperprolactinemia: Neuroendocrine regulation of prolactin secretion in patients with lesions of the hypothalamus and pituitary stalk. In: MacLeod RM, Thorner MO, Scapagnini U, eds., Prolactin. Basic and Clinical Correlates. Proceedings of the IVth International Congress on Prolactin, Padova, Italy, Liviana Press, 1985, p. 709.
38. Molitch ME, Russell EJ. The pituitary incidentaloma. Ann Intern Med. 1990;112:925.
39. Mosca L, Costanzi G, Anotonacci C, et al. Hypophyseal pathology in AIDS. Histol Histopathol. 1992;7:291.
40. Mosca L, Solcia E, Capella C, et al. Pituitary adenomas: surgical versus post-mortem findings today. In: Faglia G, Giovanelli MA, MacLeod RM, eds. Pituitary Microadenomas. New York: Academic Press; 1980, p.137.
41. Muhr C, Bergstrom K, Grimelius L, et al. A parallel study of the roentgen anatomy of the sella turcica and the histopathology of the pituitary gland in 205 autopsy specimens. Neuroradiology 1981;21:55.
42. Naidich MJ, Russell EJ. Current approaches to imaging of the sellar region and pituitary. Endocrinol Metab Clin North Am. 1999;28:XX.
43. Parent AD, Bebin J, Smith RR. Incidental pituitary adenomas. J Neurosurg. 1981;54:228.
44. Peck WW, Dillon WP, Norman D, et al. High-resolution MR imaging of microadenomas at 1.5 T: experience with Cushing disease. Am J Neuroradiol. 1988;9:1085.
45. Peyster RG, Adler LP, Viscarello RR, et al. CT of the normal pituitary gland. Neuroradiology 1986;28:161.
46. Powrie JK, Powell M, Ayers AB, et al. Lymphocytic adenohypophysitis: magnetic resonance imaging features of two new cases and a review of the literature. Clin Endocrinol. 1995;42:315.

47. Raff H, Findling J. Current approaches to the diagnosis of Cushing's disease. Endocrinol Metab Clin North Am. 1999;28:XX.
48. Reincke M, Allolio B, Saeger W, et al. The 'incidentaloma' of the pituitary gland. Is neurosurgery required? J A M A. 1990;263:2772.
49. Sano T, Kovacs KT, Scheithauer BW, et al. Aging and the human pituitary gland. Mayo Clin Proc. 1993;68:971.
50. Saris SC, Patronas NJ, Doppman JL, et al. Cushing syndrome: pituitary CT scanning. Radiology 1987;162:775.
51. Scheithauer BW, Kovacs KT, Randall RV, et al. Effects of estrogen on the human pituitary: a clinicopathologic study. Mayo Clin Proc. 1989;64:1077.
52. Schwezinger G, Warzok R. Hyperplasien und adenome der hypophyse im unselektierten sektionsgut. Zentralbi Allg Pathol 1982;126:495.
53. Schlechte J, Dolan K, Sherman B, et al. The natural history of untreated hyperprolactinemia; a prospective analysis. J Clin Endocrinol Metab. 1989;68:412.
54. Sharara FI, Chrousos GP, Patronas NJ. Watchful waiting and craniopharyngioma. Ann Intern Med 1992;117:876.
55. Shomali ME, Katznelson L. Medical therapy for gonadotroph and thyrotroph tumors. Endocrinol Metab Clin North Am. 1999;28:XX.
56. Shubiger O, Haller D. Metastases to the pituitary-hypothalamic axis. An MR study of 7 symptomatic patients. Neuroradiology 1992;34:131.
57. Siqueira MG, Guembarovski AL. Subclinical pituitary microadenomas. Surg Neurol. 1984;22:134.
58. Sisam DA, Sheehan JP, Sheeler LR. The natural history of untreated microprolactinomas. Fertil Steril. 1987;48:67.
59. Sommers SC. Pituitary cell relations to body states. Lab Invest. 1959;8:588.
60. Soule SG, Jacobs HS. The evaluation and management of subclinical pituitary disease. Postgrad Med J. 1996;72:258.
61. Susman W. Pituitary adenoma. Br Med J. 1933;2:1215.
62. Teramoto A, Hirakawa K, Sanno N, et al. Incidental pituitary lesions in 1,000 unselected autopsy specimens. Radiology 1994;193:161.
63. Von Werder K. Pituitary enlargement. Clin Endocrinol. 1996;44:299.
64. Webb SM, Ruscalleda J, Schwarzstein D, et al. Computerized tomography versus magnetic resonance imaging: a comparative study in hypothalamic-pituitary and parasellar pathology. Clin Endocrinol. 1992;36:459.
65. Weiss MH, Teal J, Gott P, et al. Natural history of microprolactinomas: six-year follow-up. Neurosurgery 1983;12:180.
66. Wolpert SM, Molitch ME, Goldman JA, et al. Size, shape and appearance of the normal female pituitary gland. Am J Neuroradiol. 1984;5:263.

THYROID

5

ULTRASONOGRAPHY, CT, MRI OF THE THYROID GLAND

Brian Gorman, M.B., B.Ch., F.R.C.R., M.B.A.
Carl C. Reading, M.D.
Mayo Medical School; Rochester, Minnesota.

INTRODUCTION

Ultrasonography, CT, and MRI may all be used to study the anatomy and pathology of the thyroid gland. Of these, however, ultrasonography is the main technique used in clinical practice for thyroid imaging, because it is noninvasive, relatively inexpensive, and very sensitive in detecting thyroid lesions. Therefore, this chapter focuses mainly on ultrasonographic imaging.

TECHNIQUES

Ultrasonography

The ultrasonographic examination of the thyroid is performed with the patient in the supine position, with the neck extended. A pad may be placed under the patient's shoulders to facilitate the examination. The examiner usually sits behind the patient. A high-frequency (7.5-13 MHz) linear array transducer is used to provide optimal near-field detail for the relatively superficial thyroid gland. Gray-scale imaging is performed primarily. Color and spectral Doppler may be used selectively to provide additional information. Scans of the neck are performed in the longitudinal and transverse planes. The ultrasonographic examination should include the lateral neck to look for lymph nodes along the jugular chains.

CT

CT is of limited value for studying the internal morphology of the thyroid. CT is used principally to image the extent of thyroid lesions and, in particular, any regional lymph node involvement. Contrast material is usually given at a rate of 2 to 3 mL/s to opacify blood vessels and to help distinguish them from enlarged nodes. If a helical scanner is used, scanning begins at 25 s, and 5-mm slices are obtained from the angle of the mandible to the superior mediastinum.

MRI

MRI also has a limited role in thyroid imaging, because it has less spatial resolution and is relatively more expensive than ultrasonography. The technique does not usually provide a specific diagnosis for thyroid nodules. The major indications for MRI are to show the extent of substernal goiter and to evaluate the extent of invasive thyroid malignancy. A dedicated neck receiver coil is used to image the thyroid and to provide optimal spatial resolution and signal-to-noise ratio. Transaxial T_1- and fast spin-echo T_2-weighted images of the neck using thin slices (3 to 5 mm) are usually obtained. Images in the coronal or sagittal plane are useful to evaluate the retrosternal extension of goiter. Using a presaturation pulse (1) may reduce artifacts from flowing blood and motion.

ANATOMY

High-frequency ultrasound demonstrates the anatomy of the thyroid, adjacent musculature, and vessels in exquisite detail (Figure 1). The sternothyroid, sternohyoid, and omohyoid muscles are seen anterior to the thyroid. The sternocleidomastoid muscle is seen lateral to the thyroid. The longus colli muscle lies posterior to the thyroid lobes. The esophagus is usually seen to the left of the midline (Figure 2). Normal thyroid parenchyma has a homogeneous echotexture. Color Doppler is helpful in identifying blood vessels within and adjacent to the thyroid.

NODULAR DISEASE

Prevalence

In North America, the incidence of thyroid nodules detected by palpation is estimated to be 0.1% per year, with a prevalence of between 4% and 7% in the general population (2). Palpable thyroid nodules are more common in women, with advancing age, in areas of iodine deficiency, and after exposure to external radiation (3,4). In 1955, Mortensen et al. (5) examined thyroid glands removed at autopsy from 821 patients who had clinically normal thyroid glands. Clinically unsuspected thyroid nodules were found in 49.5% of these patients. Most of the nodules were benign. Only 4% of the nodular glands had malignant nodules. Most of the malignant nodules were small papillary tumors that typically follow an indolent course.

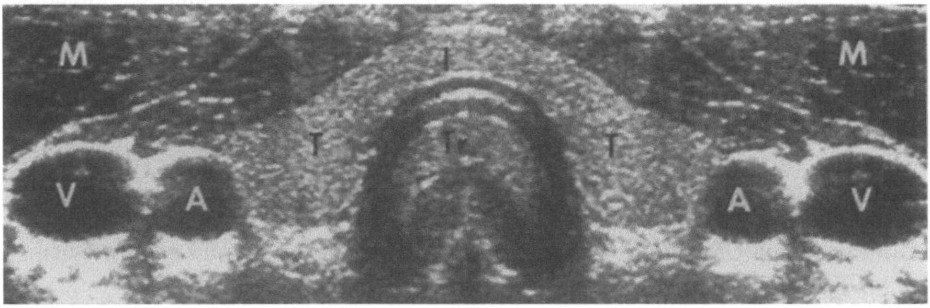

Figure 1. Normal ultrasonographic thyroid anatomy. Transverse ultrasonographic scan of the neck showing thyroid lobes (T), thyroid isthmus (I), trachea (Tr). *A*, Common carotid artery; *M*, sternocleidomastoid muscle; *V*, internal jugular vein. (From Solbiati et al. [9]. By permission of Mosby-Year Book.)

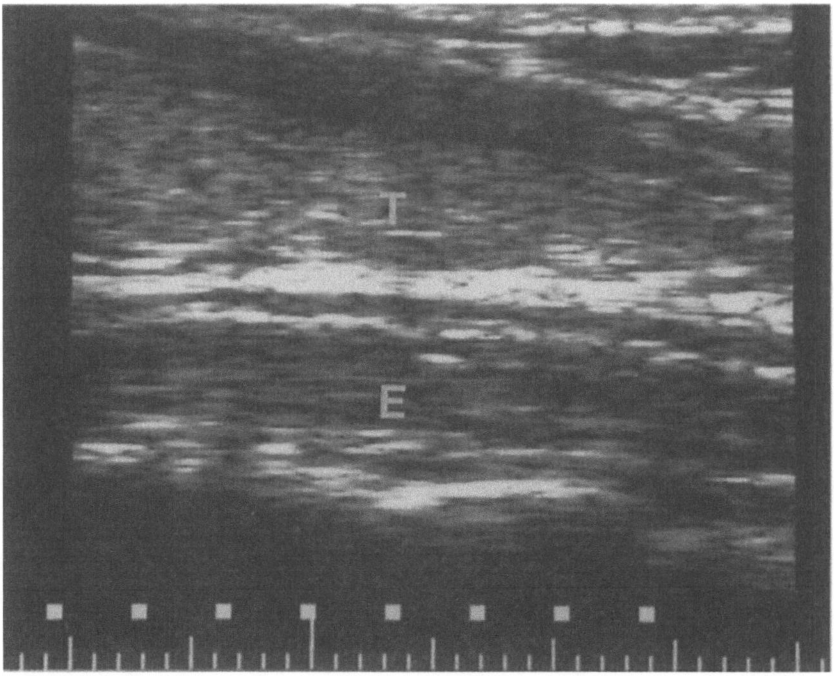

Figure 2. Normal esophagus. Longitudinal ultrasonogram of neck showing thyroid (*T*) and esophagus (*E*).

Studies of the thyroid with high-frequency ultrasound have confirmed the high prevalence of clinically unsuspected thyroid nodules (6-8). Because ultrasonography of the neck is frequently performed for clinical reasons other than a suspected thyroid lesion, incidental thyroid nodules will frequently be detected. It would be impractical, and prohibitively expensive, to extensively investigate all the nodules found incidentally. The challenge is to differentiate the small number of malignant, or potentially malignant, nodules found incidentally from the great majority of nodules that are benign.

Sonographic Features

Ultrasonographic features may help in predicting whether a thyroid nodule is benign or malignant.

Internal Contents. True epithelial simple cysts of the thyroid are extremely rare (Figure 3). Almost all cystic lesions of the thyroid seen with ultrasonography have internal debris or solid elements. Thirty percent of thyroid nodules have some cystic change (9). Most cystic thyroid nodules are benign. Cystic nodules are usually either hyperplastic nodules that have accumulated colloid or adenomas that have undergone degeneration or hemorrhage (Figure 4). Papillary thyroid cancer may produce colloid material and can present as a cystic thyroid nodule, but this is extremely rare (Figure 5) (10).

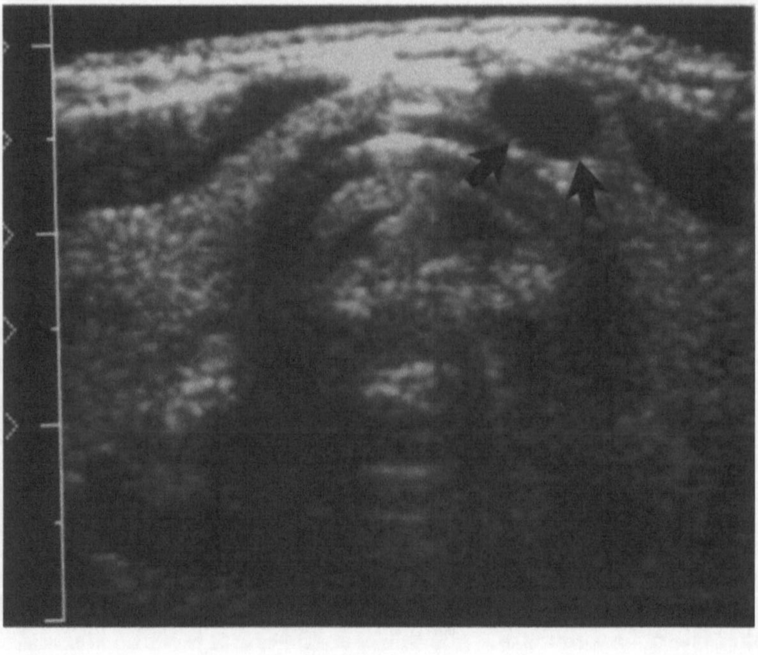

Figure 3. Simple cyst. Transverse ultrasonogram of neck showing simple cyst (arrows) in thyroid isthmus.

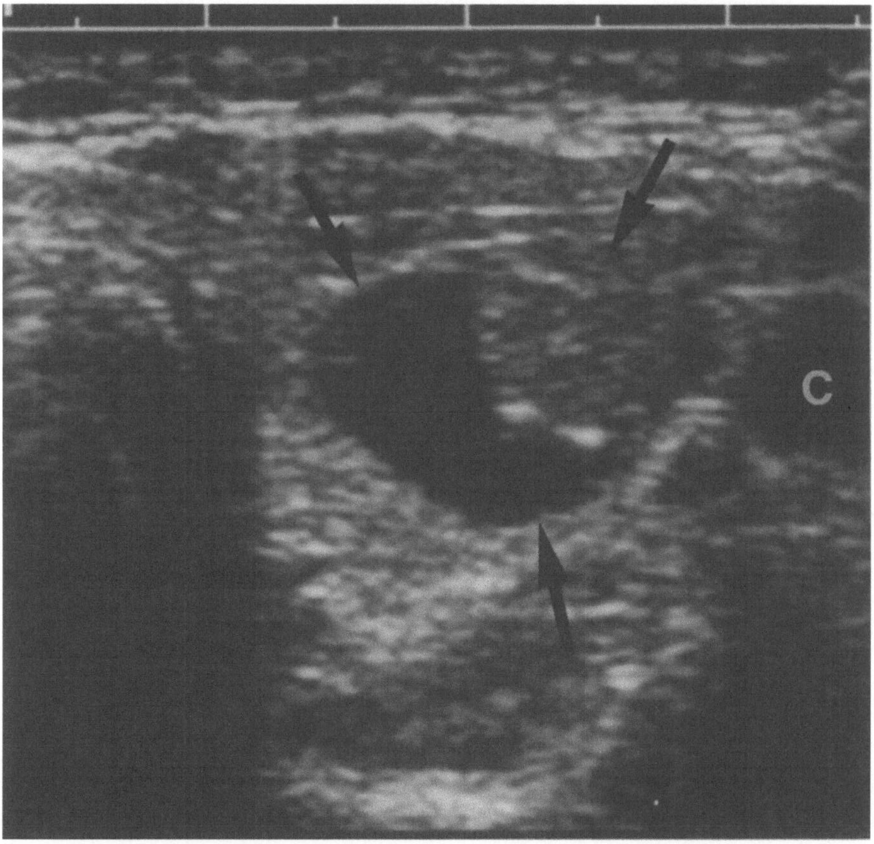

Figure 4. Benign cystic nodule. Transverse ultrasonogram of neck showing cystic thyroid nodule *(arrows)* with solid component. *C*, Common carotid artery.

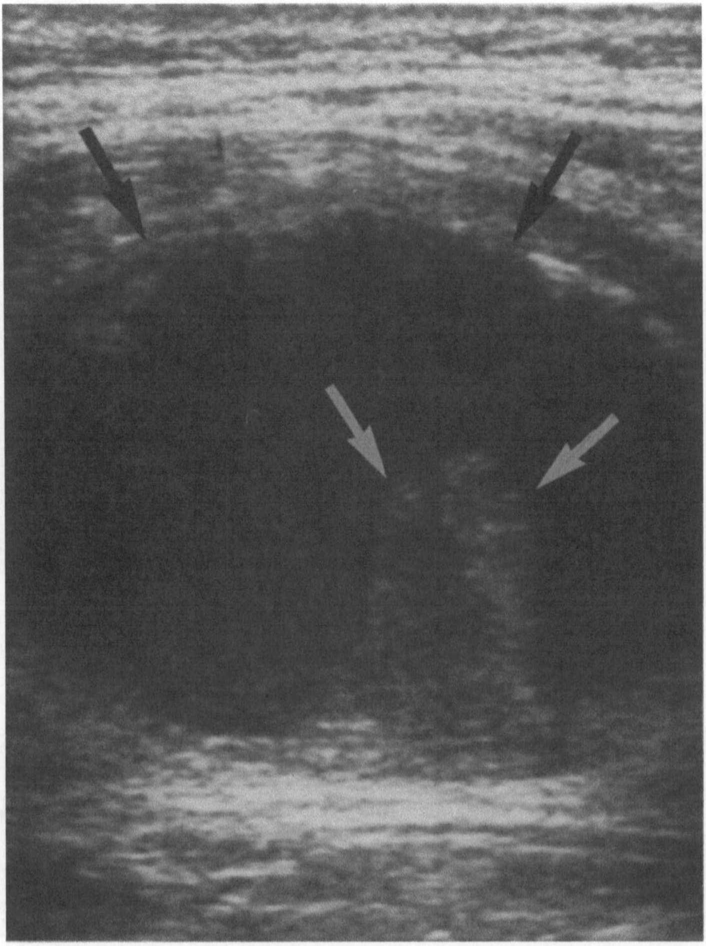

Figure 5. Cystic papillary thyroid carcinoma. Longitudinal ultrasonogram of neck showing mainly cystic thyroid nodule *(black arrows)* with solid component *(white arrows)*.

Any colloid material that is present may produce bright echoes with "comet-tail" artifacts (Figure 6). The comet tail artifacts may occur in the cystic fluid or in septations within the cystic nodule. Comet tail artifacts typically are associated with benign thyroid nodules (11). However, in contrast to thyroid nodules, cystic change in a cervical lymph node is most likely due to metastases, either from papillary thyroid cancer or squamous cell carcinoma (Figure 7).

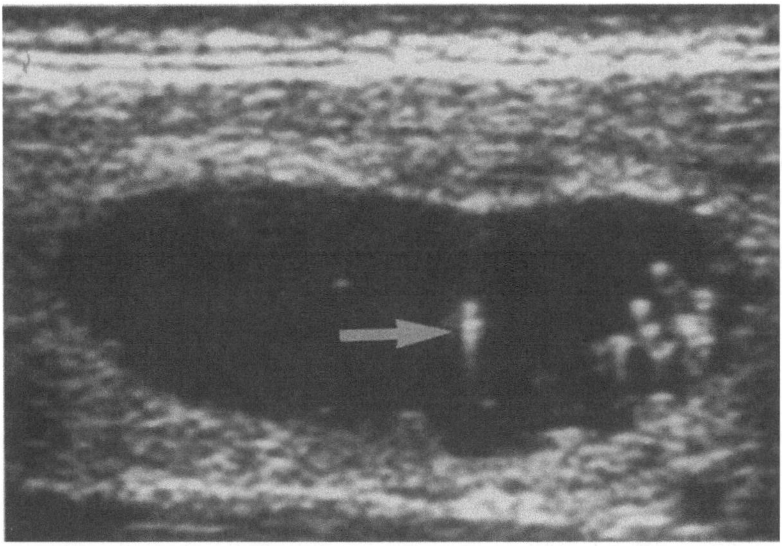

Figure 6. Benign cystic nodule with colloid crystals. Longitudinal ultrasonogram of neck showing cystic thyroid nodule with bright echogenic foci *(arrow)* due to colloid crystals.

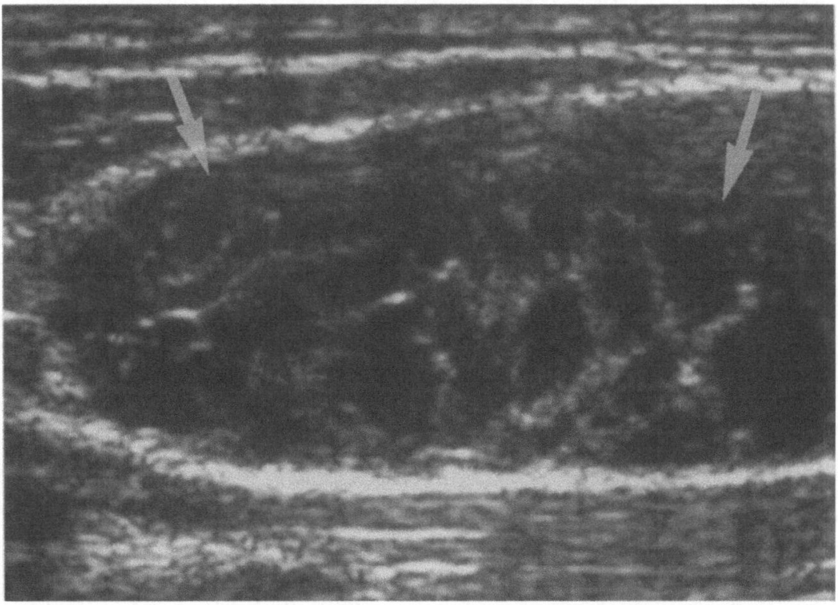

Figure 7. Lymph node with metastatic papillary thyroid carcinoma. Longitudinal ultrasonogram of neck showing lymph node with cystic change due to metastatic papillary thyroid carcinoma *(arrows)*.

Echogenicity. Most thyroid cancers are hypoechoic relative to the thyroid parenchyma. However, most hypoechoic nodules will be benign, because benign nodules are much more common than malignant nodules. A hyperechoic nodule is unlikely to be malignant (12).

Halo. Unlike liver lesions, the presence or absence of a relatively hypoechoic halo around a thyroid nodule is not helpful in distinguishing benign from malignant nodules. A peripheral halo may be seen with both benign and malignant nodules (12,13). The halo around a benign nodule is typically thin and regular. A thick, irregular halo around a nodule suggests a malignant nodule, but this appearance is rarely seen (Figure 8) and is of little use clinically.

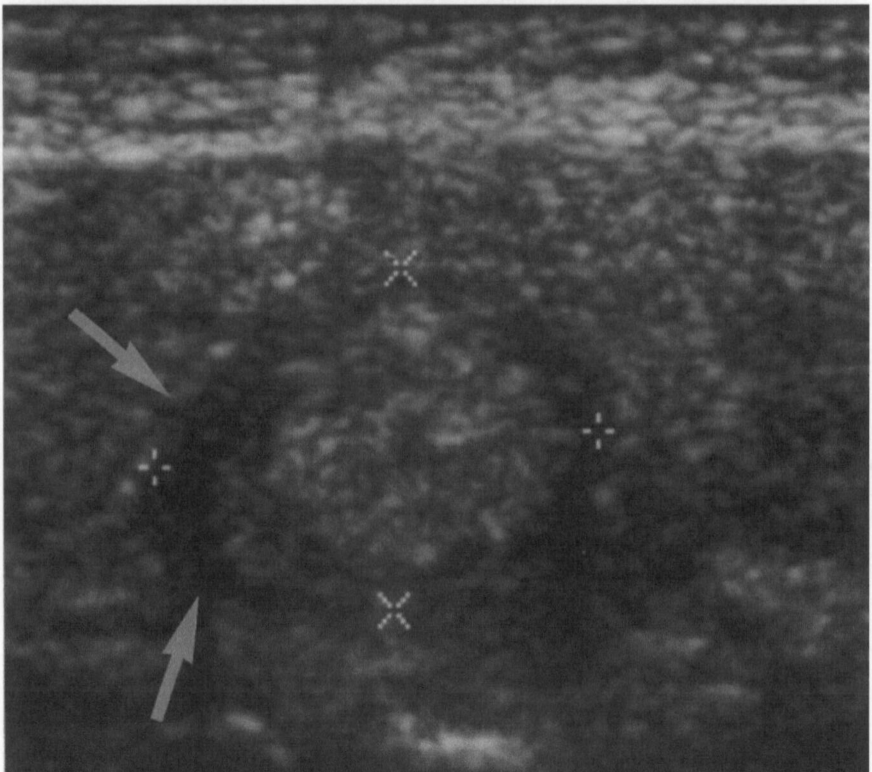

Figure 8. Papillary thyroid carcinoma. Longitudinal ultrasonogram of neck showing thyroid nodule with thick halo (arrows) due to papillary thyroid carcinoma. (From Hopkins CR, Reading CC. Thyroid and parathyroid imaging. Semin. Ultrasound CT MRI. 1995;16:279-295. By permission of WB Saunders Company.)

Calcification. About 10% to 15% of thyroid nodules contain some calcification, and this occurs in both benign and malignant nodules. The characteristics and pattern of the calcification may be helpful in distinguishing benign from malignant nodules. Peripheral, or "eggshell," calcification is a reliable, but rare, feature of benign calcification (Figure 9). When peripheral calcification is seen, a confident diagnosis of a benign nodule may be made, and no further investigation is needed.

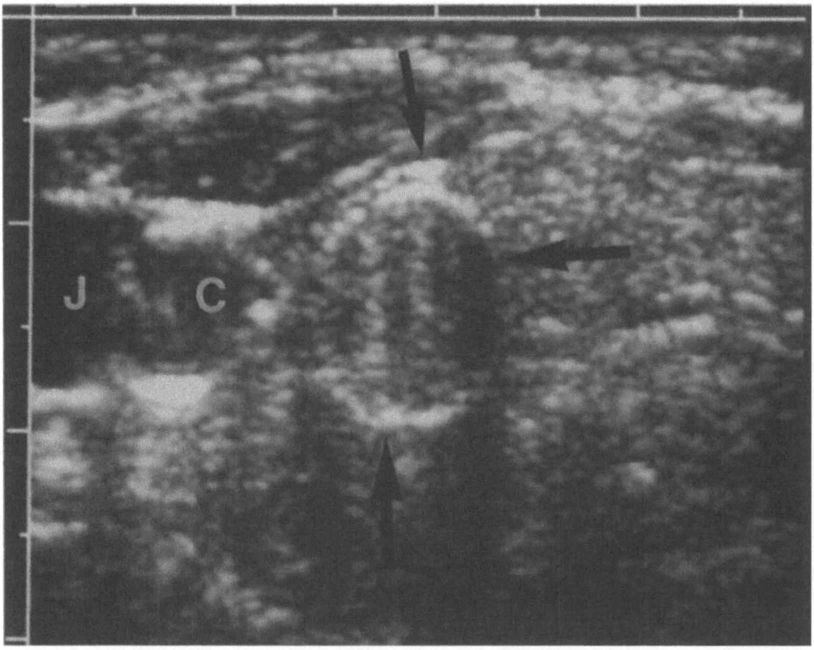

Figure 9. Benign calcified thyroid nodule. Transverse ultrasonogram of neck showing peripherally calcified benign thyroid nodule *(arrows)*. *C*, Common carotid artery; *J*, internal jugular vein.

Scattered echogenic foci occur more commonly. When these calcifications are large and coarse, the nodule is likely to be benign (Figure 10). When the calcifications are fine, they most likely are due to psammomatous calcifications associated with papillary thyroid carcinoma (Figure 11). With the better resolution of modern ultrasonographic equipment, microcalcifications are seen more frequently in papillary thyroid carcinoma (14). However, with increased resolution, calcium oxalate crystals present in benign nodules may be visible and mistaken for malignant calcifications (Figure 12). Therefore, although the sensitivity of detecting malignant microcalcifications has improved with better resolution of equipment, the specificity has decreased.

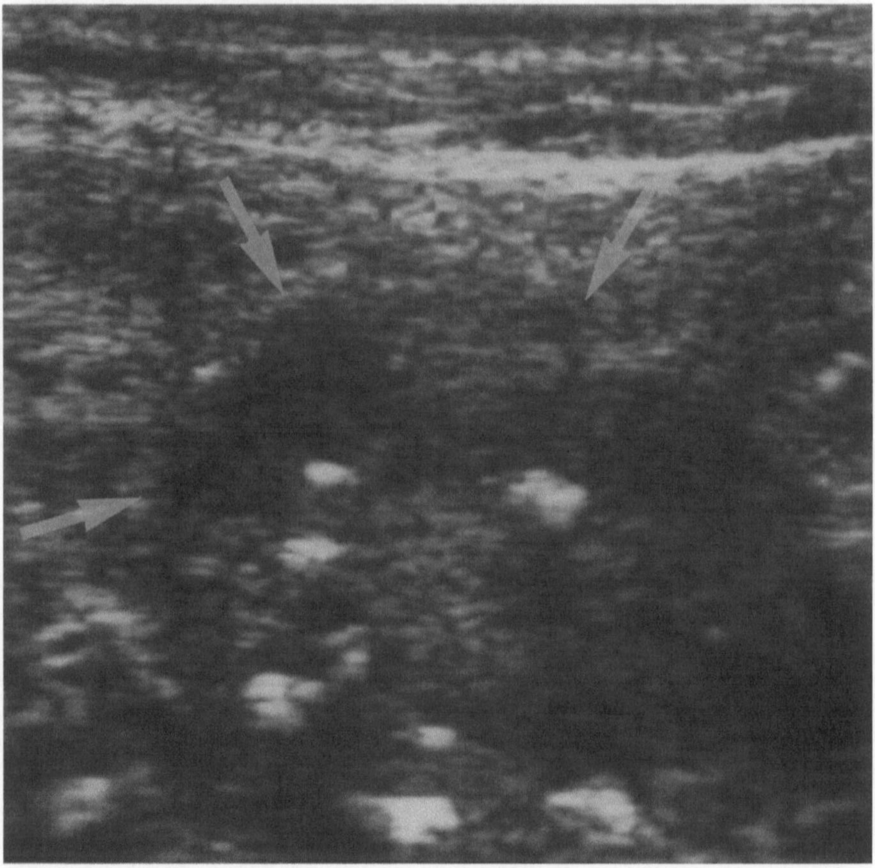

Figure 10. Benign thyroid nodule. Longitudinal ultrasonogram of neck showing benign thyroid nodule *(arrows)* containing coarse calcification.

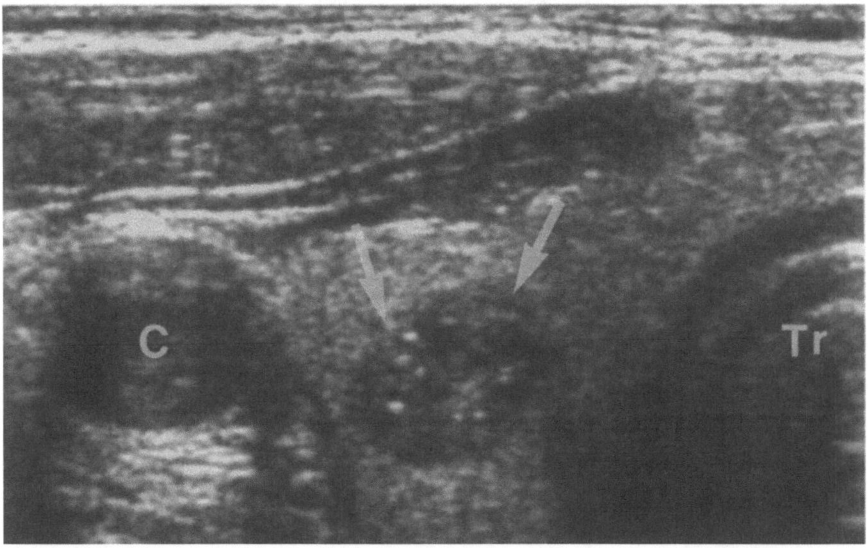

Figure 11. Papillary thyroid carcinoma. Transverse ultrasonogram of neck showing papillary thyroid carcinoma *(arrows)* containing bright echogenic foci due to psammoma calcification. *C*, Common carotid artery; *Tr*, trachea.

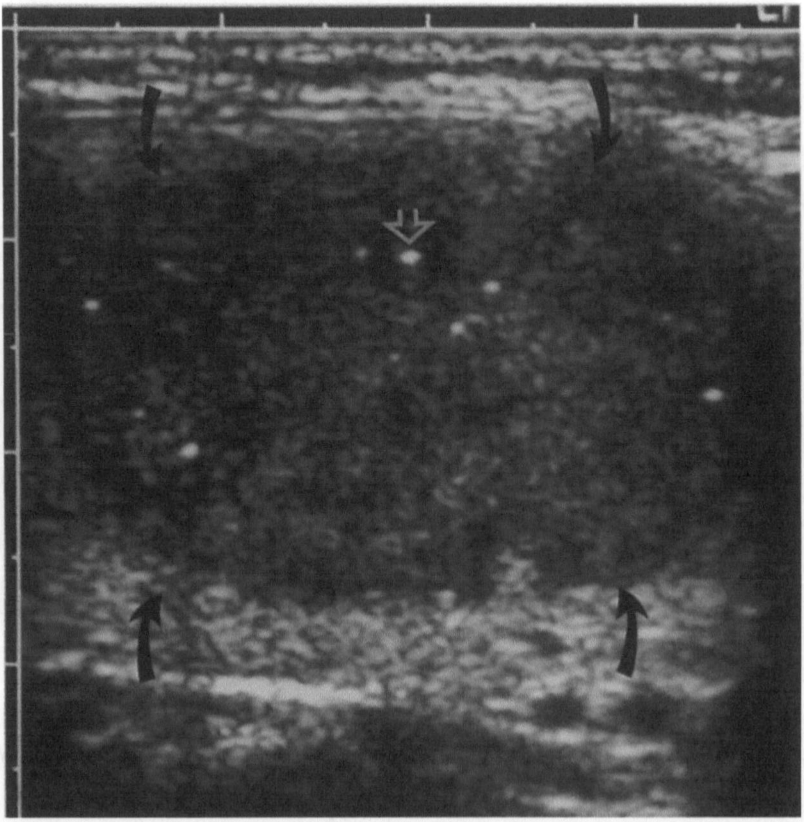

Figure 12. Benign thyroid nodule. Longitudinal ultrasonogram of neck showing benign thyroid nodule *(arrows)* with bright echogenic foci *(open arrow)* due to calcium oxalate crystals.

Color Doppler. Most hyperplastic nodules are relatively hypovascular. Most well-differentiated thyroid carcinomas are hypervascular. With color Doppler imaging, benign nodules, therefore, tend to show little internal flow and to have mainly peripheral flow (Figure 13). Malignant nodules usually show significant internal flow (Figure 14) (15-17). There is, however, too much overlap between the appearance of benign and malignant nodules on color Doppler imaging for this to be a useful discriminator (18). The increased sensitivity of modern equipment frequently shows significant internal flow in benign nodules (Figure 15).

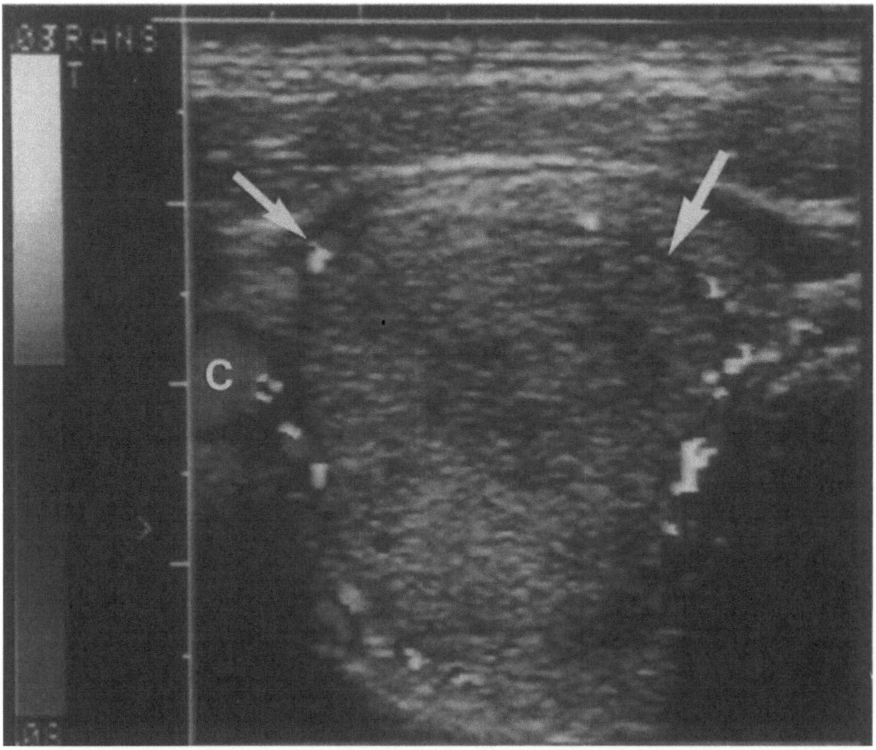

Figure 13. Benign thyroid nodule. Transverse ultrasonogram of neck with color Doppler showing mainly peripheral flow in benign thyroid nodule *(arrows)*. *C*, Common carotid artery. (Color image reproduced in black-and-white).

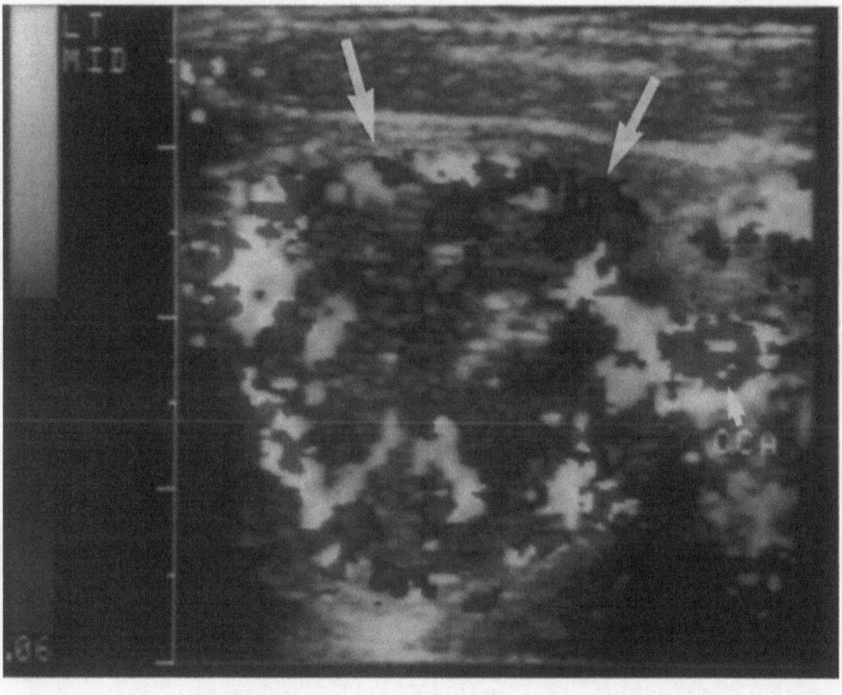

Figure 14. Papillary thyroid carcinoma. Transverse ultrasonogram of neck with color Doppler showing chaotic central flow in thyroid nodule *(arrows)*, which was a papillary carcinoma. *CCA*, common carotid artery. (From Reading CC. Palpable Neck Masses, in Bluth EI, Arger PH, Hertzberg BS, Middleton WD [eds]: Syllabus: A Special Course in Ultrasound. Oak Brook, Illinois, Radiological Society of North America, 1996, pp. 351-361. By permission of the publisher). (Color image reproduced in black-and-white).

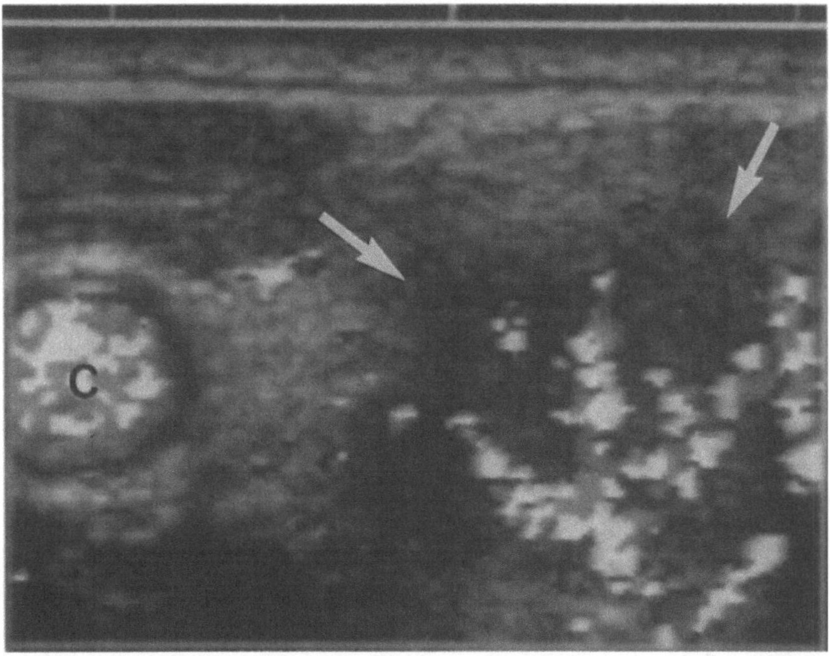

Figure 15. Benign thyroid nodule. Transverse ultrasonogram of neck with color Doppler showing benign thyroid nodule *(arrows)* with orderly central flow. *C*, Common carotid artery. (Color image reproduced in black-and-white).

Tumor Characteristics.

1. Papillary—Papillary thyroid carcinoma is typically hypoechoic on ultrasonography. Microcalcifications are extremely common (Figure 11) (14). On color Doppler imaging, papillary thyroid carcinoma typically appears hypervascular (Figure 14). Papillary thyroid carcinoma frequently metastasizes to regional lymph nodes, which may have microcalcifications or cystic change (Figure 16).

2. Follicular—No reliable sonographic features distinguish a follicular adenoma from a follicular carcinoma. Follicular neoplasm may appear hypoechoic, isoechoic, or hyperechoic relative to the surrounding thyroid parenchyma. There may be a peripheral halo, which is due to a vascular capsule (Figure 17). Metastatic lymph nodes are rare with follicular neoplasm.

3. Medullary—Medullary thyroid carcinoma typically appears hypoechoic on ultrasonography. Calcification is common and typically coarser than in papillary thyroid carcinoma. The calcification in medullary thyroid carcinoma is associated with deposits of amyloid and may be seen in lymph node or hepatic metastases (19).

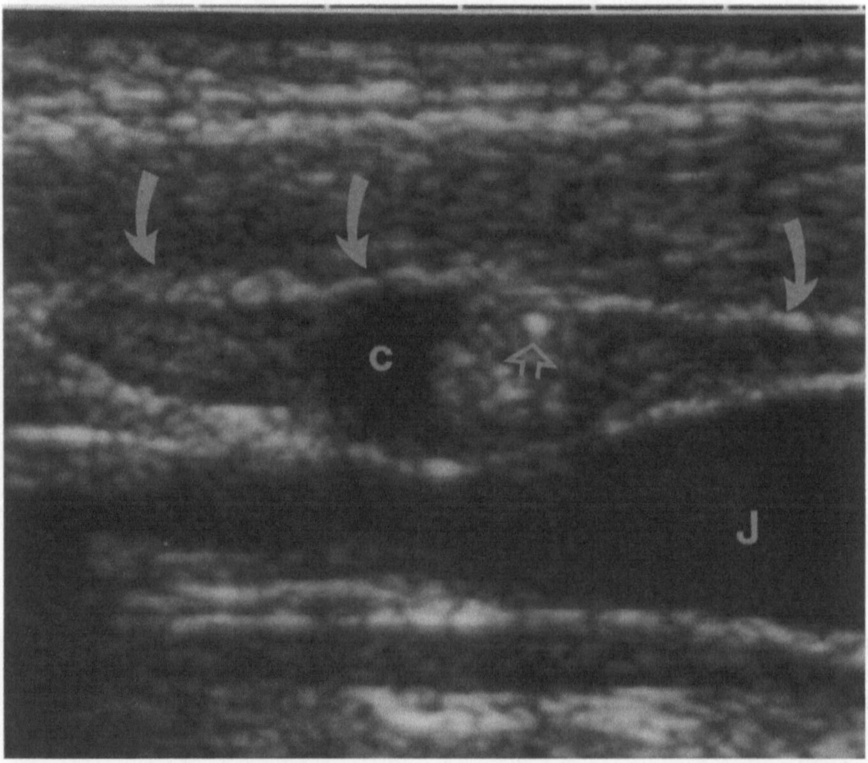

Figure 16. Lymph node with metastatic papillary thyroid carcinoma. Longitudinal ultrasonogram of neck showing lymph node *(arrows)* with cystic change *(c)* and bright echogenic foci *(open arrow)* due to psammoma calcification. *J*, Internal jugular vein.

4. Undifferentiated—Undifferentiated (anaplastic) carcinomas usually appear hypoechoic on ultrasonography. These tumors grow rapidly and may invade adjacent soft tissues or major blood vessels, usually best demonstrated on CT or MRI (Figure 18).

5. Lymphoma—Lymphoma of the thyroid is rare, and when it occurs, there is usually preexisting chronic lymphocytic thyroiditis. Lymphoma typically appears as an ill-defined hypoechoic mass that may resemble undifferentiated carcinoma (Figure 19).

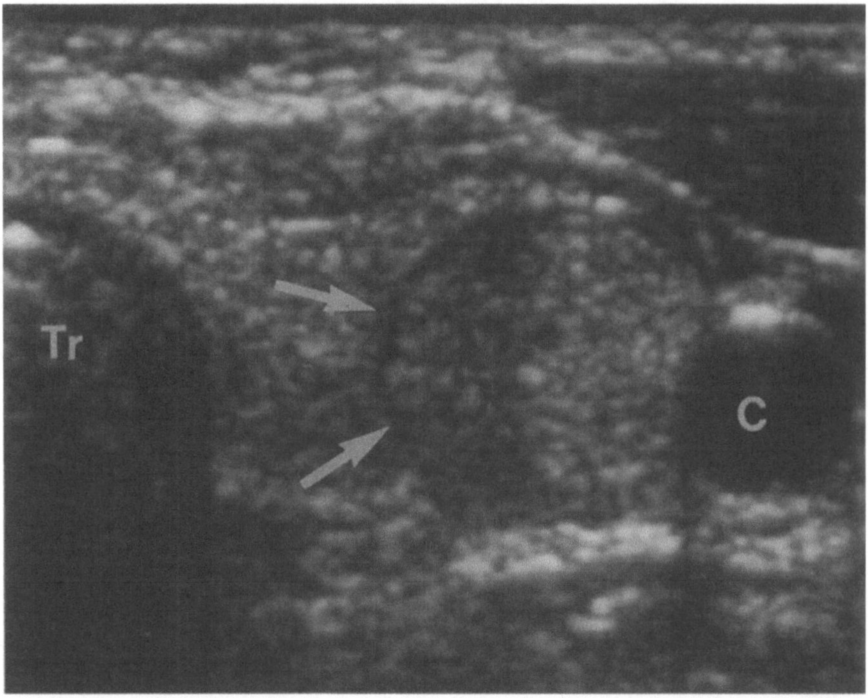

Figure 17. Benign follicular adenoma. Transverse ultrasonogram of neck showing benign follicular adenoma *(arrows)* with thin hypoechoic halo. *C*, Common carotid artery; *Tr*, trachea.

MRI Features

MRI has been used to characterize thyroid nodules. Follicular adenomas typically appear as well-circumscribed heterogeneous nodules with increased signal on T_2-weighted images. Colloid cysts and hemorrhagic cysts are characterized by homogeneous signal on T_1-weighted examinations (20). Malignant nodules may have irregular margins, but this appearance is not diagnostic because it may also occur with benign nodules (20,21). In practice, there is too much overlap in the appearance of benign and malignant nodules on MRI for it to be a useful discriminating technique.

CT Features

CT may show coarse calcification in benign nodules, but the CT characteristics of thyroid nodules are not generally helpful in distinguishing benign from malignant nodules (Figure 20). In clinical practice, thyroid nodules usually are imaged with CT only incidentally during an examination of the neck performed for some other indication.

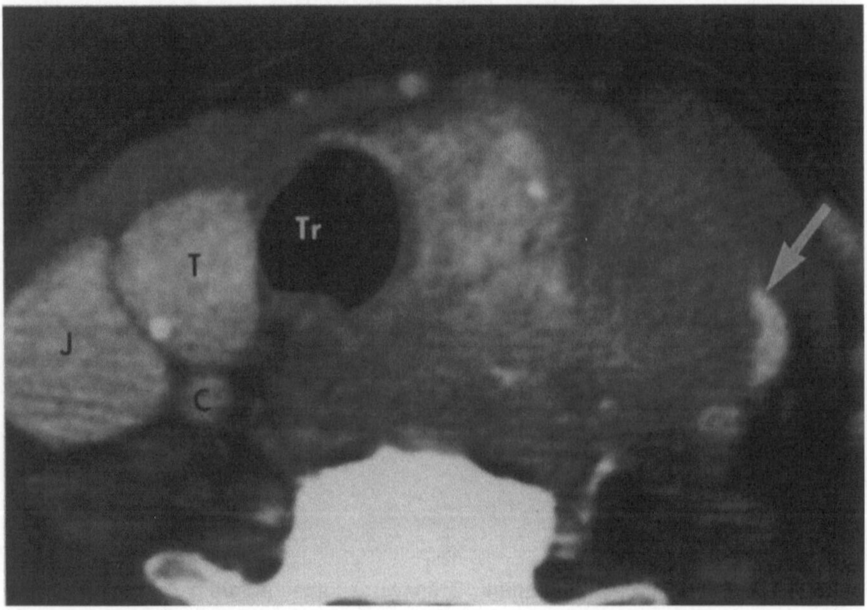

Figure 18. Undifferentiated carcinoma. Axial contrast-enhanced CT shows a mass *(arrow)* diffusely involving left lobe of thyroid retrotracheal region and left internal jugular vein, with poor definition of surrounding soft tissues. *C*, Right common carotid artery; *J*, right internal jugular vein; *T*, right lobe of thyroid; *Tr*, trachea.

GUIDED BIOPSY

Indication

Because of the lack of specificity of imaging characteristics, fine needle aspiration (FNA) biopsy has become, in many practices, the primary means of evaluating a thyroid nodule (22-25). FNA usually provides a conclusive characterization of a thyroid nodule in a relatively inexpensive and noninvasive way. The procedure is very safe, with almost no complications (26). A review of more than 18,000 palpation-guided FNA biopsies from seven large series showed mean sensitivities and specificities of 83% and 92%, respectively. The overall accuracy of cytologic diagnosis using this method is 95% (27).

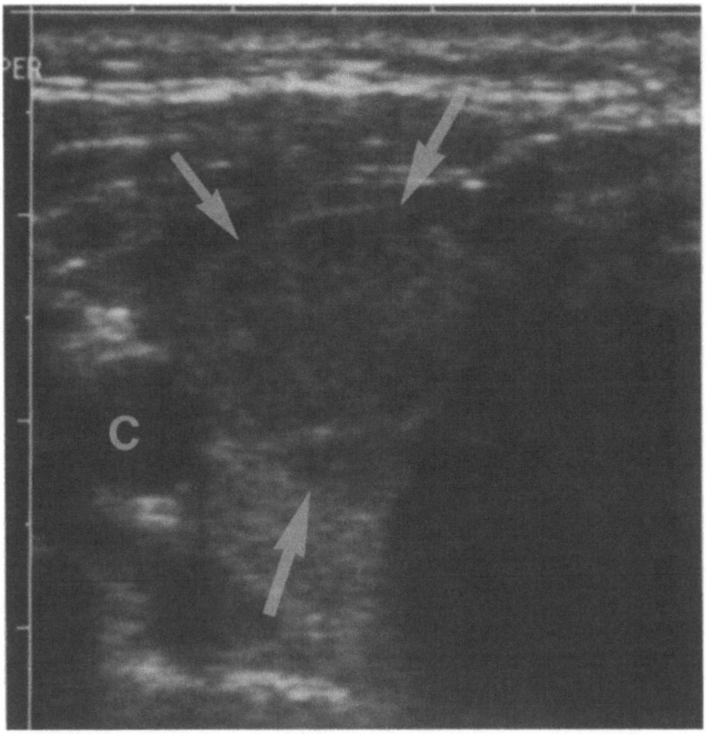

Figure 19. Thyroid lymphoma. Transverse ultrasonogram of neck showing ill-defined hypoechoic mass *(arrows)* in right lobe of thyroid due to thyroid lymphoma. *C*, Common carotid artery.

A biopsy may be performed on most nodules with palpation only, without any imaging for guidance. However, ultrasonographic guidance is useful in several circumstances. If a nodule is suspected clinically but is difficult to palpate, ultrasonography may be useful to confirm the presence of the nodule and to provide guidance for biopsy. If a patient previously has had a palpation-guided biopsy with a nondiagnostic result, ultrasonographic guidance will allow the needle to be directed into the more peripheral, cellular part of the nodule (Figure 21).

Technique

Before biopsy, the skin on the patient's neck and the transducer are cleansed with povidone-iodine solution. It is not necessary to cover the transducer with a sterile sheath. Sterile gel is used as a coupling agent. The "free-hand" technique is the preferred method for thyroid biopsies. In this technique, the transducer is held in one hand and the needle, held in the other hand, is directed into the target nodule at an oblique angle, within the image plane of the transducer. This technique allows greater flexibility than the alternative method, which is to attach a guide to the transducer.

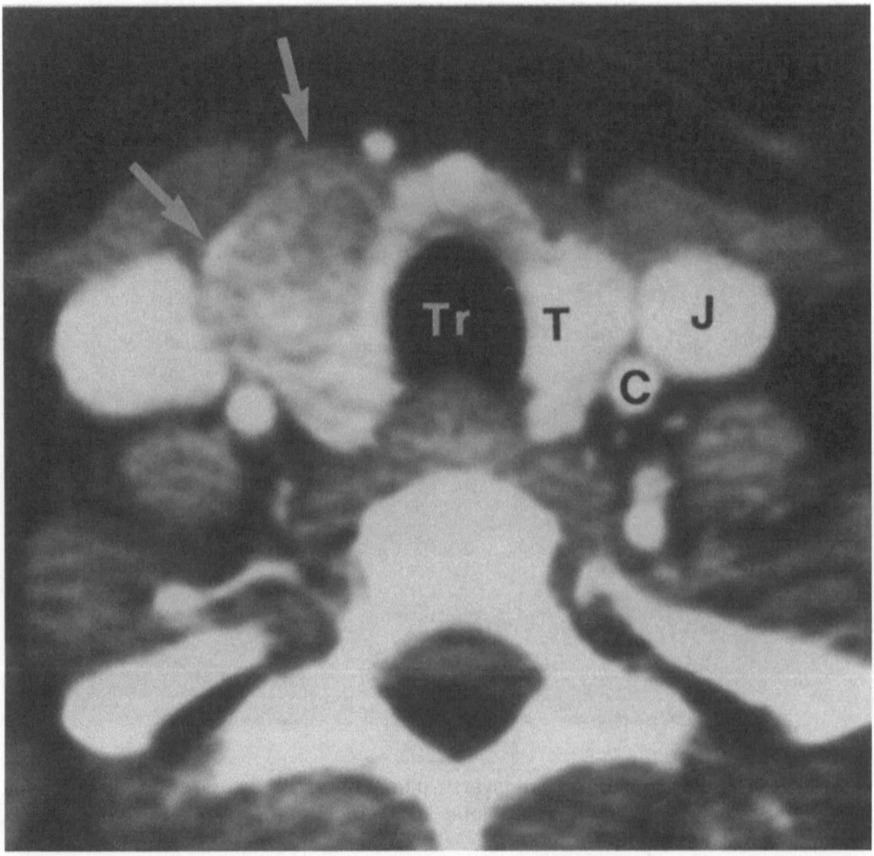

Figure 20. Papillary thyroid carcinoma. Axial contrast-enhanced CT scan showing nodule *(arrows)* in right lobe of thyroid due to papillary thyroid carcinoma. *C*, Common carotid artery; *J*, internal jugular vein; *T*, left lobe of thyroid; *Tr*, trachea.

ULTRASONOGRAPHIC-GUIDED ABLATION

Ultrasonographic guidance may be used not only for diagnostic needle aspiration but also for the therapeutic injection of ethanol to ablate thyroid nodules. Favorable results have been obtained using ultrasonographic-guided ethanol ablation of autonomous hyperfunctioning thyroid nodules, with cure in more than 90% of patients (28-30). The incidence of treatment-induced hypothyroidism is less than 1% for ethanol injection, compared with 5% to 30% for oral radioactive iodine therapy (29). Preliminary results suggest that percutaneous ethanol injection therapy with ultrasonographic guidance may be an alternative to surgical excision in the treatment of symptomatic solid, benign, non-hyperfunctioning thyroid nodules (31,32).

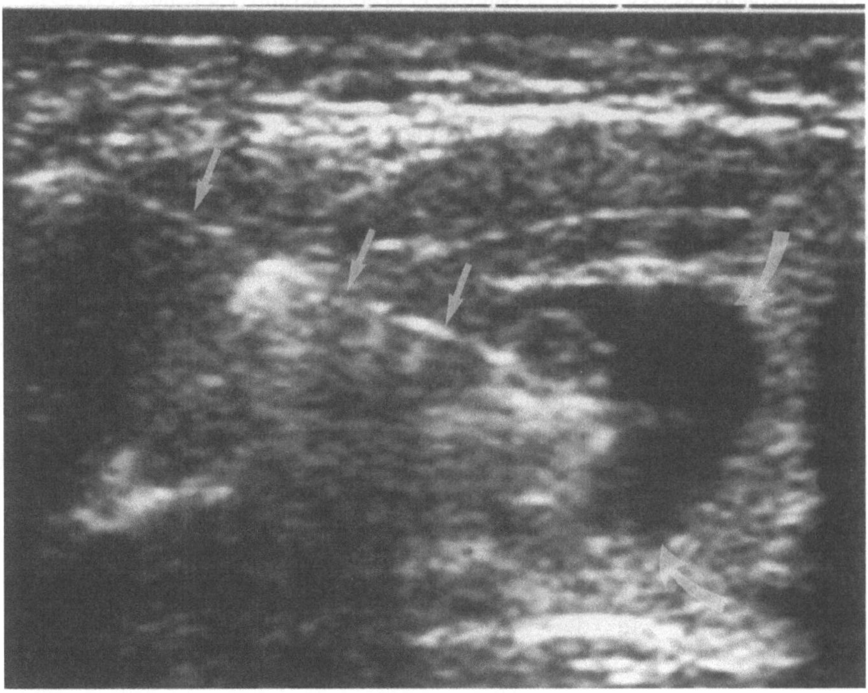

Figure 21. Biopsy of thyroid nodule. Transverse ultrasonogram of neck showing needle *(arrows)* directed into solid component of largely cystic nodule *(curved arrow).*

LYMPH NODES AND POSTOPERATIVE THYROID BED

CT, MRI, and ultrasonography may all be used to assess the presence and extent of lymph node involvement in patients with thyroid cancer and to image the neck of patients who have had a thyroidectomy to assess for tumor recurrence. Ultrasonography is especially helpful because it may be used to guide biopsy of lymph nodes or any mass in the thyroid bed. The ultrasonographic appearance of lymph nodes may be helpful in distinguishing nodes likely to be malignant from those that are benign (33-35). Benign or inflammatory nodes usually have an elongated oval shape, with the greatest dimension in the longitudinal axis, and a visible fatty hilum. In comparison, malignant nodes typically have a more rounded configuration (36,37). Early reports suggested that color Doppler is of little value in distinguishing benign from malignant nodes (38). More recently, flow patterns in lymph nodes have been described using frequency shift and power color Doppler, which may help distinguish benign from malignant nodes (39,40). Benign nodes typically show no flow or flow radiating from the hilum of the node. Malignant nodes, however, show a more chaotic pattern of flow, with spotted, peripheral, or mixed patterns.

Because there is some overlap in the appearance of benign and malignant nodes, ultrasonographic-guided biopsy is required to make a definitive diagnosis (41-43).

DIFFUSE DISEASE

Chronic Lymphocytic (Hashimoto) Thyroiditis

The most common type of thyroiditis is chronic lymphocytic (Hashimoto) thyroiditis. This is an autoimmune disorder that occurs most commonly in women. It is also the most common thyroiditis in children. Clinically, it presents as painless diffuse enlargement of the thyroid. Although patients initially may have symptoms of thyroid overactivity, they invariably become hypothyroid as the disease progresses. Ultrasonographically, chronic lymphocytic thyroiditis typically appears as enlargement of the gland, with a heterogeneous coarsened echotexture (Figure 22) (44). Multiple hypoechoic micronodules from 1 to 7 mm large may be seen (45). There may be associated local lymphadenopathy. Larger benign or malignant nodules may occur in a gland affected by chronic lymphocytic thyroiditis (46).

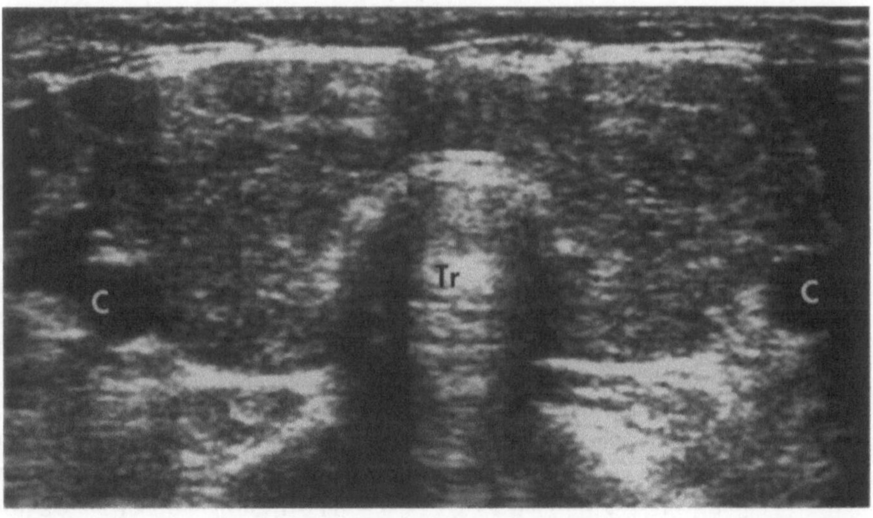

Figure 22. Hashimoto thyroiditis. Transverse ultrasonogram of neck showing diffusely enlarged heterogeneous thyroid gland. *C*, Carotid artery; *Tr*, trachea.

Patients with Hashimoto thyroiditis have an increased risk for developing lymphoma of the thyroid and may be at increased risk for developing papillary thyroid carcinoma (47-49). MRI of the thyroid in patients with chronic lymphocytic thyroiditis shows increased signal intensity, sometimes with linear low-intensity bands seen on T_2-weighted images. These low-intensity bands initially were thought to represent fibrosis (20). However, the fibrosis in Hashimoto thyroiditis may be a dense hyaline fibrosis, which has increased signal intensity on T_2-weighted imaging (50).

Graves Disease

Graves disease is a common cause of thyroid overactivity that is usually diagnosed clinically. Ultrasonographically, the thyroid appears enlarged and may be homogeneous or slightly heterogeneous because of the presence of many intraparenchymal blood vessels (Figure 23) (9). Color Doppler typically shows increased blood flow, producing a pattern called "thyroid inferno" (Figure 24) (51). Color Doppler has been used to assess the activity of Graves disease and to predict the outcome after withdrawal of medical therapy (52).

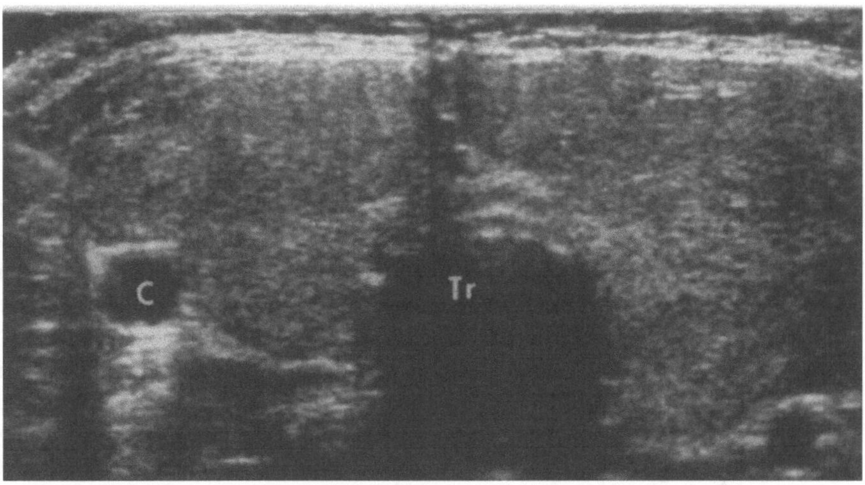

Figure 23. Graves disease. Transverse ultrasonogram of neck showing diffusely enlarged homogeneous thyroid gland. *C*, Common carotid artery; *Tr*, trachea.

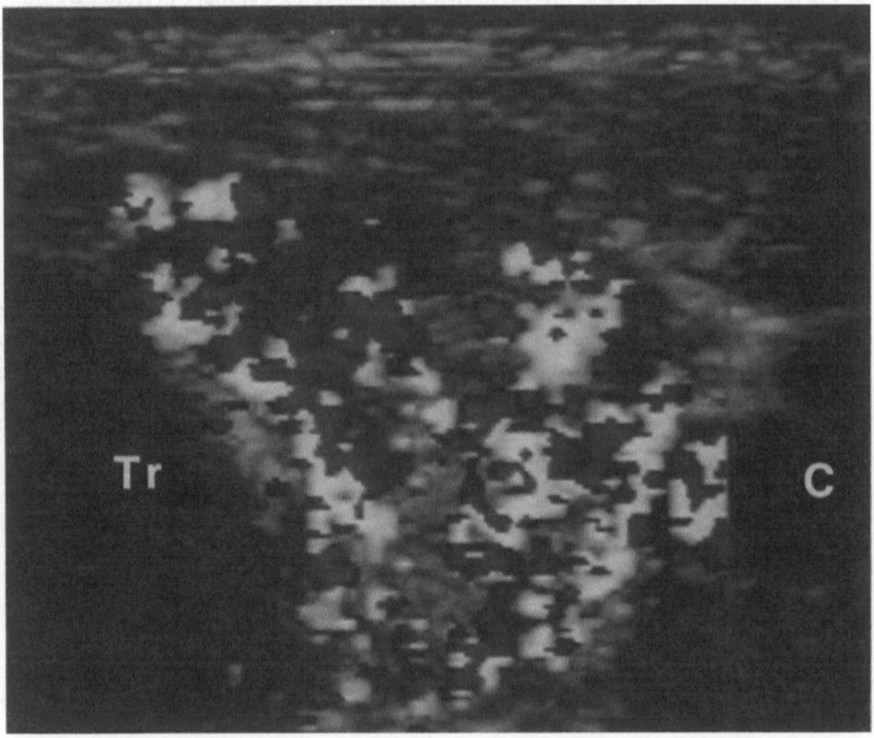

Figure 24. Graves disease. Transverse color Doppler ultrasonogram of neck showing increased flow in thyroid gland. *C*, Common carotid artery; *Tr*, trachea. (Color image reproduced in black-and-white).

Riedel Thyroiditis

Riedel thyroiditis is a chronic, inflammatory, invasive, fibrous thyroiditis that is more common in women than men. It may be associated with mediastinal or retroperitoneal fibrosis or sclerosing cholangitis (53). On ultrasonography, Riedel thyroiditis appears as a hypoechoic mass that replaces normal thyroid and infiltrates surrounding tissues and vascular structures (Figure 25). The appearance on ultrasonography and CT resembles undifferentiated invasive carcinoma (Figure 26). MRI may be helpful in distinguishing tumor from fibrous thyroiditis. The fibrous tissue in Riedel thyroiditis produces low signal on both T_1- and T_2-weighted images, but tumor appears as high signal on T_2-weighted images (54). However, open biopsy may be required to establish the diagnosis, and the main indication for imaging is to show the extent of vascular encasement.

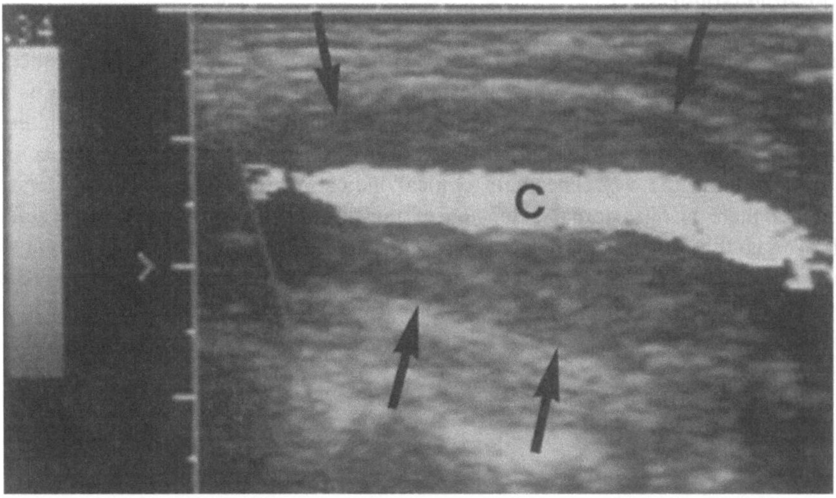

Figure 25. Riedel thyroiditis. Longitudinal ultrasonsogram of neck with color Doppler showing tissue *(arrows)* surrounding common carotid artery, *C*. (Color image reproduced in black-and-white).

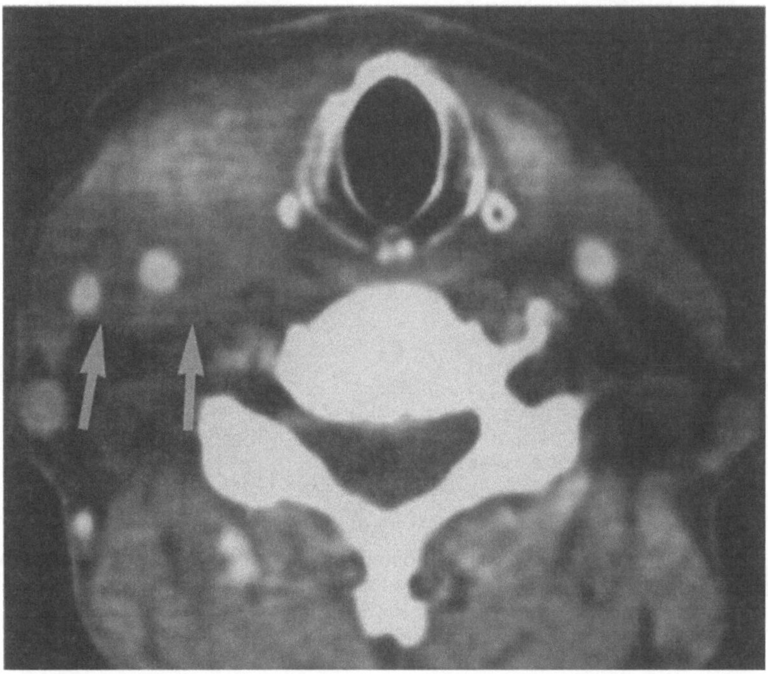

Figure 26. Riedel thyroiditis. Transverse contrast-enhanced axial CT showing tissue (arrows) enveloping the great vessels on right side of neck.

Euthyroid Goiter

Enlargement of the thyroid (goiter) may be due to hyperplasia, which can either be diffuse or nodular. Diffuse goiter is usually a clinical diagnosis, and imaging is not required unless the thyroid enlargement is asymmetrical and a thyroid nodule is suspected clinically. Some authors have used ultrasonography or CT to estimate thyroid volume (55-57). The main clinical indication for imaging is to determine whether there is retrosternal extension of the thyroid; CT or MRI is preferable to ultrasonography for this purpose (Figure 27 and 28) (58). The criteria for diagnosing mediastinal goiter with CT include continuity with the cervical gland, calcification, and high attenuation on unenhanced scan, with increased enhancement after contrast (59).

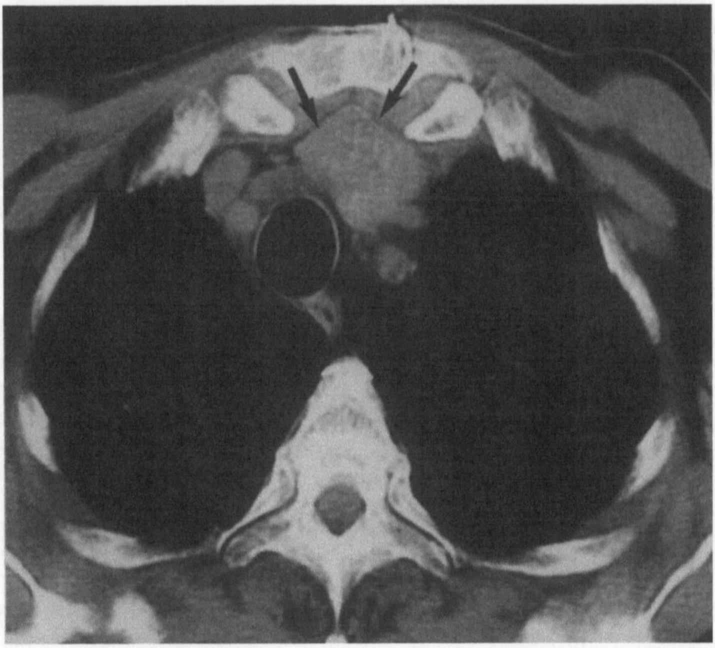

Figure 27. Multinodular goiter with retrosternal extension. Axial CT scan showing retrosternal goiter *(arrows)*.

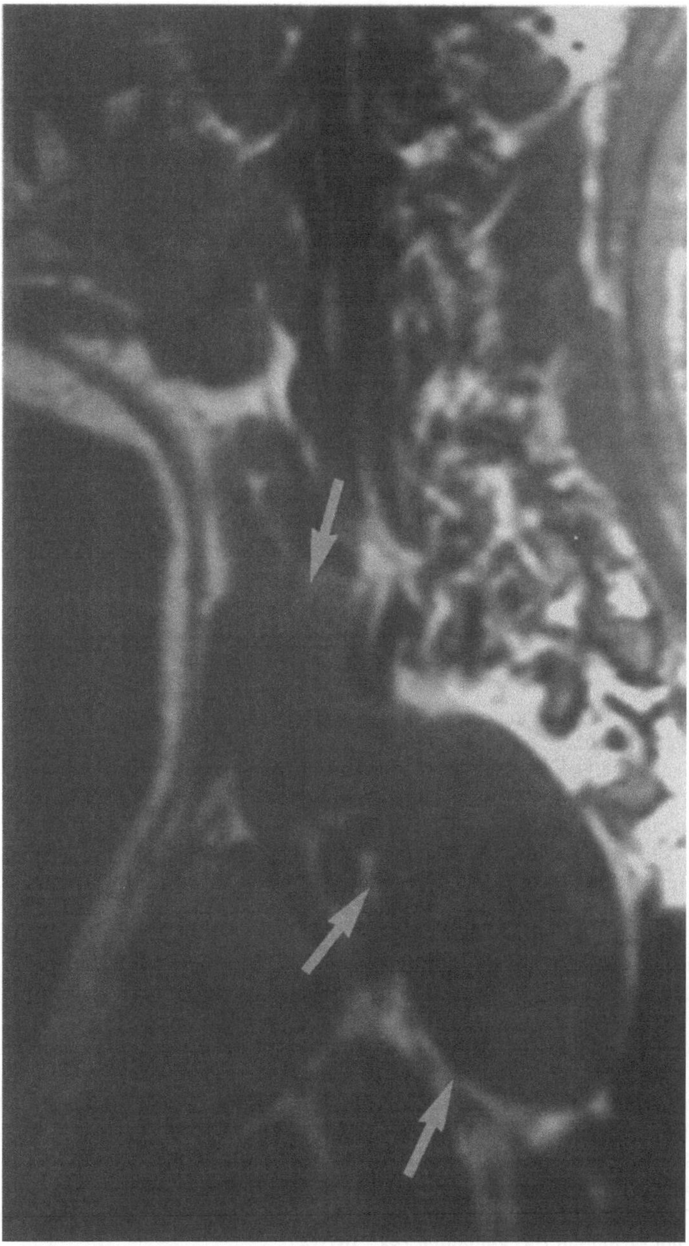

Figure 28. Multinodular goiter with retrosternal extension. Sagittal MRI showing large multinodular goiter with retrosternal extension *(arrows)*.

References

1. Felmlee JP, Ehman RL. Spatial presaturation: A method for suppressing flow artifacts and improving depiction of vascular anatomy in MR imaging. Radiology 1987:164:559.
2. Tan GH, Gharib H. Thyroid incidentalomas: Management approaches to nonpalpable nodules discovered incidentally on thyroid imaging. Ann Intern Med. 1997;126:226.
3. Rojeski MT, Gharib H. Nodular thyroid disease. Evaluation and management. N Engl J Med. 1985;313:428.
4. Kumpusalo L, Kumpusalo E, Soimakallio S, Salomaa S, Paile W, Kolmakow S, et al. Thyroid ultrasound findings 7 years after the Chernobyl accident. A comparative epidemiological study in the Bryansk region of Russia. Acta Radiol. 1996;37:904.
5. Mortensen JD, Woolner LB, Bennett WA. Gross and microscopic findings in clinically normal thyroid glands. J Clin Endocrinol Metab. 1955;15:1270.
6. Tan GH, Gharib H, Reading CC. Solitary thyroid nodule. Comparison between palpation and ultrasonography. Arch Intern Med. 1995;155: 2418.
7. Horlocker TT, Hay JE, James EM, Reading CC, Charboneau JW. Prevalence of incidental nodular thyroid disease detected during high-resolution parathyroid ultrasonography, in Medeiros-Neto G, Gaitan E (eds): Frontiers in Thyroidology. New York, Plenum Medical Book Company, vol 2, 1986, p 1309.
8. Stark DD, Clark OH, Gooding GA, Moss AA. High-resolution ultrasonography and computed tomography of thyroid lesions in patients with hyperparathyroidism. Surgery 1983;94:863.
9. Solbiati L, Charboneau JW, James EM, Hay ID. The Thyroid Gland, in Rumack CM, Wilson SR, Charboneau JW (eds): Diagnostic Ultrasound, ed 2. St Louis, Mosby, 1998, pp 703.
10. Hammer M, Wortsman J, Folse R. Cancer in cystic lesions of the thyroid. Arch Surg. 1982;117:1020.
11. Ahuja A, Chick W, King W, Metreweli C. Clinical significance of the comet-tail artifact in thyroid ultrasound. J Clin Ultrasound. 1996;24:129.
12. Solbiati L, Volterrani L, Rizzatto G, et al. The thyroid gland with low uptake lesions: Evaluation by ultrasound. Radiology 1985;155:187.
13. Propper RA, Skolnick ML, Weinstein BJ, Dekker A. The nonspecificity of the thyroid halo sign. J Clin Ultrasound. 1980;8:129.
14. Takashima S, Fukuda H, Nomura N, Kishimoto H, Kim T, Kobayashi T. Thyroid nodules: Re-evaluation with ultrasound. J Clin Ultrasound. 1995;23:179.
15. Solbiati L, Cioffi V, Ballarati E. Ultrasonography of the neck. Radiol Clin North Am. 1992;30:941.
16. Kerr L. High-resolution thyroid ultrasound: The value of color Doppler. Ultrasound Q. 1994;12:21.
17. Argalia G, D'Ambrosio F, Lucarelli F, et al. Echo Doppler in the characterization of thyroid nodular disease. Radiol Med (Torino) 1995;89:651.
18. Shimamoto K, Endo T, Ishigaki T, Sakuma S, Makino N. Thyroid nodules: Evaluation with color Doppler ultrasonography. J Ultrasound Med. 1993;12:673.
19. Gorman B, Charboneau JW, James EM, et al. Medullary thyroid carcinoma: Role of high-resolution US. Radiology 1987;162:147.
20. Gefter WB, Spritzer CE, Eisenberg B, et al. Thyroid imaging with high-field-strength surface-coil MR. Radiology 1987;164:483.
21. Noma S, Kanaoka M, Minami S, et al. Thyroid masses: MR imaging and pathologic correlation. Radiology 1988;168:759.

22. Gharib H, Goellner JR. Fine-needle aspiration biopsy of the thyroid: An appraisal. Ann Intern Med. 1993;118:282.
23. Yokozawa T, Miyauchi A, Kuma K, Sugawara M. Accurate and simple method of diagnosing thyroid nodules by the modified technique of ultrasound-guided fine needle aspiration biopsy. Thyroid 1995;5:141.
24. Sanchez RB, vanSonnenberg E, D'Agostino HB, et al. Ultrasound guided biopsy of nonpalpable and difficult to palpate thyroid masses. J Am Coll Surg.1994;178:33.
25. Santos JEC, Leiman G. Nonaspiration fine needle cytology. Application of a new technique to nodular thyroid disease. Acta Cytol. 1988;32:353.
26. Goellner JR, Gharib H, Grant CS, Johnson DA. Fine needle aspiration cytology of the thyroid, 1980 to 1986. Acta Cytol. 1987;31:587.
27. Gharib H. Fine-needle aspiration biopsy of thyroid nodules: Advantages, limitations, and effect. Mayo Clin Proc. 1994;69:44.
28. Ozdemir H, Ilgit ET, Yucel C, et al. Treatment of autonomous thyroid nodules: Safety and efficacy of sonographically guided percutaneous injection of ethanol. Am J Roentgenol. 1994;163:929.
29. Livraghi T, Paracchi A, Ferrari C, Reschini E, Macchi RM, Bonifacino A. Treatment of autonomous thyroid nodules with percutaneous ethanol injection: 4-Year experience. Radiology 1994;190:529.
30. Livraghi T, Paracchi A, Ferrari C, et al. Treatment of autonomous thyroid nodules with percutaneous ethanol injection: Preliminary results. Work in progress. Radiology 1990;175:827.
31. Goletti O, Monzani F, Lenziardi M, et al. Cold thyroid nodules: A new application of percutaneous ethanol injection treatment. J Clin Ultrasound. 1994;22:175.
32. Bennedbaek FN, Karstrup S, Hegedus L. Percutaneous ethanol injection therapy in the treatment of thyroid and parathyroid diseases. Eur J Endocrinol. 1997;136:240.
33. Rubaltelli L, Proto E, Salmaso R, Bortoletto P, Candiani F, Cagol P. Sonography of abnormal lymph nodes *in vitro*: Correlation of sonographic and histologic findings. Am J Roentgenol. 1990;155:1241.
34. Evans RM, Ahuja A, Metreweli C. The linear echogenic hilus in cervical lymphadenopathy—a sign of benignity or malignancy? Clin Radiol. 1993;47:262.
35. Vasallo P, Wernecke K, Roos N, Peters PE. Differentiation of benign from malignant superficial lymphadenopathy: The role of high-resolution US. Radiology 1992;183:215.
36. Tohnosu N, Onoda S, Isono K. Ultrasonographic evaluation of cervical lymph node metastases in esophageal cancer with special reference to the relationship between the short to long axis ratio (S/L) and the cancer content. J Clin Ultrasound. 1989;17:101.
37. Vassallo P, Edel G, Roos N, Naguib A, Peters PE. In-vitro high-resolution ultrasonography of benign and malignant lymph nodes. A sonographic-pathologic correlation. Invest Radiol. 1993;28:698.
38. Chang DB, Yuan A, Yu CJ, Luh KT, Kuo SH, Yang PC. Differentiation of benign and malignant cervical lymph nodes with color Doppler sonography. Am J Roentgenol. 1994;162:965.
39. Tschammler A, Ott G, Schang T, Seelbach-Goebel B, Schwager K, Hahn D. Lymphadenopathy: Differentiation of benign from malignant disease—color Doppler US assessment of intranodal angioarchitecture. Radiology 1998;208:117.
40. Wu CH, Chang YL, Hsu WC, Ko JY, Sheen TS, Hsieh FJ. Usefulness of Doppler spectral analysis and power Doppler sonography in the differentiation of cervical lymphadenopathies. Am J Roentgenol. 1998;171:503.
41. Boland GW, Lee MJ, Mueller PR, Mayo-Smith W, Dawson SL, Simeone JF. Efficacy of sonographically guided biopsy of thyroid masses and cervical lymph nodes. Am J Roentgenol. 1993;161:1053.

42. Lee MJ, Ross DS, Mueller PR, Daniels GH, Dawson SL, Simeone JF. Fine-needle biopsy of cervical lymph nodes in patients with thyroid cancer: A prospective comparison of cytopathologic and tissue marker analysis. Radiology 1993;187:851.
43. Sutton RT, Reading CC, Charboneau JW, James EM, Grant CS, Hay ID. US-guided biopsy of neck masses in postoperative management of patients with thyroid cancer. Radiology 1988;168:769.
44. Nordmeyer JP, Shafeh TA, Heckmann C. Thyroid sonography in autoimmune thyroiditis. A prospective study on 123 patients. Acta Endocrinol (Copenh). 1990;122:391.
45. Yeh HC, Futterweit W, Gilbert P. Micronodulation: Ultrasonographic sign of Hashimoto thyroiditis. J Ultrasound Med. 1996;15:813.
46. Takashima S, Matsuzuka F, Nagareda T, Tomiyama N, Kozuka T. Thyroid nodules associated with Hashimoto's thyroiditis: Assessment with US. Radiology 1992;185:125.
47. Kasagi K, Hatabu H, Tokuda Y, et al. Lymphoproliferative disorders of the thyroid gland: Radiological appearances. Br J Radiol. 1991;64:569.
48. Hamburger JI, Miller JM, Kini SR. Lymphoma of the thyroid. Ann Intern Med. 1983;99:685.
49. Ott RA, Calandra DB, McCall A, Shah KH, Lawrence AM, Paloyan E. The incidence of thyroid carcinoma in patients with Hashimoto's thyroiditis and solitary cold nodules. Surgery 1985;98:1202.
50. Takashima S, Fukuda H, Tomiyama N, Fujita N, Iwatani Y, Nakamura H. Hashimoto thyroiditis: Correlation of MR imaging signal intensity with histopathologic findings and thyroid function test results. Radiology 1995;197:213.
51. Ralls PW, Mayekawa DS, Lee KP, et al. Color-flow Doppler sonography in Graves disease: "Thyroid inferno." Am J Roentgenol. 1988;150:781.
52. Castagnone D, Rivolta R, Rescalli S, Baldini MI, Tozzi R, Cantalamessa L. Color Doppler sonography in Graves' disease: Value in assessing activity of disease and predicting outcome. Am J Roentgenol. 1996;166:203.
53. Malotte MJ, Chonkich GD, Zuppan CW. Riedel's thyroiditis. Arch Otolaryngol Head Neck Surg. 1991;117:214.
54. Perez FFJ, Cordido CF, Pombo FF, Mosquera OJ, Villalba MC. Riedel thyroiditis: US, CT, and MR evaluation. J Comput Assist Tomogr. 1993;17:324.
55. Hermans R, Bouillon R, Laga K, et al. Estimation of thyroid gland volume by spiral computed tomography. Eur Radiol. 1997;7:214.
56. Rasmussen SN, Hjorth L. Determination of thyroid volume by ultrasonic scanning. J Clin Ultrasound. 1974;2:143.
57. Hegedus L. Thyroid size determined by ultrasound. Influence of physiological factors and non-thyroidal disease. Dan Med Bull. 1990;37:249.
58. Naik KS, Bury RF. Imaging the thyroid. Clin Radiol. 1998;53:630.
59. Glazer GM, Axel L, Moss AA. CT diagnosis of mediastinal thyroid. Am J Roentgenol. 1982;138:495.

6

IODINE AND TECHNETIUM SCINTIGRAPHY OF THE THYROID

Dyde A. Huysmans, M.D.
Ad R. Hermus, M.D.
Catharina Hospital
Eindhoven, the Netherlands
University Hospital Nijmegen
Nijmegen, the Netherlands

INTRODUCTION

Scintigraphy of the thyroid using iodine or technetium provides information on thyroid anatomy and function. In this chapter, a short description of radionuclides, equipment and imaging techniques used for thyroid scintigraphy precedes a review of scintigraphic appearances of thyroid pathologies. Finally, the use of recombinant human thyroid-stimulating hormone (TSH) as an adjunct to radioiodine imaging of differentiated thyroid carcinoma, and the phenomenon of "stunning" of thyroid tissue by diagnostic doses of radioiodine will be discussed. Only thyroid scintigraphy using radioiodine and technetium-99m pertechnetate will be discussed here. The use of other radioisotopes such as thallium-201, technetium-99m sestamibi, fluorine-18 fluorodeoxyglucose and nonradioisotopic imaging techniques are beyond the scope of this chapter.

Physical and biological properties of iodine-123, technetium-99m pertechnetate and iodine-131

Iodine-123 (^{123}I) and technetium-99m (^{99m}Tc) pertechnetate are predominantly used for imaging the thyroid gland, whereas iodine-131 (^{131}I) is almost exclusively used for whole body scintigraphy after thyroidectomy for differentiated thyroid cancer.

Iodine-123 causes a relatively low radiation exposure of the thyroid and whole body due to its short physical half-life (13 hours) and its emission of only gamma radiation and no beta radiation. The energy of the photons emitted by ^{123}I (159 keV) is very suitable for imaging with a modern gamma camera. ^{123}I is trapped by a number of tissues, including the thyroid gland, choroid plexus, salivary glands, and gastric mucosa. In the thyroid, radioiodide is retained because of its incorporation into thyroglobulin. Therefore, imaging is possible up to 24 hours after administration of a 200 to 500 μCi oral dose of ^{123}I. ^{123}I images usually show high target-to-background ratios.

Iodine-123 is not as readily available as ^{99m}Tc pertechnetate and, in contrast to ^{99m}Tc pertechnetate, it should be administered on the day of delivery (1). Another disadvantage of ^{123}I is its relative expensiveness.

Technetium-99m pertechnetate shares with ^{123}I some favorable properties for gamma camera imaging: a short physical half-life (6 hours), the absence of beta emissions, and a suitable photon energy (140 keV). The radiation exposure from ^{99m}Tc pertechnetate to the thyroid and the whole body is even lower than that of ^{123}I, because the residence time of ^{99m}Tc pertechnetate in the thyroid is shorter than that of ^{123}I (2,3). Furthermore, ^{99m}Tc pertechnetate is cheap and available around the clock. Therefore, it is widely used for thyroid imaging.

^{99m}Tc pertechnetate is trapped by the thyroid iodide-concentrating mechanism. However, in contrast to radioiodine, it rapidly leaks out of the thyroid because it is not organified. Therefore, ^{99m}Tc pertechnetate has to be given intravenously and in higher doses (1 to 10 mCi) than those used for ^{123}I imaging. Furthermore, ^{99m}Tc pertechnetate imaging must be done earlier than ^{123}I imaging: approximately 20 minutes after administration. Because imaging is done sooner after administration of the isotope thyroid uptake is lower and background activity in surrounding tissues is higher on ^{99m}Tc pertechnetate images in comparison to ^{123}I images, resulting in a slightly inferior overall quality. Background activity from radioisotope in the esophagus due to secretion of ^{99m}Tc pertechnetate into saliva may be superimposed on the thyroid and may thereby cause confusion with interpretation. To obviate this problem the patient should drink water immediately before scintigraphy.

Discrepancies between ^{123}I and ^{99m}Tc pertechnetate scintigraphy occur (4–8). The most frequent one is that of a thyroid nodule appearing hyperfunctioning ("hot") on ^{99m}Tc pertechnetate scintigraphy but normofunctioning or hypofunctioning ("cold") on radioiodine scintigraphy. Most probably this is explained by the above mentioned fact that radioiodine is trapped and organified, whereas ^{99m}Tc pertechnetate is only trapped.

Iodine-131 has a long physical half-life (8 days) which permits scanning of patients for many days after administration of a tracer dose. This is advantageous in whole body scanning of patients with differentiated thyroid carcinoma because maximum tumor-to-background ratios in patients with thyroid cancer metastases are often reached only several days after administration of radioiodine (9).

Iodine-131 should not be used for imaging of benign thyroid diseases, because it gives a high radiation exposure to the thyroid by the emission of beta particles and because the scintigraphic images are of moderate resolution due to the high photon energy (364 keV).

Equipment and imaging techniques

A **gamma camera** is commonly used for imaging the thyroid. A planar anterior image may be complemented by anterior oblique views to further delineate the thyroid outline. Clinical examination of the patient at the time of scintigraphy is of utmost importance to mark the site of palpable lesions on the scintigram, thus avoiding interpretation errors. A number of substances (radiographic contrast media, iodine-containing medications and food ingredients) interfering with radioiodine uptake should be avoided before thyroid scintigraphy (Table 1).

Table 1 Interfering Factors in Thyroid Imaging

Factor	*Period*
Iodide	
Lugol's solution	1-3 weeks
Amiodarone	months
Pyelogram / angiogram	1-3 weeks
Cholecystogram	2-3 weeks
Bronchogram	Month
Myelogram	Year
Antithyroid drugs	
(PTU, methimazole, carbimazole)	3 days
Thyroid hormones	
L-thyroxine	4-6 weeks
Triiodothyronine	2 weeks

A pinhole collimator (aperture 2 to 5 mm) is routinely used to image the thyroid because it provides higher resolution images in comparison to those made with a parallel hole collimator. It should be realized that a pinhole collimator gives a magnification, which is dependent on the distance of the imaged structure from the pinhole. Therefore, the representation of tissues at different depths is not linear and the scintigram is not identical to the true structure.

Thyroid radioactive iodide uptake (RAIU) can be estimated from a planar anterior gamma camera image with ^{123}I (or ^{131}I). A region of interest is selected over the thyroid with corrections for background activity. The thyroid activity is compared to a standard of known activity measured in a neck phantom at the same distance from the gamma camera as the thyroid of the patient. Measurements can be done between 3 and 24 hours after ^{123}I administration. Normal values should be obtained locally because of regional variations due to differences in dietary iodine intake.

By rotating the head of a gamma camera around the patient single photon emission computed tomography (SPECT) images can be acquired. The data collected are reconstructed by a computer to obtain transverse, sagittal and coronal slices and three dimensional images.

A gamma camera is also used for whole body ^{131}I scintigraphy of patients with differentiated thyroid cancer. A high energy parallel hole collimator is needed for this purpose because the field of view of a pinhole collimator is too small. Quantification of uptake in thyroid cancer foci can be done for dosimetric purposes.

The **rectilinear scanner** has a probe with a sodium iodide crystal and a focused collimator that moves back and forth over the area of interest. In this way an image is created in lines with dots representing radioactive incidents. The image is life size, which is an advantage over a gamma camera scintigram made with a pinhole collimator. However, the accuracy of rectilinear images is considerably less than that of images obtained by a gamma camera with pinhole collimator (10). In addition, the time for imaging is longer and oblique images cannot easily be obtained. Therefore, the use of a rectilinear scanner cannot be recommended.

A **positron emission tomography (PET) camera** can be used to image the distribution of the positron-emitting agent iodine-124 (^{124}I) in the thyroid. The technique produces high-resolution images of the thyroid (11). However, PET is rarely used for thyroid imaging because of its high cost, the limited number of PET facilities, and the widespread availability of SPECT using ^{123}I or ^{99m}Tc pertechnetate. Furthermore, thyroid radiation exposure from ^{124}I is relatively high due to its relatively long physical half-life (4.2 days).

A **gamma probe** is a small handheld radiation detector, which can be used intraoperatively after administration of radioiodine (iodine-125 or iodine-131) to detect small remnants of functioning thyroid tissue or lymph node metastases of differentiated thyroid carcinoma. The gamma probe can be used intraoperatively in patients undergoing total thyroidectomy for differentiated thyroid carcinoma. (12). Furthermore, the gamma probe can be used in patients who undergo surgery for cervical metastases of thyroid carcinoma a few days after the administration of a high dose of radioiodine (13).

The normal thyroid

The lobes of the thyroid gland appear on a scintigram as two pear-shaped structures with homogeneous tracer distribution. The long axis of each lobe is approximately 5 cm and the widest transverse diameter is 2 to 3 cm. The lobes are often somewhat asymmetrical and many normal variants have been described (14). Sometimes the pyramidal lobe, which is the inferior part of the thyroglossal duct, is visualized (15,16).

Abnormal thyroid development

Thyroid hemiagenesis appears to be rare (17,18). It is most often detected by chance during evaluation of hyperthyroid patients. Scintigraphy may show a characteristic "hockey stick" image representing the remaining lobe and isthmus (18). However, when the isthmus is also missing the remaining lobe can easily be misinterpreted as an autonomously functioning nodule with suppression of the extranodular tissue.

Patients with thyroid hemiagenesis are usually euthyroid. In contrast, congenital thyroid hypofunctioning is usually present in other forms of abnormal thyroid development. These forms of abnormal thyroid development can be differentiated by thyroid scintigraphy, which should be done before thyroid hormone replacement is started. The scan may reveal no detectable thyroid tissue, ectopic thyroid tissue (19) or eutopic thyroid tissue (20).

Ectopic thyroid tissue is usually caused by abnormal descent of the thyroid during ontogenesis. It can be found at any point from the foramen cecum at the base of the tongue to the pyramidal lobe (Figure 1). Sometimes, ectopic thyroid tissue is found inferior to the normal cervical location (21).

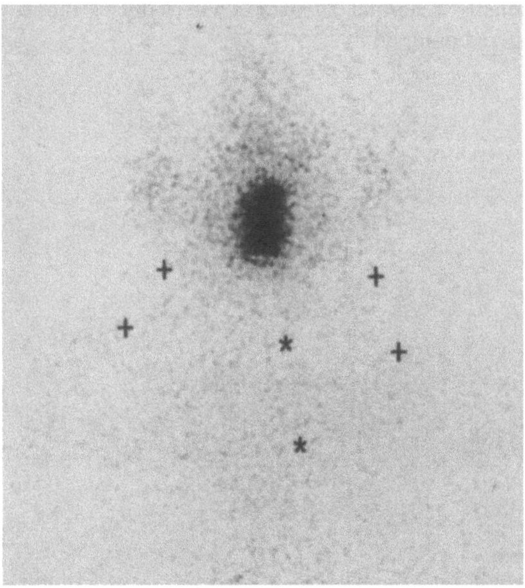

Figure 1. Iodine-123 scintigraphy in a 2-year-old child with ectopic thyroid tissue at the base of the tongue and no eutopic thyroid tissue (+ indicates lateral margin of the neck; upper * indicates hyoid; lower * indicates jugulum)

When eutopic thyroid tissue is found a perchlorate discharge test may be done to detect a disorder in thyroid hormone synthesis (22). Two hours after oral administration of a tracer dose of radioiodine RAIU is measured. Then potassium perchlorate, a competitive inhibitor of iodide uptake, is administered orally. This results in a rapid discharge of unbound (non-organified) iodide from the thyroid gland, while organified iodine is retained in the thyroid. One hour later the retention of radioiodine in the thyroid is measured. A decrease in radioiodine retention by 5-10% or more is considered indicative of an organification defect.

Sometimes ectopic thyroid tissue is diagnosed later in life in patients with a cervical midline mass. Radioiodine scintigraphy can easily differentiate such a lesion from a thyroglossal cyst, a frequent cervical midline lesion (23), which seldom contains sufficient follicular cells to be imaged (24). A rare form of ectopic thyroid tissue is the so-called struma ovarii, which can be diagnosed by scintigraphic demonstration (using ^{123}I or ^{131}I) of thyroid tissue in the pelvic region.

Graves' disease

In Graves' disease the thyroid gland is diffusely enlarged. There is homogeneously increased tracer uptake and little or no background activity. The pyramidal lobe is often visualized (Figure 2) (15). Thyroid radioiodine uptake in patients with Graves' disease is nearly always elevated between 3 and 24 hours after radioiodine administration. Occasionally a normal 24 hour RAIU value is found due to rapid turnover of the administered radioiodine.

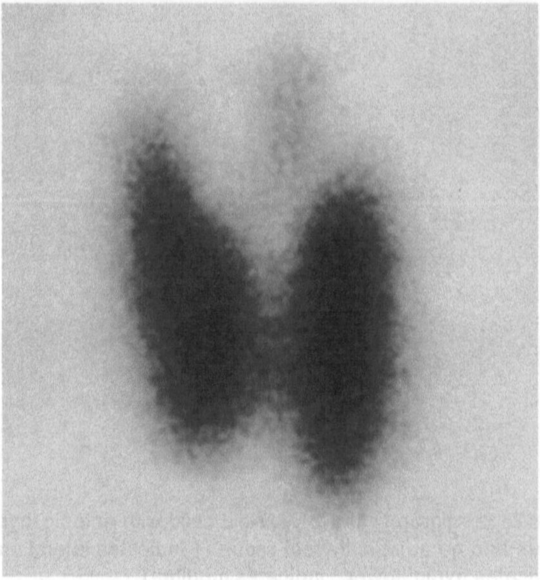

Figure 2.Iodine-123 scintigraphy in a 34-year-old woman with Graves' disease. Note the visualization of the pyramidal lobe.

In hyperthyroid patients with classical signs and symptoms of Graves' ophthalmopathy thyroid scintigraphy is not indicated. However, when the clinical picture is not characteristic a thyroid scintigram may help to differentiate Graves' disease from other forms of thyrotoxicosis, e.g. toxic nodular goiter. A RAIU measurement is especially helpful to differentiate Graves' disease from causes of thyrotoxicosis with low thyroid radioiodine uptake, e.g. subacute thyroiditis. It should be realized that the finding of an enlarged thyroid gland with homogeneously increased tracer uptake is not pathognomonic for patients with Graves' disease. It is also found in the rare patients with hyperthyroidism due to inappropriate secretion of TSH by the pituitary or due to excessive production of human chorionic gonadotropin by a hydatiform mole.

Nodular thyroid diseases

Clinically solitary thyroid nodules

A clinically solitary thyroid nodule is a discrete swelling within an otherwise palpably normal thyroid gland. With time, solitary thyroid nodules may enlarge, shrink, or even disappear spontaneously (25,26), but most do not change appreciably (27). Most of these nodules are benign colloid nodules composed of irregularly enlarged follicles containing abundant colloid. Most are actually the largest of multiple colloid nodules in small, clinically unrecognized multinodular goiter (28). Other causes of benign solitary nodules are thyroid adenomas, cysts, and thyroiditis. Approximately 5% of all solitary thyroid nodules are thyroid carcinomas (29–33).

The use of scintigraphy in the differential diagnosis of clinically solitary thyroid nodules is based on the fact that most thyroid cancers concentrate less radioiodine than normal thyroid tissue and, therefore, are usually hypo- or nonfunctional ("cold") on scintigraphy (Figure 3) (34). However, most benign nodules are also cold: In more than 5000 patients with thyroid nodules undergoing preoperative thyroid scintigraphy, 84% of nodules were cold, but subsequent thyroid surgery revealed thyroid carcinoma in only a small minority of patients with cold nodules (35). Because the majority of both benign and malignant thyroid nodules appear hypofunctional relative to the adjacent normal thyroid tissue, the finding of a cold nodule on thyroid scintigraphy has a low specificity for the diagnosis of thyroid carcinoma. On the other hand, not all thyroid carcinomas appear cold on scintigraphy. For example, a small nonfunctioning carcinoma covered by normal thyroid tissue may appear functioning due to radiation from the overlying normal tissue. Furthermore, a large carcinoma, despite its hypofunctioning, may appear to have equal activity to the adjacent thyroid tissue due to its greater mass than the surrounding normal thyroid tissue.

In patients with a small thyroid nodule SPECT imaging appears to be superior to planar imaging in defining the functional status of the nodule (36,37). PET imaging using ^{124}I allows even smaller thyroid nodules to be distinguished from the surrounding thyroid tissue than SPECT imaging using ^{123}I or ^{99m}Tc pertechnetate, because the spatial resolution of PET images is higher than that obtained by SPECT imaging (11). However, like planar scintigraphy, neither SPECT nor PET allows benign nodules to be differentiated reliably from malignant nodules. Therefore, in most cases it is unlikely that SPECT or PET imaging will add much to planar imaging in patients with a solitary thyroid nodule (36,37).

Given the low specificity of thyroid scintigraphy for the diagnosis of thyroid carcinoma, the role of this technique in the evaluation of patients with clinically solitary thyroid nodules has decreased, especially since the introduction of fine-needle aspiration biopsy (31,32,35). Most authors agree that thyroid scintigraphy is not routinely indicated in the work-up of these patients. However, thyroid scintigraphy is helpful in patients with a solitary thyroid nodule who have a low serum TSH level. In these patients thyroid scintigraphy should demonstrate hyperfunctioning of the nodule and little or no uptake in the extranodular tissue. Such autonomously functioning nodules are rarely malignant (38–41).

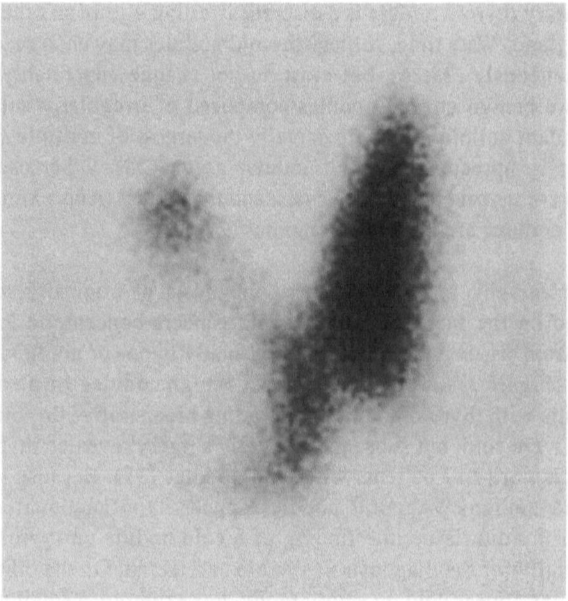

Figure 3. Iodine-123 scintigraphy in a 46-year-old man with a clinically solitary nodule in the right thyroid lobe. The palpable nodule correlated with the cold area on the thyroid image.

When there is complete suppression of extranodular tissue, a hyperfunctioning nodule should be differentiated from thyroid hemiagenesis. This can be done by several methods: ^{123}I scintigraphy with shielding of the nodule with lead (42), ultrasonography (43), thallium-201 scintigraphy (44), and ^{99m}Tc-sestamibi scintigraphy (45).

It should be realized that neither a normal serum TSH level nor a lack of suppression of uptake in extranodular tissue excludes that a clinically solitary thyroid nodule is autonomously functioning. In some euthyroid patients autonomous function of a solitary nodule can be demonstrated by a lack of suppressibility of uptake in the nodule after the administration of exogenous thyroid hormone (T_3 suppression test) (Figure 4).

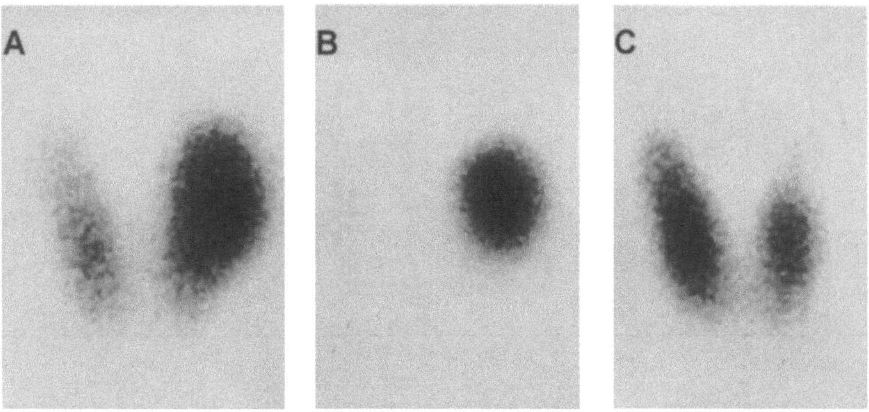

Figure 4 A: Iodine-123 scintigraphy in a 27-years-old woman (TSH level 1.0 mU/L, FT_4 12.1 pmol/L) with an autonomously functioning nodule in the upper pole of the left thyroid lobe. Note the incomplete suppression of the extranodular thyroid tissue. B: Iodine-123 scintigraphy in the same patient after TSH suppression (triiodothyronine, 75 µg daily for 10 days). Note the lack of suppression of radioiodine uptake in the nodule and the complete suppression of extranodular tissue. C: Iodine-123 scintigraphy in the same patient 6 months after radioiodine therapy. The normal extranodular tissue has resumed its function. The nodule, which was no longer palpable, shows a decreased uptake of iodine-123.

Multinodular goiter

A multinodular goiter may be defined as a structurally and functionally heterogeneous thyroid enlargement. Worldwide, such goiters are most often caused by iodine deficiency. In the early phase of goitrogenesis, the thyroid may be diffusely enlarged, but with time diffuse goiters tend to grow and become more nodular. Thyroid function often becomes more autonomous with increasing age (46,47), and euthyroidism may gradually change to subclinical hyperthyroidism, and eventually into overt hyperthyroidism.

In patients with toxic or nontoxic multinodular goiter scintigraphy with ^{123}I or ^{99m}Tc pertechnetate shows an enlarged gland with heterogeneous uptake. It can also demonstrate whether nodules are functioning or not. In patients with toxic multinodular goiter thyroid scintigraphy should be done at a suppressed serum TSH level, in order to get a good distinction of the autonomously functioning areas from the non-autonomously functioning tissue (Figure 5). In some patients who clinically have a multinodular goiter radioiodine imaging shows a fairly homogeneous tracer uptake. This may be caused by co-existent autoimmunity (48,49).

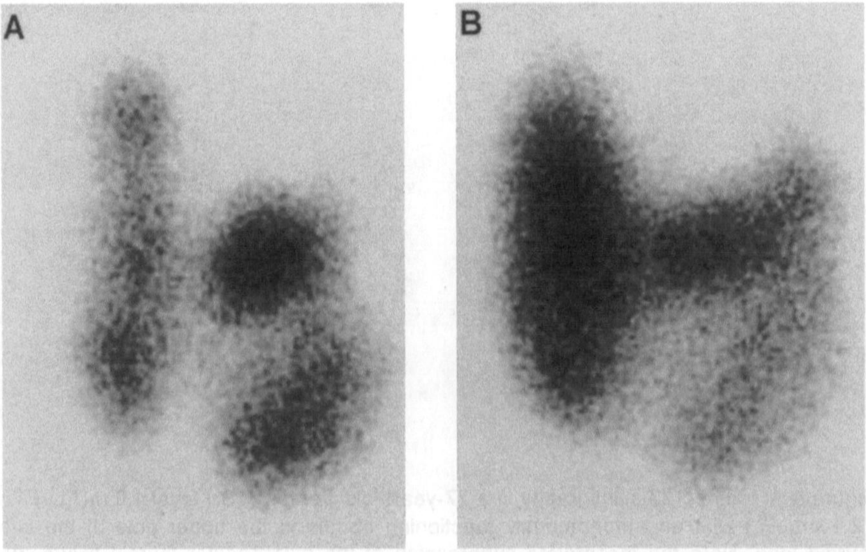

Figure 5 A: Iodine-123 scintigraphy in a 60-year-old woman with toxic multinodular goiter (serum TSH level <0.03 mU/L) B: Iodine-123 scintigraphy in the same patient during treatment with antithyroid drugs in combination with levothyroxine (serum TSH level 2.7 mU/L). Note that tracer distribution depends on serum TSH.

Most authors agree that thyroid scintigraphy is not routinely indicated in patients with multinodular goiter. The value of thyroid scintigraphy for detecting thyroid malignancy in patients with multinodular goiter is as low as in those with a clinically solitary thyroid nodule (50). Thyroid scintigraphy is helpful when an anterior mediastinal mass is seen on a chest roentgenogram or computed tomography scan. Radioiodine scintigraphy can prove that the mass consists of functional thyroid tissue. ^{99m}Tc pertechnetate scintigraphy should not be used in these cases because of its unfavorable target-to-background ratio (high background activity in the great vessels and the heart and low uptake in the thyroid (1-3%) at the usual scanning time after administration ^{99m}Tc pertechnetate) (51).

Thyroid scintigraphy (and RAIU measurement) is also of value when radioiodine therapy is considered for the reversal of hyperthyroidism or for thyroid volume reduction in a patient with a multinodular goiter. Many hyperthyroid patients with multinodular goiter have normal or even low RAIU values (52). This may make radioiodine therapy less attractive or even impossible. Successful thyroid volume reduction with radioiodine is not to be expected when large parts of the thyroid are cold on scintigraphy.

In patients with multinodular goiter the tomographic techniques (SPECT and PET) appear to be superior to planar imaging for calculating functional thyroid volume (36,53,54). However, for measuring the anatomical thyroid volume ultrasonography is superior.

Thyroiditis

In acute thyroiditis, thyroid scintigraphy shows areas of decreased activity corresponding to areas of acute inflammation or abscess formation. RAIU is usually within normal limits.

In patients presenting with subacute thyroiditis thyroid scintigraphy may give poor quality images due to diffusely depressed uptake or may show focal defects. In general RAIU is depressed. As the inflammation subsides, the depressed RAIU slowly returns to normal. This may take from a few weeks to a few months. Subacute thyroiditis must be differentiated from other forms of thyrotoxicosis with low thyroid radioiodide uptake, such as exogenous thyroid hormone administration (factitious thyrotoxicosis), struma ovarii, metastatic thyroid carcinoma with thyroid hormone overproduction, and iodine-induced thyrotoxicosis. Iodine-induced thyrotoxicosis is most frequent in patients over 50 years of age with a multinodular goiter.

In patients with Hashimoto's thyroiditis thyroid scintigraphy often shows a heterogeneously enlarged gland similar to that of a multinodular goiter (55). Most often there is hypothyroidism with a decreased 24-hour RAIU value. However, in the early phase of Hashimoto's thyroiditis patients may be thyrotoxic and the thyroid scintigram may appear similar to that in patients with Graves' disease and RAIU may be elevated (55). Like in Hashimoto's thyroiditis lymphomas in the thyroid show areas of irregularly decreased activity (56). 24-hour RAIU is commonly normal.

Radioiodine whole body scintigraphy after thyroidectomy for differentiated thyroid carcinoma

Five to 15% of patients treated for differentiated thyroid carcinoma will develop a local recurrence and/or neck metastases and 10 to 15% will have distant metastases during follow-up (57). In patients who have been treated for differentiated thyroid carcinoma by (near-)total thyroidectomy radioiodine whole body scintigraphy can show the presence of residual normal thyroid tissue or thyroid carcinoma tissue in the neck or elsewhere in the body. It can also help to determine whether treatment with ^{131}I is useful. Dosimetric calculations can be made using scintigraphic measurements and radioactivity measurements in blood and urine samples in order to determine the therapeutic amount of radioiodine to be administered (58,59). The introduction of serum thyroglobulin measurements has allowed for a decrease in the frequency of radioiodine whole body scintigraphy, especially in patients at low risk for recurrence of the disease (57).

Some patient preparations are important to optimize the sensitivity of radioiodine whole body scintigraphy. A high serum TSH level (more than 30 mU/L) is needed to optimally stimulate radioiodine uptake in residual normal thyroid tissue and in thyroid carcinoma tissue (60). After (near-)total thyroidectomy this is usually reached within 4 to 6 weeks (61). In patients who use thyroid hormone this can be reached by discontinuation of exogenous thyroid hormone medication: levothyroxine (L-T4) should be stopped for 4 to 6 weeks (62) and levotriiodothyronine (L-T3), because of its shorter half-life, for 10 to 14 days (61,63). Serum TSH levels should always be verified as being at least 30 mU/l before imaging is carried out. A low-iodine diet may be of value, especially in areas of high iodine intake, to increase radioiodine uptake in residual normal thyroid tissue and in thyroid carcinoma tissue by lowering the plasma inorganic iodine level (64). The degree of iodine restriction varies among diets, but most important recommendations are no iodized or sea salt, eggs, milk and dairy products, seafood and bread containing iodate conditioners, and restaurant meals (65). The diet is started at least one week before administration of the radioiodine, and is continued for 3 to 7 days after radioiodine therapy. By using a low-iodine diet excretion of urinary iodide can be reduced to less than 50 µg/day (65). Of course, radiographic contrast agents and iodine-containing medications should also be avoided.

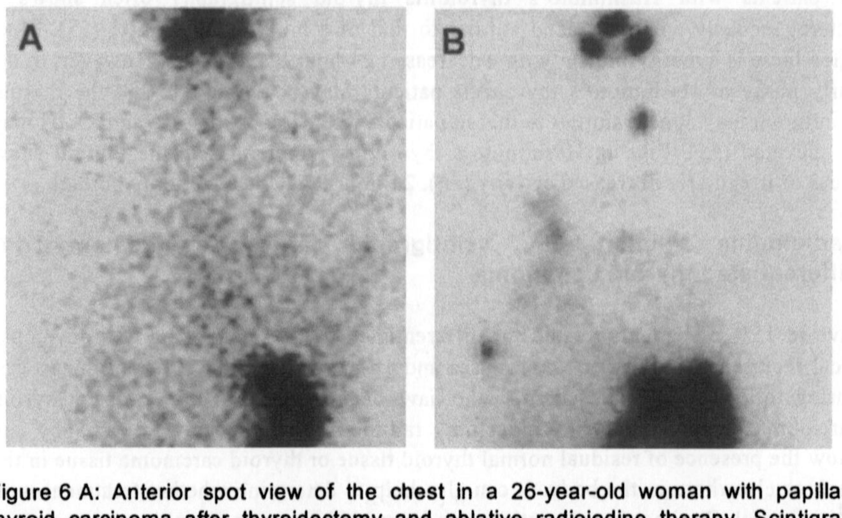

Figure 6 A: Anterior spot view of the chest in a 26-year-old woman with papillary thyroid carcinoma after thyroidectomy and ablative radioiodine therapy. Scintigram obtained 72 hours after administration of 5 mCi of iodine-131. B: Anterior spot view of the chest in the same patient obtained 7 days after therapeutic administration of 150 mCi of iodine-131. The spot in the neck and the lung metastases are only visible on the post-therapy scintigram.

^{131}I is preferred over ^{123}I for diagnostic whole body scintigraphy, because maximum target-to-background ratios usually occur at 48 to 72 hours and imaging for as long as 7 days may be required in some instances (9). This is only possible with iodine-131 with its long physical half-life.

Anterior and posterior whole body scintigrams with a minimum of 50,000 counts per image are made. Because of the poor resolution of these images and lack of anatomic landmarks, markers, e.g. suprasternal and xiphoid, should be used. Additional spot views of the neck and other regions of concern, with uptake measurements, are recommended. For spot views of the neck the superior resolution of a pinhole collimator may be useful in determining whether foci of radioiodine accumulation are within or outside the thyroid bed.

The dose of ^{131}I to be used for whole body scintigraphy is the subject of debate. There is evidence that larger doses (5 to 10 mCi, or even higher) are able to visualize lesions better and allow lesions which are not visible at lower doses (1 to 2 mCi) to be detected (66,67). Whole body scintigraphy done approximately 7 days after administration of a therapeutic dose of ^{131}I, may show lesions, which were not visible during diagnostic scintigraphy (Figure 6) (67–71). In contrast to scintigrams obtained 2 to 3 days after a diagnostic dose, scintigrams obtained 7 days after a therapeutic dose often show homogeneous uptake in the liver. This is due to concentration and metabolization of radioactive thyroid hormones in the liver (72). For liver visualization there must be sufficient functioning normal or carcinomatous thyroid tissue and there must be enough time for incorporation of the radioiodine into thyroid hormones, release of the radioactive hormones, and subsequent concentration of these hormones in the liver (73). In contrast, focal lesions in the liver that concentrate radioiodine are likely to be metastases.

The uptake of radioiodine in residual normal thyroid tissue is usually greater than that in thyroid carcinoma tissue (74,75). Pulmonary lesions can be macroscopic and focal but can also be microscopic and diffuse (76). In approximately 20% to 30% of patients with pulmonary metastases detected by radioiodine whole body scintigraphy, these metastases are not visible on chest radiographs (77–79). Most skeletal metastases are visible on radioiodine whole body scintigraphy. Skeletal foci may be single (in approximately 30% of patients), but are often multiple (79). The most frequent site of skeletal metastases is the spine (approximately 40% of lesions). Other sites are the skull (approximately 25%) and somewhat less often the ribs, pelvis, sternum, long bones, scapulae and claviculae (varying from 4 to 15%) (80). Metastases of undifferentiated thyroid carcinoma will be missed because their capacity to take up radioiodine is too low. Also Hürthle cell carcinomas and their metastases are often poorly iodine-concentrating (76,81). Avoidable causes for false negative results are a low serum TSH level or iodine contamination by high intake of iodine or radiographic contrast. Rarely, false positive results can be caused by uptake of ^{131}I, e.g. in inflammatory lung disease (82), in a Meckel's diverticulum (83), in a renal cyst (84) and in benign and malignant nonthyroidal tumors (85–87). Avoidable causes of false positives are contamination of the patient or clothes, with radioactive secretions, such as saliva, urine, sweat or mucus and misinterpretation of radioiodine uptake in organs that physiologically accumulate iodine, such as salivary glands or thymus (88–90).

Use of recombinant human TSH as an adjunct to radioiodine whole body scintigraphy of differentiated thyroid carcinoma

Diagnostic radioiodine whole body scintigraphy for detecting residual or recurrent thyroid carcinoma in thyroidectomized patients is traditionally done after withdrawal of thyroid hormone therapy, subjecting the patient to hypothyroidism for several weeks. The hypothyroid state often results in discomfort and morbidity and therefore has a major negative impact on the quality of life. Moreover, in some patients, especially those with intracranial or intraspinal metastases, serious complications can occur due to accelerated tumor growth (91–93). An elegant solution to these problems is whole body scintigraphy after the administration of recombinant human TSH (rhTSH). rhTSH, which has recently become available, makes it possible to conduct radioiodine whole body scintigraphy without discontinuing thyroid hormone therapy.

The use of rhTSH has now been investigated in two phase III studies. In the first phase III trial (94), 127 patients with thyroid cancer underwent radioiodine whole body scintigraphy (using 2 to 4 mCi ^{131}I) by two techniques: first after receiving two doses of 0.9 mg of rhTSH administered with an interval of 24 hours while thyroid hormone therapy was continued and second after the withdrawal of thyroid hormone therapy while no rhTSH was administered. In 62 of the 127 patients radioiodine whole body scintigrams by one or both techniques were positive. The scintigrams obtained after administration of rhTSH were equivalent to the scintigrams obtained after withdrawal of thyroid hormone in 41 of these 62 patients (66%), superior in 3 (5%), and inferior in 18 (29%). When the 65 patients with negative whole body scintigrams by both techniques were included, the two scintigrams were equivalent in 106 patients (83%). Eight patients (13% of those with at least one positive scintigram) were treated with radioiodine on the basis of superior scintigrams obtained after withdrawal of thyroid hormone therapy. As expected, patients had more symptoms of hypothyroidism and dysphoric mood states after withdrawal of thyroid hormone than after administration of rhTSH. In the second phase III study (Genzyme Inc., data on file) a total of 229 patients with differentiated thyroid carcinoma were treated with rhTSH and randomized in either one of the two dosing regimens, i.e., 0.9 mg of rhTSH administered every 24 hours for two doses (arm 1) or 0.9 mg of rhTSH administered every 72 hours for three doses (arm 2). This study also formally examined the utility of rhTSH in TSH-stimulated thyroglobulin testing and the value of the combination of radioiodine whole body scintigraphy and thyroglobulin testing after administration of rhTSH for detecting thyroid carcinoma. For the second phase III study a higher scanning dose of iodine-131 (4 mCi) was chosen based on results of an evaluation conducted in a subset of patients of the first phase III study that indicated that the clearance rate of radioiodine was greater in the euthyroid state than when patients were hypothyroid. Furthermore, stricter scintigraphy protocols were used for acquiring whole body scintigrams and a more clinically relevant definition of equivalent scans was used. Furthermore, in this trial more patients with metastatic disease were enrolled. The results of the trial showed that the rhTSH scan was rated either equivalent to or better than the withdrawal scan in 92% and 93% of patients in arm 1 and arm 2, respectively. Furthermore, this study revealed that in both dosing regimens the combination of radioiodine whole body scintigraphy and thyroglobulin testing after administration of rhTSH did not miss any patients with metastatic disease. Overall, it can be concluded that the combination of radioiodine imaging and thyroglobulin testing after administration of rhTSH is as effective as the currently accepted "gold standard", which is radioiodine whole body scintigraphy and thyroglobulin testing following withdrawal of thyroid hormone therapy. With the use of rhTSH the morbidity associated with hypothyroidism using the current "gold standard" can be avoided.

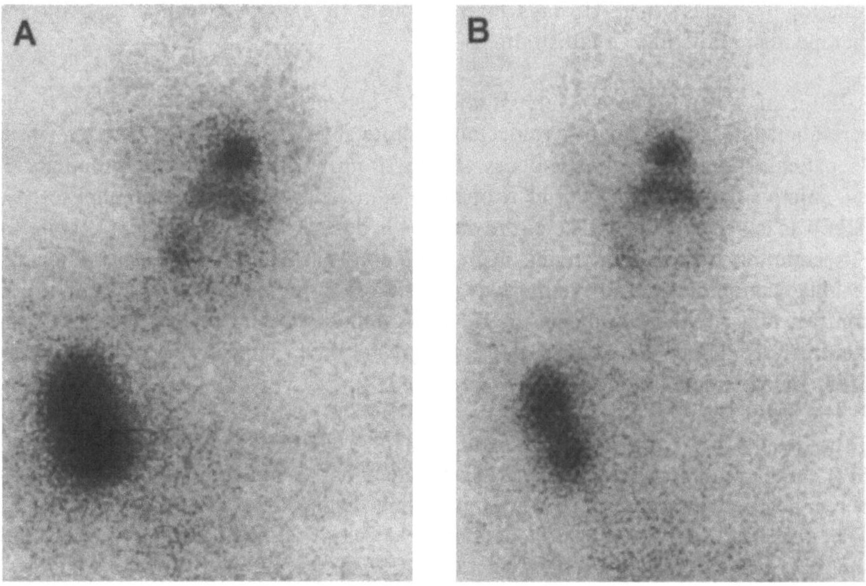

Figure 7 A: Anterior spot view of the chest in a patient with metastatic thyroid carcinoma. Scintigram obtained 2 days after administration of 2 mCi of iodine-131 which was given 24 hours after rhTSH administration (0.9 mg for 2 times with an interval of 24 hours) B: Anterior spot view of the chest in the same patient. Scintigram obtained 2 days after administration of iodine-131, which was given after withdrawal of thyroid hormone therapy (serum TSH level greater than 25 mU/L). Both scans show abnormal foci of iodine-131 activity in the right superior thorax and physiologic activity in the nasopharynx. Reproduced from Ladenson, et al. (94) with the permission of the publisher.

The phenomenon of "stunning" of thyroid tissue by diagnostic doses of iodine-131

Diagnostic doses of ^{131}I may decrease the uptake of a subsequent therapeutic dose of ^{131}I after (near-)total thyroidectomy. This phenomenon is called "stunning" of thyroid tissue. The phenomenon of stunning was first studied in 1986 by Jeevanram et al. (95), but it has drawn more attention in recent years. Jeevanram et al. studied 52 patients who had undergone (near-)total thyroidectomy for differentiated thyroid carcinoma and who had a more than 5% uptake of radioiodine in the thyroid bed. Diagnostic doses were 0.1 to 5 mCi of iodine-131. Patients were divided in three subgroups on the basis of the estimated absorbed dose in the residual thyroid tissue (below 17.5 Gy, 17.5 to 35 Gy, and higher than 35 Gy). In these three groups the ratio of the 72-hour uptake of the subsequently administered ablative dose of radioiodine to the 72-hour uptake of the diagnostic dose averaged 0.76, 0.37, and 0.25, respectively. The decrease in uptake of the ablative dose did not correlate with the time interval (ranging from less than 10 days to more than 40 days) between diagnostic and therapeutic radioiodine administration.

Park et al. (96) retrospectively studied 26 patients with differentiated thyroid carcinoma after (near-)total thyroidectomy before ablative radioiodine therapy. These 26 patients received diagnostic doses of 3 to 10 mCi ^{131}I. In 20 (77%) the uptake of the ablative dose (100 to 200 mCi) of radioiodine administered some hours to days later was lower than the uptake of the diagnostic dose on visual judgement (Figure 8). Fifteen of 24 (63%) foci in the neck, including normal thyroid tissue remnants, residual tumor tissue, and lymph node metastases in the neck, showed stunning, in contrast to 1 of 11 (9%) distant foci. These authors also found that the higher the administered diagnostic activity of ^{131}I, the greater the chance of a decrease in uptake of the therapeutic dose of ^{131}I.

These results were confirmed by Sisson, et al. (97) and Leger, et al. (98). Sisson et al. (97) compared the percentage uptake in the neck of a therapeutic dose (Rx) with the percentage uptake in the neck of the preceding diagnostic dose (Dx) of iodine-131. The ratio Rx/Dx was 0.36 with diagnostic doses of 2 mCi (n=22) and 0.56 with diagnostic doses of 1 mCi (n=9). Leger et al. (98) measured 2-hour ^{123}I uptake in neck foci in 17 patients with differentiated thyroid carcinoma after (near-)total thyroidectomy before administration of a diagnostic dose of 5 mCi ^{131}I and in 12 of these patients 12 to 84 days later, immediately before ablative radioiodine therapy. The second uptake (1.97% ± 0.71%) was significantly lower than the first one (3.76% ± 1.50%). In 5 of 17 patients post-therapy images showed no foci in contrast to the preceding diagnostic images.

Stunning of thyroid tissue by diagnostic doses of ^{131}I may diminish the success of subsequent thyroid ablation. Park et al. (99) compared the success of subsequent ablative radioiodine therapy in 25 patients imaged with ^{131}I (3 to 10 mCi) and 40 patients imaged with iodine-123 (300 μCi). Follow-up after 1 year showed less successful ablations in the iodine-131-imaging group than in the iodine-123-imaging group (60% versus 75%), although the difference was not significant (p=0.271).

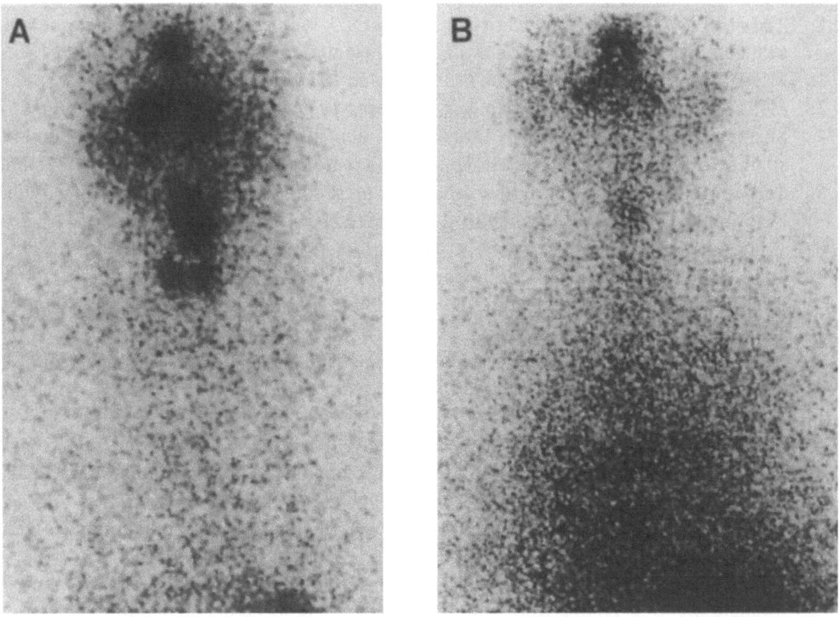

Figure 8 A: Anterior spot view of neck and chest in a 37-year-old woman with papillary carcinoma who had a total thyroidectomy and received 106 mCi of ^{131}I 1 year previously. Scintigram obtained 2 days after administration of 10 mCi of iodine-131. Note the uptake by the pyramidal lobe and two small foci in the thyroid bed. B: Anterior spot view of neck and chest in the same patient. Scintigram obtained 2 days after administration of 100 mCi of ^{131}I. Note that there is less uptake in the lesions in comparison with the diagnostic scintigram. Reproduced from Park, et al. (96) with the permission of the publisher.

In the light of the stunning phenomenon, it seems prudent, in case ^{131}I is chosen for diagnostic whole body scintigraphy after (near-)total thyroidectomy before ablative radioiodine therapy, to use a low dose (e.g. 1 to 2 mCi). Alternatively, ^{123}I can be used. Park et al. (99) found no stunning in 14 patients with differentiated thyroid carcinoma after (near-)total thyroidectomy who got ablative radioiodine therapy after diagnostic whole body scintigraphy with 300 μCi ^{123}I. Furthermore, ^{123}I (300 μCi) was found to be not significantly less accurate than ^{131}I (3 to 10 mCi) whole body scintigraphy in this setting (90% versus 93% accuracy, respectively). A third alternative is to omit whole body scintigraphy preceding ablative radioiodine therapy.

For the follow-up of patients after thyroid ablation with radioiodine we recommend ^{131}I because of its superior diagnostic accuracy (see before) and because there is up till now no evidence of clinically significant stunning of thyroid carcinoma metastases.

References

1. Zeissman H, Fahey F, Gochoco J. Impact of radiocontaminants in commercially available iodine-123: dosimetric evaluation. J Nucl Med 1986;27:428.
2. MIRD: Dose Estimate Report No. 5. J Nucl Med 1975;16:857.
3. MIRD: Dose Estimate Report No. 8. J Nucl Med 1977;17:74.
4. Shambaugh GE III, Quinn JL, Oyasu R, et al. Disparate thyroid imaging: Combined studies with sodium pertechnetate Tc-99m and radioactive iodine. JAMA 1974;228:866.
5. Turner JW, Spencer RP. Thyroid carcinoma presenting as a pertechnetate "hot" nodule, but without 131I uptake: case report. J Nucl Med 1976;17:22.
6. Erjavec M, Movrin T, Auersperg M, Golough R. Comparative accumulation of 99mTc and 131I in thyroid nodules: case report. J Nucl Med 1977;18:346.
7. Ryo UY, Vaidya PV, Schneider AB, et al. Thyroid imaging agents: a comparison of I-123 and Tc-99m pertechnetate. Radiol 1983;148:829.
8. Kusic Z, Becker DV, Saenger EL, et al. Comparison of technetium-99m and iodine-123 imaging of thyroid nodules: correlation with pathologic findings. J Nucl Med 1990;31:393.
9. Briele B, Hotze A, Grunwald F, Overbeck B, Biersack HJ. Increased sensitivity of whole-body scintigraphy with I-131 for the detection of iodine-accumulating metastases by means of delayed imaging. Nucl Med 1990;29:264.
10. Sostre S, Ashare AB, Quinones JD, et al. Thyroid scintigraphy: pinhole images versus rectilinear scans. Radiology 1978;129:759.
11. Flower MA, Irvine AT, Ott RJ, et al. Thyroid imaging using positron emission tomography – a comparison with ultrasound imaging and conventional imaging in thyrotoxicosis. Br J Radiol 1990;63:325.
12. Lennquist S, Persliden J, Smeds S. The value of intraoperative scintigraphy as a routine procedure in thyroid carcinoma. World J Surg 1988;12:586.
13. Ricard M, Regal R, Schlumberger M, et al. Détection peropératoire du I-125 et du I-131 au moyen d'une sonde portable. J Méd Nucl Bioph (Paris) 1990;14:151.
14. Hurley PJ, Strauss HW, Pavoni P, et al. The scintillation camera with pinhole collimator in thyroid imaging. Radiology 1971;101:133.
15. Levy HA, Sziklas JJ, Rosenberg RJ, Spencer RP. Incidence of a pyramidal lobe on thyroid scans. Clin Nucl Med 1982;7:560.
16. Siraj QH, Aleem N, Inam-Ur-Rehman A, Qaisar S, Ahmad M. The pyramidal lobe: a scintigraphic assessment. Nucl Med Commun 1989;10:685.
17. Hamburger JI, Hamburger SW. Thyroid hemiagenesis. Arch Surg 1970;100:319.
18. Melnick JC, Stemkowski PE. Thyroid hemiagenesis (hockey stick sign): a review of the world literature and a report of four cases. Clin Endocrinol Metab 1981;52:247.
19. Katz AD, Zager WJ. The lingual thyroid. Arch Surg 1971;102:582.
20. Brooks PT, Archard ND, Carty HML. Thyroid screening in congenital hypothyroidism: a review of 41 cases. Nucl Med Commun 1988;9:613.
21. Rieser GD, Ober KP, Cowan RJ, Cordell AR. Radioiodide imaging of struma cordis. Clin Nucl Med 1988;13:421.
22. Baschieri L, Benedetti G, DeLuca F, et al. Evaluation and limitations of the perchlorate test in the study of thyroid function. J Clin Endocrinol Metab 1963;23:786.
23. Knight PJ, Hamoudi AB, Vassy LE. The diagnosis and treatment of midline neck masses in children. Surgery 1983;93:603.
24. Noyek AM, Friedberg J. Thyroglossal duct and ectopic thyroid disorders. Otolaryng Clin N Am 1981;14:187.
25. Cheung PSY, Lee JMH, Boey JH. Thyroxine suppressive therapy of benign solitary thyroid nodules: a prospective randomized study. World J Surg 1989;13:818.

26. Kuma K, Matsuzuka F, Kobayashi A, et al. Outcome of long standing solitary thyroid nodules. World J Surg 1992;16:583.
27. Vander JB, Gaston EA, Dawber TR. The significance of nontoxic thyroid nodules. Final report of a 15-year study of the incidence of thyroid malignancy. Ann Intern Med 1968;69:537.
28. Tan GH, Gharib H, Reading CC. Solitary thyroid nodule. Comparison between palpation and ultrasonography. Arch Intern Med 1995;155:2418.
29. Sheppard MC, Franklyn JA. Management of the single thyroid nodule. Clin Endocrinol 1992;37:398.
30. Ridgway EC. Clinician's evaluation of a solitary thyroid nodule. J Clin Endocrinol Metab 1992;74:231.
31. Mazzaferri EL. Management of a solitary thyroid nodule. N Engl J Med 1993;328:553.
32. Gharib H, Goellner JR. Fine-needle aspiration biopsy of the thyroid: an appraisal. Ann Intern Med 1993;118:282.
33. Singer PA. Evaluation and management of the solitary thyroid nodule. Otolaryngol Clin North Am 1996;29:577.
34. Sisson DB, Bartold SP, Bartold SL. The dilemma of the solitary thyroid nodule: Resolution through decision analysis. Semin Nucl Med 1978;8:59.
35. Ashcraft MW, Van Herle AJ. Management of thyroid nodules. II. Scanning techniques, thyroid suppressive therapy, and fine needle aspiration. Head Neck Surg 1981;3:296.
36. Chen JJS, LaFrance ND, Allo MD, et al. Single photon emission computed tomography of the thyroid. J Clin Endocrinol Metab 1988;66:1240.
37. Krausz Y, Wilk M, Saliman F, Chisin R. Role of high-resolution pinhole tomography in the evaluation of thyroid abnormalities. Thyroid 1997;7:847.
38. Ghose MK, Genuth SM, Abellera RM, et al. Functioning primary thyroid carcinoma and metastases producing hyperthyroidism. J Clin Endocrinol Metab 1971;33:639.
39. Landgarten S, Spencer RP. A study of the natural history of "hot" nodule. Yale J Biol Med 1973;46:259.
40. Livadas DP, Kotoulas OB, Bouropoulos V, et al. The coexistence of thyroid malignancy with autonomous hot nodules of the thyroid. Clin Nucl Med 1977;2:350.
41. Nagai GR, Pitts WC, Basso L, et al. Scintigraphic hot nodules and thyroid cancer. Clin Nucl Med 1987;12:123.
42. Rizzi G, Argiro G, Gentile L, et al. Use of the 99mTc scintiscan with lead-shield on the hot nodule in the diagnosis of adenomatous adenoma. Nucl Med Comm 1987;8:217.
43. Cornelius EA. Combined nuclear medicine and ultrasound studies in the evaluation of suppressed thyroid tissue. Clin Nucl Med 1983;8:8.
44. Corstens F, Huysmans D, Kloppenborg P. Thallium-201 scintigraphy of the suppressed thyroid: an alternative for iodine-123 scanning after TSH. J Nucl Med 1988;29:1360.
45. Ramanathan P, Patel RB, Subrahmanyan N, et al. Visualization of suppressed thyroid tissue by technetium-99m-tertiary butyl isonitrile: an alternative to post-TSH stimulation scanning. J Nucl Med 1990;31:1163.
46. Wiener JD. Long-term follow-up in untreated Plummer's disease (autonomous goiter). Clin Nucl Med 1987;12:198.
47. Berghout A, Wiersinga WM, Smits NJ, Touber JL. Interrelationships between age, thyroid volume, thyroid nodularity, and thyroid function in patients with sporadic nontoxic goiter. Am J Med 1990;89:602.
48. Grubeck-Loebenstein B, Derfler K, Kassal H, et al. Immunological features of nonimunogenic hyperthyroidism. J Clin Endorinol Metab 1985;60:150.
49. Kraiem Z, Glaser B, Yigla M, Pauker J, Sheinfeld M. Toxic, multinodular goiter: a variant of autoimmune hyperthyroidism. J Clin Endocrinol Metab 1987;65:659.
50. Hermus AR, Huysmans DA. Treatment of benign nodular thyroid disease. New Engl J Med 1998;338:1438.

51. Park H, Tarver RD, Siddiqui AR, et al. Efficacy of thyroid scintigraphy in the diagnosis of intrathoracic goiter. Am J Radiol 1987;148:527.
52. Hamburger JI, Hamburger SW. Diagnosis and management of large toxic multinodular goiters. J Nucl Med 1985;26:888.
53. Webb S, Flower MA, Ott RJ , et al. Single photon emission computed tomography and volume estimation of the thyroid using fan-beam geometry. Br J Radiol 1986;59:951.
54. Ott RJ, Batty V, Webb S, et al. Measurement of radiation dose to the thyroid using positron emission tomography. Br J Radiol 1987;60:245.
55. Ramtoola S, Maisey MN, Clarke SEM, Fogelman I. The thyroid scan seen in Hashimoto's thyroiditis: the great mimic. Nucl Med Commun 1988;9:639.
56. Hamburger JL, Miller JM, Kini SR. Lymphoma of the thyroid. Ann Intern Med 1983;99:685.
57. Schlumberger MJ. Papillary and follicular thyroid carcinoma. N Engl J Med 1998;338:297.
58. Benua RS, Cicale NR, Sonenberg M, et al. The relation of radioiodine dosimetry to results and complications in the treatment of metastatic thyroid cancer. Am J Roentgenol 1962;87:171.
59. Maxon HR, Thomas SR, Hertzberg VS, et al. Relation between effective radiation dose and outcome of radioiodine therapy for thyroid cancer. N Engl J Med 1983;309:937.
60. Edmonds CJ, Hayes S, Kermode JC, et al. Measurement of serum TSH and thyroid hormones in the management of treatment of thyroid carcinoma with radioiodine. Br J Radiol 1977;50:799.
61. Hilts SV, Hellman D, Anderson J, et al. Serial TSH determination after T3 withdrawal or thyroidectomy in the therapy of thyroid carcinoma. J Nucl Med 1979;20:928.
62. Beierwaltes WH. Radioiodine in the therapy of thyroid carcinoma. In: Spencer RP, ed. Therapy in nuclear medicine. New York: Grune & Stratton, 1978:101.
63. Goldman JM, Line BR, Aamodt RL, et al. Influence of triiodothyronine withdrawal time on 131-I uptake postthyroidectomy for thyroid cancer. J Clin Endocrinol Metab 1980;50:734.
64. Maxon HR, Thomas SR, Boehringer A, et al. Low iodine diet in I-131 ablation of thyroid remnants. Clin Nucl Med 1983;8:124.
65. Lakshmanan M, Schaffer A, Robbins J, et al. A simplified low iodine diet in I-131 scanning and therapy of thyroid cancer. Clin Nucl Med 1988;13:866.
66. Ramanna L, Waxman A, Brachman MB, et al. Treatment rationale in thyroid carcinoma: Effect of scan dose. Clin Nucl Med 1985;10:687.
67. Waxman A, Ramanna L, Chapman N, et al. The significance of I-131 scan dose in patients with thyroid cancer: Determination of ablation: concise communication. J Nucl Med 1981;22:861.
68. Nemec J, Röhling S, Zamrazil V, Pohunková D. Comparison of the distribution of diagnostic and thyroablative I-131 in the evaluation of differentiated thyroid cancers. J Nucl Med 1979;20:92.
69. Pacini F, Lippi F, Formica N, et al. Therapeutic doses of iodine-131 reveal undiagnosed metastases in thyroid cancer patients with detectable serum thyroglobulin levels. J Nucl Med 1987;28:1888.
70. Clark OH, Hoelting T. Management of patients with differentiated thyroid cancer who have positive serum thyroglobulin levels and negative radioiodine scans. Thyroid 1994;4:501.
71. Sherman SI, Tielens ET, Sostre S, et al. Clinical utility of post-treatment radioiodine scans in the management of patients with thyroid carcinoma. J Clin Endocrinol Metab 1994;78:629.
72. Rosenbaum RC, Johnston GS, Valente WA. Frequency of hepatic visualization during I-131 imaging for metastatic thyroid carcinoma. Clin Nucl Med 1988;13:657.

73. Zeissman HA, Bahar H, Fahey FH, Dubiansky V. Hepatic visualization on iodine-131 whole-body thyroid cancer scans. J Nucl Med 19487;28:1408.
74. Ronga G, Fiorentino A, Paserio E, et al. Can iodine-131 whole-body scan be replaced by thyroglobulin measurement in the post-surgical follow-up of differentiated thyroid carcinoma? J Nucl Med 1990;31:1766.
75. Simpson WJ. Radioiodine and radiotherapy in the management of thyroid cancers. Otolaryngol Clin North Am 1990;23:509.
76. Samaan NA, Schultz PN, Haynie TP, et al. Pulmonary metastasis of differentiated thyroid carcinoma: Treatment results in 101 patients. J Clin Endocrinol Metab 1985;65:376.
77. Maheshwari YK, Hill CS Jr, Haynie TP III, et al. 131I therapy in differentiated thyroid carcinoma: M.D. Anderson Hospital experience. Cancer 1981;47:664.
78. Brown AP, Greening WP, McCready VR, et al. Radioiodine treatment of metastatic thyroid carcinoma: The Royal Marsden Hospital experience. Br J Radiol 1984;57:323.
79. Schlumberger M, Tubiana M, De Vathaire F, et al. Long-term results of treatment of 283 patients with lung and bone metastases from differentiated thyroid carcinoma. J Clin Endocrinol Metab 1986;63:960.
80. Hermann M, Kober F, Keminger K. Die Fernmetastasierung der Struma maligna: Eine retrospektive Studie über 892 Fälle. Onkologie 1987;10:350.
81. Mazzaferri EL. Thyroid carcinoma. In: Mazzaferri EL, Samaan NA, eds. Endocrine Tumors. Boston, Blackwell Scientific Publications, 1993.
82. Hoschl R, Choy DH-L, Gandevia B. Iodine-131 uptake in inflammatory lung disease: a pitfall in treatment of thyroid carcinoma. J Nucl Med 1988;29:701.
83. Caplan RH, Gunderson GA, Abellera RM, Kisken WA. Uptake of iodine-131 by a Meckel's diverticulum mimicking metastatic thyroid cancer. Clin Nucl Med 1987;12:760.
84. Brachman MB, Rothman BJ, Ramanna L. False-positive iodine-131 body scan caused by a large renal cyst. Clin Nucl Med 1988;13:416.
85. Fernandez-Ulloa M, Maxon HR, Mehta S, et al. Iodine-131 uptake by primary lung adenocarcinoma: misinterpretation of I-131 scan. JAMA 1976;23:857.
86. Preisman RA, Halpern SE, Shishido R, et al. Uptake of I-131 by a papillary meningioma. Am J Roentgenol 1977;129:349.
87. Sing-Yung W, Kollin J, Coogley E, et al. I-131 total-body scan: localization of disseminated gastric adenocarcinoma. Case report and survey of literature. J Nucl Med 1984;25:1204.
88. Greenler DP, Klein HA. The scope of false-positive iodine-131 images for thyroid carcinoma. Clin Nucl Med 1989;14:111.
89. Bakheet SM, Hammami MM. False-positive radioiodine whole-body scan in thyroid cancer patients due to unrelated pathology. Clin Nucl Med 1994;19:325.
90. McDougall IR. Whole body scintigraphy with radioiodine. A comprehensive list of false-positives with some examples. Clin Nucl Med 1995;20:868.
91. Maloof F, Vickery AL, Rapp B. An evaluation of various factors influencing the treatment of metastatic thyroid carcinoma with 131I. J Clin Endocrinol Metab 1956;16:1.
92. Sfakianakis GN, Skillman TG, George JM. Thyroxine withdrawal in thyroid cancer. Ohio State Med J 1975;71:79.
93. Goldberg LD, Ditchek NT. Thyroid carcinoma with spinal cord compression JAMA 1981;245:953.
94. Ladenson PW, Braverman LE, Mazzaferri EL, et al. Comparison of administration of recombinant human thyrotropin with withdrawal of thyroid hormone for radioactive iodine scanning in patients with thyroid carcinoma. New Engl J Med 1997;337:888.

95. Jeevanram RK, Shah DH, Sharma SM, Ganatra RD. Influence of initial large dose on subsequent uptake of therapeutic radioiodine in thyroid cancer patients. Nucl Med Biol 1986;13:277.
96. Park HM, Perkins OW, Edmondson JW, Schnute RB, Manatunga A. Influence of diagnostic radioiodines on the uptake of ablative dose of iodine-131. Thyroid 1994;4:49.
97. Sisson J, Shapiro B, Shulkin B, Gross M, Spaulding S. Effects of diagnostic dosages of 131-I on uptake of therapeutic 131-I by thyroid cancer. Thyroid 1997;7 (suppl 1):S-3 (abstract)
98. Leger FA, Izembart M, Dagousset F, et al. Decreased uptake of therapeutic doses of iodine-131 after 185-MBq iodine-131 diagnostic imaging for thyroid remnants in differentiated thyroid carcinoma. Eur J Nucl Med 1998;25:242.
99. Park HM, Park YH, Zhou XH. Detection of thyroid remnant/metastasis without stunning: an ongoing dilemma. Thyroid 1997;7:277.

7

SOMATOSTATIN RECEPTOR SCINTIGRAPHY IN THYROIDAL DISEASES

Eric P. Krenning, M.D.
Wouter W. de Herder, M.D.
Wilmar M. Wiersinga, M.D.
Dik J. Kwekkeboom, M.D.
University Hospital Rotterdam, Rotterdam, the Netherlands
Academic Medical Center, University of Amsterdam, Amsterdam, the Netherlands

INTRODUCTION

Tissues, which express somatostatin receptors, can be visualized with [^{111}In-DTPA^{0}] octreotide scintigraphy. With this technology the presence of the subtypes 2 and 5 of the five somatostatin receptors can be demonstrated in vivo. The first use of [^{111}In-DTPA^{0}] octreotide scintigraphy in the thyroid field with the exception of malignant thyroid diseases, was in 1991 when we extended our research of octreotide scintigraphy from (neuro-)endocrine tumors to granulomatous and autoimmune diseases (1-3). By coincidence, at that time, we found that in sarcoidosis and rheumatoid arthritis [^{111}In-DTPA^{0}]octreotide scintigraphy showed intense uptake in involved areas (3,4).

In this chapter we will discuss the clinical relevance of octreotide scintigraphy in patients with thyroidal diseases.

Auto-immune diseases

*[^{111}In-DTPA^{0}]octreotide scintigraphy in **thyroidal** Graves' disease*

In 1992 Chang and co-workers reported a favorable effect of octreotide treatment on the signs and symptoms of Graves' ophthalmopathy (5). They hypothesized that octreotide, a potent long-acting somatostatin analogue, may inhibit local synthesis of insulin-like growth factor-1 (IGF-1) by orbital fibroblasts, thereby reducing glycosaminoglycan production. The hypothesis is theoretically supported by the presence of immunoreactivity to IGF-1 in extraocular muscles and fat cells (6), and by the suppression of IGF-1 in serum by octreotide. At the same time, we used radiolabeled octreotide in patients with Graves' disease on the premise that activated lymphocytes express somatostatin receptors (1).

Postema et al. (2) injected 220 MBq [^{111}In-DTPA^{0}]octreotide iv as a bolus, and obtained planar anterior-camera images of the neck 5 and 24 h after injection. Thyroidal radiolabeled octreotide accumulation was expressed as percentage of the injected dose by the region of interest method on planar anterior images corrected for background (region adjacent to the thyroid on the same image). The results are summarized in Table 1. If thyroidal uptake of radiolabeled octreotide was set at 100% at 5h post-injection, the uptake at 24h post-injection decreased to 68±19% in patients with Graves' disease, similar to that in controls (58±12%). This decrease was significantly less than the decrease in blood pool radioactivity (from 100% to 15±4%), indicating specific uptake in the thyroid gland.

Table 1. Thyroidal [^{111}In-DTPA^{0}]octreotide accumulation ♣

Subjects	Treatment	Thyroid function	TBII	34h Thyroidal octreotide uptake*
Controls	None	euthyroid	absent	0.03%
Graves' hyperthyroidism	None	hyperthyroid	present	0.17%
Graves' hyperthyroidism	Methimazole	euthyroid	present	0.14%
Graves' hyperthyroidism	^{131}I, Thyroxine	euthyroid	present	0%
Primary hypothyroidism	Thyroxine	euthyroid	absent	0.003%

* figures are median values expressed as percentage of injected dose
♣ data reproduced with permission of Postema et al. (2)

Thyroidal octreotide uptake is low in controls and relatively high in untreated Graves' hyperthyroidism. The [^{111}In-DTPA^{0}]octreotide scintigram thus provides a faint image of the thyroid gland in the absence of thyroid disease, but a nice thyroidal image can be obtained in Graves' disease, which cannot be fully explained by the large thyroid gland in Graves' disease (2). In untreated Graves' hyperthyroidism the thyroidal octreotide uptake is positively related to serum FT4, T3 and TBII (TSH binding inhibitory immunoglobulins), suggesting a relationship with the severity of Graves' hyperthyroidism (2). The correlation is, however, no longer observed in Graves' hyperthyroid patients who have been rendered euthyroid by methimazole treatment: they still have a relatively high thyroidal octreotide uptake (2,7,8) and clearly demonstrable concentrations of TBII in serum. It has therefore been speculated that the [^{111}In-DTPA^{0}]octreotide scintigraphy visualizes the lymphocytic infiltrate in the thyroid of patients with Graves' disease, reflecting the activity rather than the severity of the disease. This assumption was supported by the finding that cultured human lymphocytes express distinct subsets of somatostatin receptors (9): human T-cells and myeloma cells had an average of 144 and 1295 high affinity somatostatin receptors per cell respectively, with corresponding Kd values of 3pM and 5pM. The presence of somatostatin receptors is also evident from the visualization of pathological lesions by somatostatin receptor scintigraphy in patients with malignant lymphoma, granulomatous inflammation, and rheumatoid arthritis (10). In these processes, not only activated T-lymphocytes and monocytes but also local veins are candidates for expression of somatostatin receptors (10), as might be the case in the thyroid gland in Graves' disease. One argument against this explanation could be that almost no thyroidal octreotide uptake was observed in patients with autoimmune hypothyroidism with goiter (10), in whom a lymphocytic infiltrate of the thyroid gland is a hallmark of the disease. The negative [^{111}In-DTPA^{0}]octreotide scintigrams in the Graves' patients rendered hypothyroid by ^{131}I (in whom TBII was still present), also does not necessarily falsify the given explanation as TBII can be produced extrathyroidally in the lymphatic system.

Of much interest are recent findings suggesting expression of somatostatin receptors on thyroid follicular epithelial cells themselves (10). This might explain the thyroidal [^{111}In-DTPA^{0}]octreotide uptake observed in patients with a TSH-producing pituitary adenoma (Figure 1), thyroid adenoma, endemic goiter, or differentiated nonmedullary thyroid cancer (8,10) . The common denominator of these conditions is thyroid growth, either autonomous in thyroid adenomas and cancer or mediated via the TSH receptor in TSH-producing pituitary adenoma and Graves' disease. It is tempting to speculate that thyroid growth itself is associated with an increased expression of somatostatin receptors on thyrocytes, explaining the visualization with [^{111}In-DTPA^{0}]octreotide scintigraphy. In this respect it is of interest to note a direct inhibitory effect of somatostatin on growth (but not on differentiation) of human thyroid follicular cells in vitro, probably by a mechanism not entirely cAMP dependent (11). Recently, it has been shown by somatostatin autoradiography that indeed follicular cells or thyrocytes express somatostatin receptors (12).

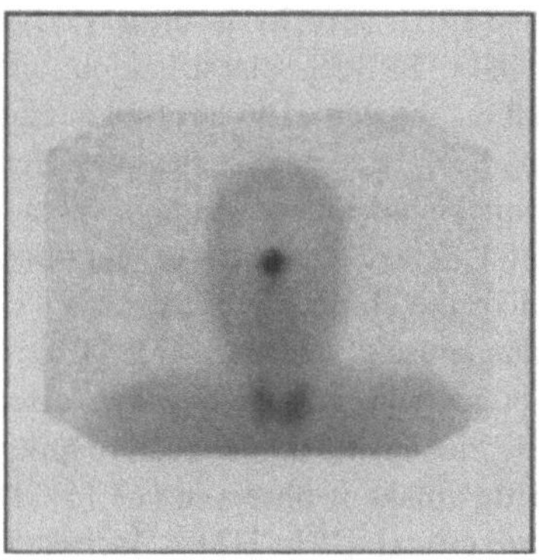

Figure 1. Somatostatin receptor imaging in a patient with a TSH-producing pituitary adenoma. There is clear uptake in the pituitary adenoma and diffuse uptake in the enlarged thyroid, which is high if compared to euthyroid patients

In summary, upregulation of somatostatin receptors on thyrocytes, local veins and/or thyroidal immune cells are presumably responsible for a positive [^{111}In-DTPA^{0}]octreotide scintigram in Graves' disease (12). The present limited data suggest that thyroidal octreotide uptake in Graves' disease might be related at least partly to the activity of the auto-immune disease rather than to the hyperthyroid state itself. Persistent thyroidal [^{111}In-DTPA^{0}]octreotide uptake as observed in Graves' patients taking methimazole would then indicate still active autoimmune thyroid disease; the implication is that a positive thyroidal [^{111}In-DTPA^{0}]octreotide scintigram increases the chance of recurrent hyperthyroidism after discontinuation of methimazole treatment. A cost-benefit analysis will be necessary when clinical application is suggested if this predictive value of thyroidal [^{111}In-DTPA^{0}]octreotide scintigraphy is proven in a controlled trial.

[^{111}In-DTPA^{0}]octreotide scintigraphy in ***orbital*** *Graves' disease*

The first orbital [^{111}In-DTPA^{0}]octreotide scans in Graves' disease have been reported since 1991 (1,2). If peak activity in the orbit 5h after injection of radiolabeled octreotide is set at 100%, a decrease to 40±4% is found at 24h, significantly different from the decrease in blood pool radioactivity (from 100% at 5h to 15±4% at 24 h). The cause of specific orbital uptake is unknown. An attractive hypothesis is that orbital uptake in Graves' disease is caused by the expression of somatostatin receptors on activated T-lymphocytes, thus visualizing the lymphocytic infiltrate in retrobulbar tissues. Alternative explanations cannot, however, be excluded like binding to receptors on other cell types (e.g. eye muscle cells, fibroblasts, endothelial cells) or local blood pooling due to venous stasis by the auto-immune orbital inflammation. Systemic hypercirculation seems only partly responsible, as evident from the rather low orbital uptake in Graves' hyperthyroid patients without clinical signs of ophthalmopathy (2).

Some studies report a relationship between orbital [^{111}In-DTPA^{0}]octreotide accumulation and the severity of Graves' ophthalmopathy, with higher uptake values in more severe eye disease (2,13); severity in these studies is indicated by a higher class or grade in the NO SPECS classification of eye signs in Graves' ophthalmopathy. Other authors, however, do not find a relationship with severity (14-16). In contrast, the activity of the eye disease is always found to be related to orbital [^{111}In-DTPA^{0}]octreotide uptake whenever studied. This is evident from a direct relationship between orbital uptake and various parameters of disease activity in Graves' ophthalmopathy like the clinical activity score (2,16) and the T2 relaxation time of the inferior rectus muscle on MRI (7). Orbital [^{111}In-DTPA^{0}]octreotide accumulation is greater in patients with active eye disease than in patients with inactive eye disease (13,14); the uptake in the inactive group is close to that in control subjects in whom no specific uptake is observed (13,15). These data strongly suggest the notion that a positive orbital [^{111}In-DTPA^{0}]octreotide scintigram in Graves' ophthalmopathy indicates active eye disease in which - in contrast to the inactive end-stage of the disease with fibrosis - immunosuppressive treatment might be of therapeutic benefit. Indeed, successful immunosuppression (be it with prednisone, orbital irradiation or intravenous immunoglobulin) is associated with a fall in orbital

[^{111}In-DTPA^{0}]octreotide uptake (13,16).

Orbital [^{111}In-DTPA^{0}]octreotide scintigraphy could thus be applied in clinical practice to select patients with Graves' ophthalmopathy who will benefit from immunosuppression. To this end one must know the predictive value of orbital [^{111}In-DTPA^{0}]octreotide uptake for the outcome of immunosuppressive treatment; such data are, however, scarce, as are data about the precision and accuracy of the technique. There are wide differences between various studies in the administered dose of [^{111}In-DTPA^{0}]octreotide, the time interval after injection for determining the orbital uptake, the selection of orbital slices for quantification of the orbital uptake, and the method of correction for background radioactivity (Table 2). The earlier studies used larger doses of radiolabeled octreotide (as usual in the visualization of neuroendocrine tumors), and preferred to determine orbital uptake 24h post injection (2,15,17) with SPECT. Moncayo et al. (16), however, applied a rather low ^{111}In-dose and measured orbital uptake after a time interval of only 2 hours, arguing that 1) the low dose decreases the radiation burden and the cost of the examination, 2) a short time interval is optimal in view of the kinetics of somatostatin binding to lymphocytic receptors (showing maximal binding after 120 min in vitro) and of the effective half-life of the radioligand in the orbits starting 4h after iv application. In disagreement, Krassas and Dumas (18) state that a low ^{111}In-dose might cause problems in count statistics, and that 2h after injection 12% of the dose is still in the blood pool causing high background uptake; furthermore, the radiation burden received from a high dose of 222 MBq is 16 mSv, in the same order as that from chest computed tomography or angiography. It must be admitted that the difference in orbital octreotide uptake between patients with active and inactive eye disease is smaller at 24h than at 4h after injection of a low dose (13,19,20). The inference is that for discrimination purposes a 4h time interval is preferred when a low dose is chosen. On the other hand, any remaining orbital radioactivity at 24h after administering a high dose might represent to a greater degree specific tissue binding, possibly enhancing the predictive value of the [^{111}In-DTPA^{0}]octreotide scintigram. Future studies should take this specific point into account. Another technical bias is the selection of orbital regions of interest, which may result in considerable intra- and inter-observer variation. SPECT images are obviously required, and measuring uptake in a number of orbital slices from SPECT images is of great advantage in the quantification of results (Figure 2).

Correction for background activity has originally been performed by using the temporal skull area (2,17). Uptake in this area may vary considerable, ascribed to additional radioactivity in the intracranial venous sinuses and parotid gland. These additional areas should be neglected when using the temporal skull area for background subtraction. Alternatively the occipital skull area can be used. Brain itself is used to measure background (13,14,15), but seems less suitable to correct for blood pool radioactivity.

Patients with very active eye disease are bound to respond favorably to immunosuppression; the activity of the eye disease in such cases is clinically evident at first glance, and would not require further assessment with [^{111}In-DTPA^{0}]octreotide scintigraphy. In many patients with moderately severe ophthalmopathy, however, it is not at all clear whether or not the eye disease is still in the active stage and whether or not the patient will benefit from immunosuppression. Under these circumstances orbital [^{111}In-DTPA^{0}]octreotide scintigraphy might be used as a predictor for outcome of immunosuppression. This will require calculation of the orbital to skull uptake ratio, preferably using quantitative measurements in well-defined regions of interest of SPECT slices. The first study in this respect is that of Krassas and co-workers (17) who observed the following orbital to skull uptake ratio's 24h after 244 MBq [^{111}In-DTPA^{0}]octreotide: controls, 1.00±0.003; Graves' disease without eye disease 1.25±0.003; Graves' ophthalmopathy responding or not responding to immunosuppression with sc. octreotide, 1.85±0.09 and 1.45±0.05 respectively (pre-treatment values). In all 13 eyes improving with treatment the ratio was 1.65, whereas 9 of 11 'nonresponding eyes' had a ratio of <1.65.

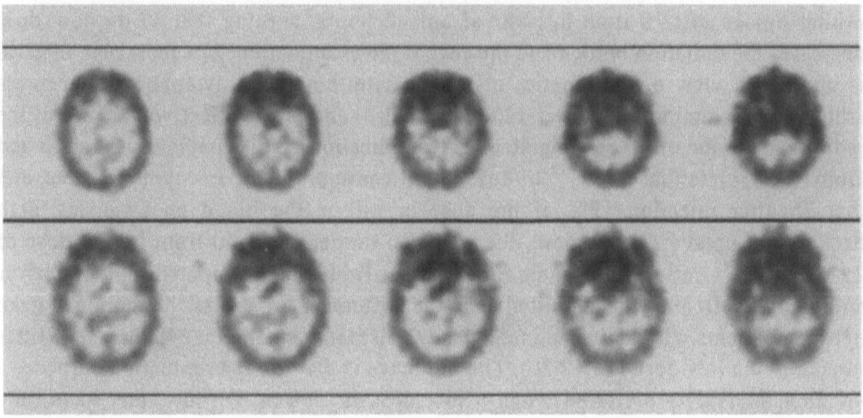

Figure 2. Somatostatin receptor imaging in a patient with Graves' ophtalmopathy. Transversal SPECT images 4 h pi (upper row) and 24 h pi (lower row). Images run from cranial to caudal. In the middle 3 images the pituitary can be seen, together with uptake in the orbits.

It remains to be seen if orbital [^{111}In-DTPA^{0}]octreotide scintigraphy will become a widely applied tool in the management of Graves' ophthalmopathy patients. First, its technique is demanding in terms of accuracy required for prediction. Each institution should develop its own cut-off values in this respect. Second, it is an expensive method. Third, it is not specific for a certain disease since more diseases are known by their increased expression of somatostatin receptors, i.e. positive orbital [^{111}In-DTPA^{0}]octreotide scans may also be obtained in patients with orbital meningioma, malignant lymphoma, pseudotumor orbitae, orbital myositis, sarcoidosis, Wegener's granulomatosis, necrotising scleritis, sinusitis and infections of the nasal mucosa (10,13,14,16). Fourth, orbital [^{111}In-DTPA^{0}]octreotide scintigraphy does not allow precise orbital imaging, i.e. evaluation of eye muscle swelling and apical crowding still requires imaging with CT- or MRI-scans. Fusion of orbital [^{111}In-DTPA^{0}]octreotide scintigrams with these techniques might increase our understanding in the pathophysiology of Graves' ophthalmopathy.

Thyroid and Pituitary tumors

*[^{111}In-DTPA^{0}] octreotide scintigraphy in **differentiated** thyroid cancer*

Well-differentiated thyroid cancer of follicular epithelial-cell origin refers to papillary and follicular carcinomas. Papillary carcinoma accounts for about 70% of thyroid carcinomas, whereas follicular carcinoma represents 15% (21,22). Papillary carcinomas more frequently metastasize to regional nodes, whereas follicular tumors more often have distant metastases (23).

In our clinics, the follow-up of patients after surgical removal of the tumor consists of the following: scintigraphic visualization of thyroid remnants after the injection of 370 MBq ^{123}I, 4 weeks after thyroidectomy, followed by ablation with 1850 MBq or 5550 MBq ^{131}I, followed a week later by total body scanning. Depending on the referring internist, renewed withdrawal of suppression with L-Thyroxine is either performed within 2 years after institution of such therapy, or is sustained until serum thyroglobulin (Tg) levels become detectable. After 4 weeks, measurement of Tg and thyroid stimulating hormone (TSH), and ^{123}I total body scanning are performed again. When metastases or recurrence are visualized or Tg levels are detectable, therapy with 5550 MBq ^{131}I is instituted, followed by post-therapy scanning.

During L-thyroxine therapy withdrawal, patients experience a period of discomfort due to hypothyroidism (24). Besides, in a certain percentage of patients with recurrent or metastatic disease, the tumors may not concentrate ^{131}I (25-27). This is correlated with the absence of immunoreactive cytoplasmic thyroglobulin and thyroxine (25) and relates in part to the diagnostic dose of ^{131}I that is used (28). There is a low rate (2%) of dedifferentiation of papillary and follicular thyroid cancer but when this happens, therapeutic options are very limited (23,27).

Although papillary and follicular thyroid cancer do not belong to the group of classical neuroendocrine tumors, the majority of patients with these cancers show uptake of the radiolabeled somatostatin analogue octreotide (29). Histologically differentiated thyroid cancers that do not take up radioiodine, may show accumulation of radiolabeled octreotide (24,30-32). Most likely, the reason for the visualization of differentiated thyroid carcinoma is the presence of somatostatin receptors on follicular cells, as demonstrated in vitro (12).

The usual follow-up of patients with differentiated thyroid carcinoma consists of whole-body radioiodine scintigraphy and serum Tg monitoring. The sensitivity of radioiodine scintigraphy for the detection of persistent or metastatic thyroid carcinoma is 50-70%, dependent on the diagnostic dose of ^{131}I used (25-28). In a recent unpublished study, using radioiodine scintigraphy, we found tumor localization's in 17 of 25 (68%) patients with differentiated thyroid carcinoma. Whole-body scintigraphy after ^{131}I therapy was more sensitive for tumor detection than ^{123}I scintigraphy 4 weeks after withdrawal of thyroxine suppression. [^{111}In-DTPA^{0}]octreotide scintigraphy demonstrated abnormal accumulation of radioactivity in 18 of these 25 (72%) patients. More importantly, in 24% of all patients, tumor sites

accumulated radiolabeled octreotide but not radioiodine (Figure 3). These data are in agreement with a recent study by Baudin et al. (30), who showed that [^{111}In-DTPA^{0}]octreotide scintigraphy was positive during hormone suppression in 80% of their patients with well-differentiated thyroid cancer and elevated serum Tg levels. Besides, in 12 of 16 (75%) patients who had a negative ^{131}I total body scan, tumor sites were visualized during [^{111}In-DTPA^{0}]octreotide scintigraphy (30). Recently, however, contrary results and conclusions were reported by Garin et al. (33), in a study to the contribution of [^{111}In-DTPA^{0}]octreotide scintigraphy in the tumor localization in 16 patients with suspected recurrence of differentiated thyroid carcinoma without iodine uptake. They found positive results in only 3 patients and concluded that [^{111}In-DTPA^{0}]octreotide scintigraphy had no important contribution in these patients. Their findings may be questioned, however, as their imaging protocol with a relatively low injected dose, short counting times (5-10 min), and no SPECT imaging, seems inadequate. Also, as the authors themselves suggest, their criteria for the interpretation of the scintigrams (i.e. the tumors had to be recognized on early scans, 4 h p.i.) are probably too restricted.

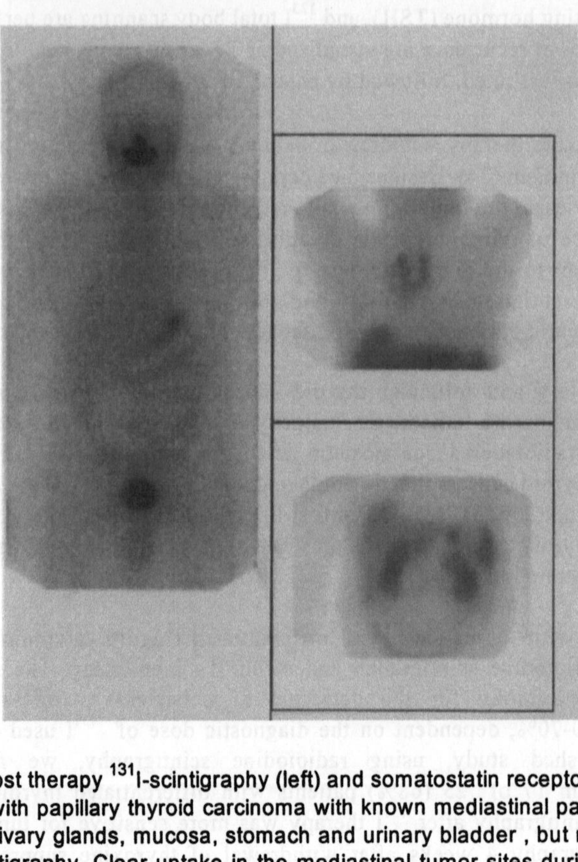

Figure 3. Post therapy ^{131}I-scintigraphy (left) and somatostatin receptor imaging (right) in a patient with papillary thyroid carcinoma with known mediastinal pathology. Normal uptake in salivary glands, mucosa, stomach and urinary bladder , but no tumor uptake with ^{131}I-scintigraphy. Clear uptake in the mediastinal tumor sites during somatostatin receptor imaging (right upper panel), and normal uptake in the liver, spleen and kidneys (right lower panel).

One of our aims was to study whether it is necessary to withdraw patients from L-thyroxine therapy in order to get optimal information from [^{111}In-DTPA^{0}]octreotide scintigraphy. In the 6 patients in whom a direct comparison was made before and after withdrawal, essentially the same information was obtained. Although the number of patients that we studied is small, these data seem to imply that upregulation of somatostatin receptor expression on follicular cells by thyrotropin, as previously hypothesized (24), is unlikely and does not seem to play a role.

From these studies, it can also be concluded that [^{111}In-DTPA^{0}]octreotide scintigraphy can be used in order to visualize tumor sites in patients with differentiated thyroid cancer that does not concentrate radioiodine. In patients with metastasized differentiated thyroid cancer, the only available treatment, apart from thyroxine suppression therapy and palliative external radiotherapy, is ^{131}I therapy. In our recent study, [^{111}In-DTPA^{0}]octreotide scintigraphy was positive in 6 of 8 patients with a negative radioiodine scan. In some patients, this could open new therapeutic options: operation, if the number of observed lesions is limited, or, alternatively, treatment with high doses of either [^{111}In-DTPA^{0}]octreotide or [^{90}Y-DOTA^{0},Tyr^{3}]-octreotide (DOTA: 1,4,7,10-tetraazacyclododecane-N,N',N",N"'-tetraacetic acid) if the uptake is sufficient. Such treatment may be rewarding in patients with progressive disease, as has already been shown in patients with progressive neuroendocrine tumors (34-38). Also, there may be a role for radiolabeled somatostatin analogue therapy in patients who are in poor health, and in whom thyroxine withdrawal and ^{131}I therapy cannot be performed, as suggested by Baudin et al. (30).

Conclusions: (1) In patients with metastatic differentiated thyroid carcinoma, tumor sites can be visualized using [^{111}In-DTPA^{0}]octreotide scintigraphy; (2) There is no need to withdraw patients from thyroxine suppression in order to perform [^{111}In-DTPA^{0}]octreotide scintigraphy; (3) In some patients whose lesions do concentrate radiolabeled octreotide but not radioiodine, the use of somatostatin analogues labeled with ^{111}In or 90Y can provide new therapeutic options.

[^{111}In-DTP^{0}]octreotide scintigraphy in ***medullary*** *thyroid cancer*

Medullary thyroid carcinoma (MTC) accounts for about 4 to 9% of all thyroid carcinomas (39,40). MTC occurs in a sporadic form and as part of the multiple endocrine neoplasia (MEN) syndrome. At presentation, about 50% of the patients have nodal spread of the cancer, whereas in 10-20% distant metastases are present (39,41).

Treatment of MTC consists of total thyroidectomy alone or in combination with neck dissection. Recurrence occurs in about 50% of the patients (39,42), and is often preceded by elevated serum calcitonin (CT) and/or carcino-embryonic antigen (CEA) concentrations (42,43). Five-year survival in patients with metastatic disease is 40%, and results of radiotherapy and chemotherapy are poor (39,44,45). Initial results of treatment with somatostatin or with the somatostatin analogue octreotide have been disappointing: no effect on CT levels and tumor growth was reported after doses of 100 μg octreotide/day) (46), and no effect on CT levels after infusion of 180 μg octreotide in 4 hr (47). However, high dosages of somatostatin (11 μg/min) could accomplish a lowering of CT levels in 12 of 15 patients (48), and it was reported that long-term treatment with octreotide in high dosages (up to 2000 μg/day) in 3 patients with MTC improved symptoms and lowered serum CT and CEA concentrations (49). MTC arises from the parafollicular C-cells of the thyroid. These cells are derived from the neural crest and have amine precursor uptake and decarboxylation (APUD) characteristics. We reported the initial results of [^{111}In-DTPA^{0}]octreotide scintigraphy in 17 patients with MTC in comparison with conventional imaging techniques, and correlated the in vivo somatostatin receptor status with serum tumor markers, in vitro tumor somatostatin content, and the in vitro somatostatin receptor status (50,51).

Tumor localization's were demonstrated in 11 of 17 (65%) patients with MTC. In 5 of these, tumor sites that were positive during in vivo somatostatin receptor imaging, were shown to possess specific binding sites with in vitro somatostatin receptor autoradiography. A somatostatin receptor positive tumor invaded lymph node in 1 patient, measuring 2*1*0.5 cm, was not visualized in vivo. This may have been due either to the size of the lesion, the (low) density of somatostatin receptors, or a combination of these. Recently, it has been reported that the size of MTC tumors affects the result of [^{111}In-DTPA^{0}]octreotide scintigraphy. Indeed, smaller lesions can be missed, a finding underlining the issue that [^{111}In-DTPA^{0}]octreotide scintigraphy has to be carried out carefully, also because this type of tumor show a lower accumulation of the radioligand than other types of neuro-endocrine tumors (52).

In 7 patients, in 2 of whom the liver was the only known site of tumor spread, liver metastases were not recognized during planar [^{111}In-DTPA^{0}]octreotide scintigraphy. The same was true for thyroid nodules in another patient. An explanation for the failure to demonstrate these lesions during octreotide scintigraphy, might be that these tumor sites were somatostatin receptor negative. However, this seems unlikely in at least some of the patients, since other tumor sites in the same patients readily accumulated labeled octreotide. It is more probable that the normal uptake of radioactivity in both the thyroid and the liver during octreotide scintigraphy, prevents the detection of tumor spots that accumulate about as much radioactivity as does the surrounding tissue in these organs. Therefore, if tumor deposits are suspected in the liver or thyroid, the results of [^{111}In-DTPA^{0}]octreotide scintigraphy should be evaluated in combination with those of, for instance, ultrasound. Also SPECT of the liver region with [^{111}In-DTPA^{0}]octreotide gives a much better information than planar imaging with regard to the presence of liver metastases. Recently, Krausz et al discussed the importance of SPECT of neck and mediastinum to localize focal lesions (53). Previously, Dorr et al reported on the discrepancy between planar and SPECT results in favor of SPECT to localize neck and mediastinum metastases (54). Behr et al discussed the so called "chimney sign" as manifestation of typically metastasizing (occult) MTC to bilateral mediastinal lymph nodes. This sign was also observed in patients without previous external beam irradiation of the mediastinum, questioning other reports, which ascribed this sign to radiation-induced pneumonitis (55-57).

In our series, in 2 patients only part of the tumor localization's were detected during [^{111}In-DTPA^{0}]octreotide scintigraphy. Reubi et al. (58) reported somatostatin receptors to be preferentially located on differentiated tumor parts of MTC. The failure to visualize part of the tumor localization's in the same patient during octreotide scintigraphy, might therefore indicate tumor de-differentiation of metastases that are not visualized.

Part of MTC contain and secrete somatostatin. Immunohistochemical stains for somatostatin have been reported to be positive in scattered cells in the majority of primary MTC (48,58), and in a minority of metastatic lesions (48). Plasma somatostatin is elevated in only few patients (48,59). Because of the possibility that endogenous production of somatostatin, and subsequent occupancy of tumorous somatostatin receptors by locally produced somatostatin, gives rise to a failure to visualize these tumors during in vivo somatostatin receptor imaging, we investigated the presence of somatostatin by immunohistochemistry on removed tumor tissue. In 1 of 5 patients whose tumors were visualized in vivo, and in neither of 2 patients whose tumors were not visualized, immunohistochemistry for somatostatin on tumor specimens was positive. Therefore, endogenous somatostatin production does not seem to influence the outcomes of in vivo somatostatin receptor imaging.

Serum CT and CEA concentrations are used as tumor markers in MTC. In the follow-up of patients with MTC, progressive disease and poor prognosis are correlated with a rise in serum CEA (60), while serum CT levels follow a non-parallel course (43). In our series, neither serum CT nor CEA concentrations differed significantly between patients whose tumors were visualized during [^{111}In-DTPA^{0}]octreotide scintigraphy, and those whose tumors were not. The ratio of CT over CEA levels, however, was significantly higher in patients in whom [^{111}In-DTPA^{0}]octreotide scintigraphy was successfully applied. This may mean that somatostatin receptor positive MTC have a slower progression, which is in accordance with the results of an in vitro study in MTC (58), which reports a preferential labeling for somatostatin receptors on highly differentiated tumor regions. Because we performed a cross-sectional study in patients with MTC, we cannot correlate the in vivo somatostatin receptor status with disease progression or alterations in tumor marker levels. Longitudinal studies in patients with newly diagnosed MTC are required to answer the interesting question whether in the follow-up patients with tumors showing de-differentiation and terminal disease progression these tumors are ultimately accompanied by a loss of somatostatin receptors. Apparently, progressive disease of MTC per se goes not always hand in hand with non-visualization of tumors with [^{111}In-DTPA^{0}]octreotide scintigraphy (52).

The successful detection of MTC tumor sites using ^{123}I- or ^{131}I-MIBG scintigraphy has been reported in 15-60% of the cases (61-63). In our series, MIBG scintigraphy indicated tumor localization's in 2 of 3 patients whose tumor was not visualized during [^{111}In-DTPA^{0}]octreotide scintigraphy. It must be emphasized, however, that in these 2 patients, who had hereditary MTC, no pathologic confirmation of the present lesions was obtained, and that the observed abnormalities on MIBG scintigraphy could therefore also be due to pheochromocytoma. Also, MIBG scintigraphy was negative in 4 patients whose tumors did accumulate labeled octreotide in vivo. The reason for the discrepancy between these 2 radionuclide imaging techniques remains as yet unclear. Rufini et al, comparing the two techniques in seven patients with known tumor localization's, also reported a higher sensitivity for [^{111}In-DTPA^{0}]octreotide scintigraphy (63).

Long-term high dose octreotide treatment in patients with MTC has been reported. Mahler et al. (49) reported in a 6 to 17 months treatment study a beneficial effect on symptoms and a lowering of CT and CEA levels by 45 to 80% in 3 patients with metastatic MTC, who were treated with up to 2000 µg octreotide daily. However, the suppression of serum tumor markers became less pronounced as therapy lasted longer. Modigliani et al. (64) observed a decrease of serum CT, but not CEA concentrations, in 4 of 14 patients with MTC, who were treated with 500 µg octreotide per day for 3 months. In a third study with a treatment interval of 3 to 19 months and octreotide doses ranging between 100 and 1000 µg 2 out of the 7 patients showed a remission lasting 12 months (65). Also, favorable effects have been reported with a combination of octreotide with rIFN-alpha-2b (66). Unfortunately, these study did not use the [^{111}In-DTPA^{0}]octreotide scintigram as a baseline measure of the somatostatin receptor (density-)status. Beneficial effects of octreotide treatment may be expected in patients with MTC who have tumors bearing (the highest density of) somatostatin receptors. Apart from its merit in tumor localization, one of the major advantages of octreotide scintigraphy in MTC may be that octreotide scintigraphy can be used to select those patients who have somatostatin receptor (subtypes 2 and 5) positive tumors, i.e. patients who could potentially benefit from octreotide treatment.

In conclusion: 1. In the majority of patients with metastatic MTC, tumor sites can be visualized using [^{111}In-DTPA^{0}]octreotide scintigraphy, especially above the diaphragm. However, if this technique is performed only with planar imaging (maximum speed 3 cm/min !), it is less sensitive than when SPECT is included in order to detect liver metastases, to identify the intrathyroidal tumor and possibly intra-thoracic metastases; 2. The visualization of MTC during in vivo somatostatin receptor imaging correlates with the in vitro presence of somatostatin receptors, subtypes 2 and 5; 3. The immunohistochemical presence of somatostatin in the tumor does not seem to influence the outcomes of in vivo somatostatin receptor imaging; 4. Higher serum CT over CEA ratios in patients whose MTC is visualized during octreotide scintigraphy might imply that somatostatin receptors are present on more differentiated MTC; 5. In patients with metastasized MTC in whom octreotide therapy is considered, [^{111}In-DTPA^{0}]octreotide scintigraphy can be used to select those patients who have somatostatin receptor positive tumors; 6. The same holds true for the treatment with radiolabeled octreotide analogues. Recently, trials with radiolabeled octreotide analogues for MTC have started. The preferred radionuclides are those emitting ß-particles because of their better crossfire than for instance the Auger electrons of ^{111}In (35). Especially, because of the heterogeneous distribution of somatostatin receptors in MTC the larger particle range of ß-particles, which are endocytosed in receptor-positive cells, are capable to irradiate neighboring cells without expression of somatostatin receptors.

[^{111}In-DTPA^{0}]octreotide scintigraphy of ***TSH-producing pituitary adenomas***

Most secreting adenomas and approximately half of nonfunctioning pituitary adenomas express somatostatin receptors as has been shown by in vitro studies, in vivo by somatostatin receptor scintigraphy (Figure 1) and response to somatostatin analogues therapy (66-69). Also, most of TSH-producing pituitary adenomas are somatostatin receptor positive and octreotide is an effective treatment for the hyperthyroidism induced by TSH-secreting adenomas. TSH levels almost always decrease with this kind of therapy, and thyroid hormone levels revert to normal in about 75% of patients. Even partial tumor shrinkage has been reported to occur in one third of patients receiving long-term octreotide treatment. The combination of [^{111}In-DTPA^{0}]octreotide scintigraphy and MRI allows the computation of a somatostatin receptor density index (= tumor uptake corrected for tumor volume) that predicts which patients may benefit from somatostatin analogue treatment (69).

References

1. Krenning EP, Oei HY, Kooij PPM, et al. Thyroid and orbital radiolabeled somatostatin accumulation in Graves' disease and Graves' ophthalmopathy. J Nucl Med 1992;33 (suppl. 5): 894.
2. Postema PTE, Krenning EP, Wijngaarde R, et al. [111In-DTPA-D-Phe1] Octreotide scintigraphy in thyroidal and orbital Graves' disease: a parameter for disease activity? J Clin Endocrinol Metab 1994;79:1845.
3. Vanhagen PM, Krenning EP, Reubi JC, et al. Somatostatin analogue scintigraphy in granulomatous diseases. Eur J Nucl Med 1994;21:497.
4. Vanhagen PM, Markusse HM, Lamberts SWJ, Kwekkeboom DJ, Reubi JC, Krenning EP. Somatostatin receptor imaging: The presence of somatostatin receptors in rheumatoid arthritis. Arthritis Rheum 1994;37:1521.
5. Chang TC, Kao SCS, Huang KM. Octreotide and Graves' ophthalmopathy and pretibial myxoedema. Brit Med J 1992;304:158.
6. Hansson HA, Petruson B, Schottner A. Somatomedin-C in pathogenesis of malignant exophthalmus of endocrine origin. Lancet 1986;ii:218.
7. Kahaly G, Diaz M, Just M, Beyer J, Lieb N. Role of octreoscan and correlation with MR imaging in Graves' ophthalmopathy. Thyroid 1995;5:107.
8. Becker W, Schrell U, Buchfelder M, Hensen J, Wendler J, Gramatzki M, Wolf F. Somatostatin receptor expression in the thyroid demonstrated with ^{111}In-octreotide scintigraphy. Nucl Med 1995;34:100.
9. Sreedharan SP, Kodama KT, Peterson KE, Goetzl EJ. Distinct subsets of somatostatin on cultured human lymphocytes. J Biol Chem 1989;264;949.
10. Krennning EP, Kwekkeboom DJ, Pauwels S, Kvols LK, Reubi JC. Somatostatin receptor scintigraphy. In: Freeman LM (editor) Nuclear Medicine Annual, Raven Press, New York, 1995:1.
11. Uberti ECD, Hanau S, Rossi R et al. Somatostatin reduces 3H-thymidine incorporation and c-myc but not thyroglobulin ribonucleic acid levels in human thyroid follicular cells in vitro. Endocrinology 1991;72:1364.
12. Reubi JC, Waser B, Friess H, Krenning EP, Buchler M, Laissue J. Regulatory peptide receptors in goiters of the human thyroid. J Nucl Med 1997;38 (suppl): 266P.
13. Kahaly G, Dinz M, Haka K, Beyer J, Bockisch A. Indium-111-pentetreotide scintigraphy in Graves' ophthalmopathy. J Nucl Med 1995;36:550.
14. Durak I, Durak H, Ergin M, Yürekli Y, Kaynak S. Somatostatin receptors in the orbit. Clin Nucl Med 1995;20:237.
15. Bohuslavziki KH, Oberwöhrmann S, Brenner W et al. 111In-octreotide imaging in patients with long-standing Graves' ophthalmopathy. Nucl Med Commun 1995;16:912.
16. Moncayo R, Baldnisera I, Decristoforo C, Kendler D, Donnemiller E. Evaluation of immunological mechanisms mediating thyroid-associated ophthalmopathy by radionuclide imaging using the somatostatin analog ^{111}In-octreotide. Thyroid 1997;7:21.
17. Krassas GE, Dumas A, Pontikides N, Kaltsas Th. Somatostatin receptor scintigraphy and octreotide treatment in patients with thyroid eye disease. Clin Endocrinol 1995;42:571.
18. Krassas, Dumas A; and Moncayo R. Octreoscan in Graves' ophthalmopathy. Thyroid 1997;7:805.
19. Gerding MN, van der Zant FM, van Royen EA, et al. Octreotide-scintigraphy is a disease-activity parameter in Graves' ophthalmopathy. Clin Endocrinol 1999;50:373.
20. Wiersinga WM, Gerding MN, Prummel MF, Krenning EP. Octreotide scintigraphy in thyroidal and orbital Graves' disease. Thyroid. 1998;8:433.

21. Hedinger C, Williams ED, Sabin LH. The WHO histological classifications of thyroid tumors: a commentary on the second edition. Cancer 1989;63:908.
22. Robbins J, Merino MJ, Boice JD. Thyroid cancer: a lethal endocrine neoplasm. Ann Intern Med 1991;115:133.
23. Maxon HR, Smith HS. Radioiodine-131 in the diagnosis and treatment of metastatic well-differentiated thyroid cancer. Endocrinol Metab Clin North Am 1990;19:685.
24. Postema PT, de Herder WW, Reubi JC, et al. Somatostatin receptor scintigraphy in non-medullary thyroid cancer. Digestion 1996;57(Suppl 1):36.
25. Batge B, Dralle H, Padberg B. Histology and immunocytochemistry of differentiated thyroid carcinomas do not predict radioiodine uptake: a clinicomorphological study of 62 reccurent or metastatic tumors. Virchows Arch 1992;421:521.
26. Maheshwari YK, Hill CS, Haynie T. I-131 therapy in differentiated thyroid carcinoma: M.D. Anderson Hospital experience. Cancer 1981;47:664.
27. Mallin WH, Elgazzar AH, Maxon III HR. Imaging modalities in the follow-up of non-iodine avid thyroid carcinoma. Am J Otolaryngol 1994;15:417.
28. Brown AP, Greening WP, McCready VR. Radioiodine treatment of metastatic thyroid carcinoma. Br J Radiol 1984;57:323.
29. Krenning EP, Kwekkeboom DJ, Reubi JC. Peptide receptor scintigraphy in oncology. In: Murray, Ell (Eds). Nuclear Medicine in clinical diagnosis and treatment, 2nd ed. Churchill Livingstone, London, 1998;859.
30. Baudin E, Schlumberger M, Lumbroso J, Travagli JP, Caillou B, Parmentier C. Octreotide scintigraphy in patients with differentiated thyroid carcinoma: contribution for patients with negative radioiodine scan. J Clin Endocrinol Metab 1996;81:2541.
31. Tenenbaum F, Lumbroso J, Schlumberger M, Caillou B, Fragu P, Parmentier C. Radiolabeled somatostatin analog scintigraphy in differentiated thyroid carcinoma. J Nucl Med 1995;36:807.
32. Kölby L, Wängberg B, Ahlman H, et al. Somatostatin receptor subtypes, octreotide scintigraphy, and clinical response to octreotide treatment in patients with neuroendocrine tumors. World J Surg 1998;22:679.
33. Garin E, Devillers A, Le Cloirec J, et al. Use of indium-111 pentetreotide somatostatin receptor scintigraphy to detect recurrent thyroid carcinoma in patients without detectable iodine uptake. Eur J Nucl Med 1998;25:687.
34. Krenning EP, Kooij PPM, Pauwels S, et al. Somatostatin receptor scintigraphy and radionuclide therapy. Digestion 1996;57(suppl 1):57.
35. Krenning EP, de Jong M, Kooij PPM, et al. Radiolabelled somatostatin analogue(s) for peptide receptor scintigraphy and radionuclide therapy. Ann Oncology 1999; 10 (suppl. 2): S23.
36. Otte A, Jermann E, Behe M, et al. DOTATOC: a powerful new tool for receptor-mediated radionuclide therapy. Eur J Nucl Med 1997;24:792.
37. Otte A, Mueller-Brand J, Dellas S, Nitzsche EU, Herrmann R, Maecke HR. Yttrium-90-labelled somatostatin-analogue for cancer treatment. Lancet 1998;351:417.
38. McCarthy KE, Woltering EA, Espenan GD, Cronin M, Maloney TJ, Anthony LB. In situ radiotherapy with 111In-pentetreotide: initial observations and future directions. Cancer J Sci Am 1998;4:94.
39. Saad MF, Ordonez NG, Rashid RK, Guido JJ, Hill CS Jr., Hickey RC, Samaan NA. Medullary carcinoma of the thyroid. Medicine 1984;63:319
40. Jensen MH, Davis RK, Derrick L. Thyroid cancer: a computer-assisted review of 5287 cases. Otolaryngol Head Neck Surg 1990;102:51.
41. Rougier P, Parmentier C, Laplanche A, et al. Medullary thyroid carcinoma: prognostic factors and treatment. Int J Radiation Oncology Biol Phys 1983;9:161.
42. Rougier P, Calmettes C, Laplanche A, Travagli JP, Lefevre M, Parmentier C, Milhaud G, Tubiana M. The values of calcitonin and carcinoembryonic antigen in the treatment

and management of nonfamilial medullary thyroid carcinoma. Cancer 1983;51:855.
43. Saad MF, Fritsche HA Jr., Samaan NA. Diagnostic and prognostic values of carcinoembryonic antigen in medullary carcinoma of the thyroid. J Clin Endocrinol Metab 1984;58:889.
44. Samaan NA, Schultz PN, Hickey RC. Medullary thyroid carcinoma: prognosis of familial versus sporadic disease and the role of radiotherapy. J Clin Endocrinol Metab 1988;67:801.
45. Petursson SR. Metastatic medullary thyroid carcinoma. Cancer 1988;62:1899.
46. Jerkins TW, Sacks HS, O'Dorisio TM, Tuttle S, Solomon SS. Medullary carcinoma of the thyroid, pancreatic nesidioblastosis and microadenosis, and pancreatic polypeptide hypersecretion: a new association and clinical and hormonal responses to long-acting somatostatin analog SMS 201-995. J Clin Endocrinol Metab 1987;64:1313.
47. Modigliani E, Chayvialle JA, Cohen R, et al.. Effect of a somatostatin analog (SMS 201-995) in perfusion on basal and pentagastrin-stimulated calcitonin levels in medullary thyroid carcinoma. Horm Metab Res 1988;20:773.
48. Pacini F, Elisei R, Anelli S, Basolo F, Cola A, Pinchera A. Somatostatin in medullary thyroid cancer. Cancer 1989;63:1189.
49. Mahler C, Verhelst J, De Longueville M, Harris A. Long-term treatment of metastatic medullary thyroid carcinoma with the somatostatin analogue octreotide. Clin Endocrinol 1990;33:261.
50. Kwekkeboom DJ, Reubi JC, Lamberts SWJ, et al. In vivo somatostatin receptor imaging in medullary thyroid carcinoma. J Clin Endocrinol Metab 1993;76:1413.
51. Kwekkeboom DJ, Lamberts SW, Habbema JD, Krenning EP. Cost-effectiveness analysis of somatostatin receptor scintigraphy. J Nucl Med. 1996;37:888.
52. Tisell LE, Ahlman H, Wängberg B, et al. Somatostatin receptor scintigraphy in patients with medullary thyroid carcinoma. Br J Surgery 1997;84:543.
53. Krausz Y, Rosler A, Guttmann H, et al. Somatostatin receptor scintigraphy for early detection of regional and distant metastases of medullary carcinoma of the thyroid. Clin Nucl Med. 1999;24:256.
54. Dorr U, Wurstlin S, Frank-Raue K, et al. Somatostatin receptor scintigraphy and magnetic resonance imaging in recurrent medullary thyroid carcinoma: a comparative study. Horm Metab Res Suppl. 1993;27:48.
55. Behr TM, Gratz S, Markus PM, et al. Enhanced bilateral somatostatin receptor expression in mediastinal lymph nodes ("chimney sign") in occult metastatic medullary thyroid cancer: a typical site of tumour manifestation. Eur J Nucl Med 1997;24:184.
56. Baudin E, Lumbroso J, Schlumberger M, Leclere J, Giammarile F, Gardet P, Roche A, Trafagli JP, Parmentier C. Comparison of octreotide scintigraphy and conventional imaging in medullary thyroid carcinoma. J Nucl Med 1996;37:912
57. Stoffel M, Jamar F, Donckier J, et al. Increased uptake of indium-111 pentetreotide up to 10 years after external thoracic irradiation: report of two cases. Eur J Nucl Med 1996;23:723.
58. Reubi JC, Chayvialle JA, Franc B, Cohen R, Calmettes C, Modigliani E. Somatostatin receptors and somatostatin content in medullary thyroid carcinomas. Lab Invest 1991;64:567.
59. Modigliani E, Alamowitch C, Cohen R, et al. The intratumoral immunoassayable somatostatin concentration is frequently elevated in medullary thyroid carcinoma. Cancer 1990;65:224-228.
60. Busnardo B, Girelli ME, Simioni N, Nacamull D, Bosetto E. Nonparallel patterns of calcitonin and carcinoembryonic antigen levels in the follow-up of medullary thyroid carcinoma. Cancer 1984;53:278.
61. Troncone L, Rufini V, Montemaggi P, Danza FM, Lasorella A, Mastrangelo R. The diagnostic and therapeutic utility of radioiodinated metaiodobenzylguanidine (MIBG).

Eur J Nucl Med 1990;16:325.
62. Skowsky WR, Wilf LH. Iodine 131 metaiodobenzylguanidine scintigraphy of medullary carcinoma of the thyroid. South Med J 1991;84:636.
63. Rufini V, Salvatori M, Saletnich I, et al. Radiolabeled somatostatin analog scintigraphy in medullary thyroid carcinoma and carcinoid tumor. Q J Nucl Med 1995;39:140.
64. Modigliani E, Cohen R, Joannidis S, et al. Results of long-term continuous subcutaneous octreotide administration in 14 patients with medullary thyroid carcinoma. Clin Endocrinol 1992;36:183.
65. Frank-Raue k, Raue F, Ziegler R. Therapie des metastasierten medullären schilddrüsenkarzinoms mit dem somatostatinanalogon octreotide. Med Klin 1995;90:63.
66. Lupoli G, Cascone E, Arlotta F, Vitale G, Celentano L, Salvatore M, Lombardi G. Treatment of advanced medullary thyroid carcinoma with a combination of recombinant interferon alpha-2b and octreotide. Cancer 1996;78:1114.
67. Chanson P, Weintraub BD, Harris AG. Octreotide therapy for thyroid-stimulating hormone-secreting pituitary adenomas. A follow-up of 52 patients. Ann Intern Med 1993;119:236.
68. Polak M, Bertherat J, Li JY, et al. A human TSH-secreting adenoma: endocrine, biochemical and morphological studies. Evidence of somatostatin receptors by using quantitative autoradiography. Clinical and biological improvement by SMS 201-995 treatment. Acta Endocrinol 1991;124:479.
69. Duet M, Ajzenberg C, Benelhadj S, et al. Somatostatin receptor scintigraphy in pituitary adenomas: a somatostatin receptor density index can predict hormonal and tumoral efficacy of octreotide in vivo. J Nucl Med 1999;40:1252-1256.

ADRENAL

8
IMAGING OF THE ADRENAL GLANDS

Lukas C. van Dijk, M.D.
Gabriel P. Krestin, M.D.
University Hospital Rotterdam
Rotterdam, the Netherlands

INTRODUCTION

The adrenal glands are composed of the cortex and the medulla. The cortex develops from the mesoderm and consists of three layers: from outside inwards the zona glomerulosa producing mineralocorticoids, zona fasciculata producing glucocorticoids and zona reticularis producing androgens. The medulla develops from ectodermal cells of the neural crest. These sympathic chromaffine cells invade the cortex of the adrenal gland and form the catecholamines producing medulla.

The adrenal glands descend during embryological development, while the kidneys ascend. The final position of the adrenals is independent of ectopia or absence of the kidneys. Their location is between the anterior (Gerota) and posterior (Zuckerkandl) renal fascia in the antero-superior part of the perirenal space. The right adrenal gland is located superior from the upper pole of the right kidney, posterior to the inferior vena cava, medial to the right hepatic lobe and lateral to the crus of the diaphragm. The left adrenal gland is located antero-medial from the upper pole of the kidney, lateral from the crus, postero-lateral from the aorta and posteromedial from the pancreatic tail. The form of the adrenal glands is usually linear on the right, on the left inverted V; Y or triangular shapes are more common. The normal diameter is about 8 mm on the left and 6 mm on the right and should not exceed 1 cm. The length is about 3-5 cm.

Modern imaging techniques, particularly Computed Tomography (CT) and magnetic resonance imaging (MRI) allows accurate depiction of the normal adrenal glands and of most pathologic alterations. Both the adrenal cortex and the medulla have high lipid content and therefore cannot be differentiated from one another. Mainly because of this high lipid content in the normal adrenal glands and benign adenomas, MRI and to some extent CT can often provide accurate differentiation between benign and malignant lesions and thereby obviate the need for biopsies in many cases. Since benign non-hyperfunctioning adrenal adenomas are by far the most common reason for adrenal enlargement it is important to make the distinction from malignancy. Even in patients with known malignant disease 50% or less of the adrenal masses are metastases (1-3). In this chapter the currently available radiological imaging modalities useful for adrenal imaging will be discussed and subsequently imaging strategies for the different clinical problems will be suggested according to the current published literature. For practical reasons a distinction between adrenal endocrinopathies and non-hyperfunctioning adrenal masses will be made.

Imaging modalities

Conventional radiographs and angiography.

Although some of the classical conventional techniques are still being used, their role has become very limited. Soft tissue masses can be detected on plain radiographs only if they have reached a size of at least 5 cm. Tomographic imaging and the administration of renally excreted intravenous contrast improves the delineation of a soft tissue mass from the kidney and the surrounding structures. Deformation of the upper pole of the kidney and a change of the axis and position of the kidney are secondary signs of adrenal enlargement. Before CT-scanning became available plain radiographs with CO_2-insufflation into the retroperitoneum was used to improve delineation of retroperitoneal structures (4).

Retrograde venography often combined with selective venous sampling used to be the method of choice for investigation of hormone producing adrenal abnormalities. Using this technique adenomas with a diameter of 1.0 to 1.5 cm could be detected (4). A possible complication of venography was rupture of the vein due to contrast extravasation, sometimes resulting in subsequent adrenal insufficiency. Venous sampling is currently still used in specialized centers in case of failure of modern imaging methods to undoubtedly localize an aldosterone-hypersecreting mass (5).

Arteriography of the feeding arteries was used to detect adrenal tumors, especially hyperfunctional pheochromocytomas. Following an overview aortography the suprarenal superior, medial and inferior arteries have to be selectively catheterized. A serious complication of adrenal arteriography however, is the provocation of a hypertensive crisis in patients with an active pheochromocytoma. β-blockers administered before the angiography may prevent such an incident.

Ultrasonography

Normal adrenal glands are usually visible using ultrasonography only in children or very slender patients. Depending on the size of the patient, the quality of the equipment and the quality and perseverance of the investigator, adrenal abnormalities can be detected if they have reached a size of about 3 cm. The right adrenal gland is positioned behind the inferior vena cava and the liver and cranio-anterior to the upper pole of the right kidney. The left adrenal gland can be found left from the aorta and cranioventral of the upper pole of the left kidney. Usually it is more difficult to visualize the adrenal gland on the left. In adults the normal adrenal gland is as echogenic as the surrounding retroperitoneal fat. In newborn the cortex is non-echogenic and the marrow echogenic. If a pancreatic lesion should be differentiated from an adrenal lesion, it should be born in mind that pancreatic lesions are located ventrally from the splenic vessels whereas adrenal masses are located dorsally. Generally it is not possible to distinguish different kinds of adrenal pathology using ultrasound. Any enlargement of the adrenal gland detected with ultrasound should be dealt with according to the clinical context. The accuracy of ultrasound for detection of adrenal masses was 70% in an older prospective study compared to 90% accuracy for CT (6). Although we are not aware of exact figures concerning the accuracy of ultrasound examination using modern equipment, ultrasound should not be considered as the sole method to exclude adrenal enlargement in adults.

Computed Tomography (CT)

The adrenal glands are almost always identifiable using modern CT-scanners (Figure 1). The density on CT is determined by the fact that nearly 90% of the weight of an adrenal glands is made up by cholesterol and cholesterol derivates. Density measurements on non-contrast enhanced CT are an essential part of the evaluation of enlarged adrenal glands, since low attenuation values strongly suggest a benign adenoma. On unenhanced CT scans different thresholds of Hounsefield values have been suggested varying from 0 to 18 (7-16). Boland et al. have summarized the results of several studies and showed the effects of different thresholds on sensitivity and specificity for characterization of an adrenal mass (17). According to Boland et al. a threshold of 10 Hounsefield units provides a high specificity of about 98% and an acceptable sensitivity of about 71% (17).

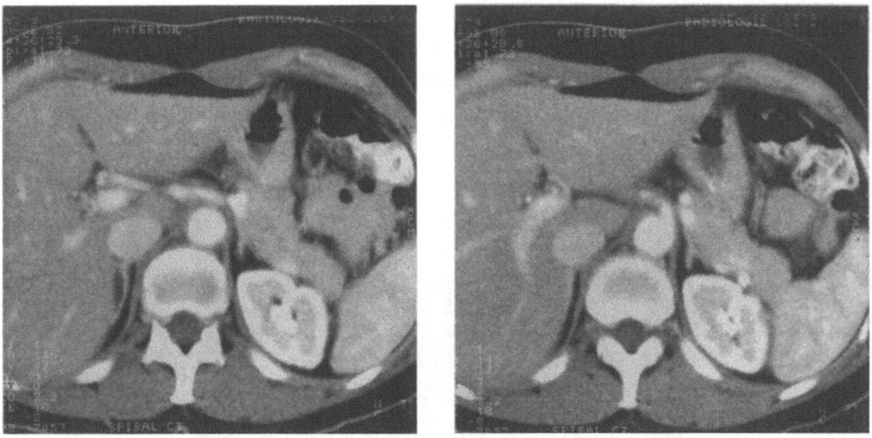

Figure 1. Spiral CT with intravenous contrast of normal adrenal glands.

Administration of intravenous contrast medium does not significantly increase the accuracy of detection and classification of adrenal masses, since both malignant and benign enlarged adrenals can show enhancement. If intravenous contrast has already been administered and attenuation values of an adrenal abnormality cannot rule out malignancy, a second CT-scan can be performed, using the different washout times of adenomas and metastases. One hour after a bolus of 150 cc of contrast, the mean decrease of attenuation of adenomas was 74% compared to 31% for metastases (18). More recent publications show that a delayed CT scan can be obtained only 10–15 minutes after contrast administration with still preserved accuracy. In three studies, Hounsefield unit measurements in adrenal masses in these slightly delayed enhanced CT's resulted in specificity values of 95 – 96% and sensitivity values of 92 – 96% for differentiating adenomas from non-adenomas (16,19,20). The rather large differences in threshold values [24 – 52] in the reports published up to now suggest that each center should establish its own threshold values for their delayed contrast enhanced CT scans.

Magnetic resonance imaging (MRI)

MRI offers unique imaging possibilities especially for enlarged adrenal glands. Excellent soft tissue contrast and the possibility to image in other planes than the transverse plane make this technique often superior in comparison to CT. To some extent MRI allows tissue characterization obviating cytological puncture or biopsy in most cases.

Delineation of the adrenal glands is usually excellent using spin-echo T1- and T2- or fast (turbo) T2-weighted spin-echo sequences. If available, phased-array coils should be used to increase the signal to noise ratio compared to the standard body-coil. Since the adrenals are moving during respiration, motion compensation techniques should be used with non-breath-hold sequences. To ensure adequate detection of small adrenal lesions slice thickness should be 5mm or less with an interleaved technique or an interslice gap of not more than 1-2 mm. In plane resolution should be <1.5 mm. The required in plane resolution can be achieved with a field of view of about 30 cm and a 256x192 matrix. For phased-array coils averaging of 2 excitations will ensure a sufficient signal to noise ratio, if a body coil is used 3–4 excitations will often be necessary (Figure 2).

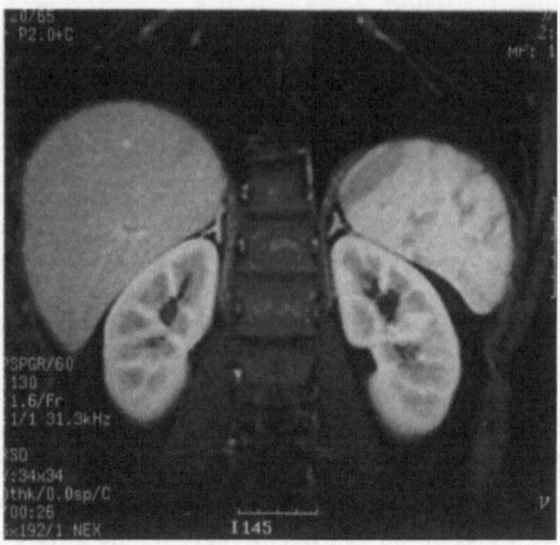

Figure 2. Coronal contrast-enhanced T1-weighted spin echo MRI scan of normal adrenal glands.

Both on T1- and T2-weighted spin-echo sequences, normal adrenal tissue is hypo- or isointense compared to liver tissue. A T2-weighted spin-echo sequence can be used to assess the etiology of adrenal lesions. Usually a multi-echo technique with a TR of 1500-2500 ms and a TE of 30–50 and 80–100 ms is used. By acquiring images with at least 4-6 different echo times the absolute T2-value of tissues can be calculated (21). Fast or Turbo T2-weighted spin echo sequences offer a significant reduction of acquisition time and thereby of motion artifacts. However calculation of the absolute T2-values of different tissues is not possible with this technique. On fast or turbo T2-sequences fat appears very bright. This bright signal potentially obscures adrenal pathology (also bright) and therefore fat suppression is appropriate. Fat suppression can be used in both T1- and T2-weighted sequences. This eliminates chemical shift artifacts and because of the expanded grayscale, small differences in tissue contrast are better appreciated (22). Using fat suppression, the normal adrenal gland is isointense on T1-weighted images and hyperintense on T2-weighted images. Disadvantages of fat suppression, however, are a reduced number of sections per acquisition and possible inhomogenicity of fat suppression throughout the image (23). As an alternative to spin-echo and fast or turbo T2-weighted spin-echo sequences, a fast gradient-echo sequence with relative T2-weighting (TR 60 ms/TE 30 ms/ flip angle 150) can be used. The main advantage of this technique is the short acquisition time thereby allowing breath-hold imaging (23).

Several MR sequences have been proposed to specifically address the distinction between adenoma versus non-adenoma. Currently Chemical Shift Imaging is considered the most effective of these techniques. Another technique proposed to make this differentiation is dynamic contrast-enhanced gradient echo imaging.

Chemical Shift Imaging (CSI) is based on the fact that benign adrenal lesions like adenomas contain intracellular lipids up to 90% of their weight (24)(Figure 3). On the other hand, malignant lesions like metastases usually contain none or only small amounts of lipids. The resonance frequency of protons in fat at 1.5 Tesla is 210 Hz higher than the frequency of protons in water. Every 2.1 ms after an excitation pulse fat and waterprotons are either in or out of phase. A gradient echo sequence with a TE of 2.1 ms (opposed phase) and 4.2 ms (in phase) is used to acquire the images. Signal intensity of the opposed phase images will be lower for lipid containing tissues, since the protons in water and the protons in fat in this tissue will be out of phase, resulting in a diminished signal compared to tissues containing no fat (25-28). Obviously signal intensity scaling has to be unchanged between the in- and opposed phase images or relative signal intensities have to be used, relating the signal intensity of the lesion to the signal intensity of the spleen or the liver. In a prospective study analyzing patients with adrenal masses and a known primary malignancy, Schwartz et al found a sensitivity of 80% and a specificity of 100% for benign lesions using a cut-off value of adrenal mass-to-spleen ratio of 0.55 (29). Scanning parameters for CSI can be TR 100-150 ms/ TE 2.1ms opposed phase and 4.2 ms in phase with a flip angle of 45°. In other than 1.5 Tesla systems the imaging parameters have to be changed according to the magnetic field strength.

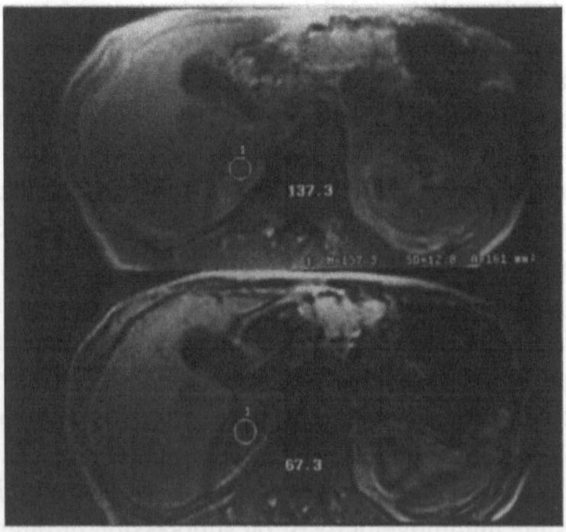

Figure 3. Chemical Shift Imaging (CSI) of a myelolipoma with significant signal decrease (67.3 on opposed phase compared to 137.3 on in phase image) on the opposed phase images.

Dynamic contrast-enhanced gradient echo imaging uses the differences in contrast enhancement characteristics of benign and malignant adrenal abnormalities (22,30,31). Although recent studies show considerable overlap between adenomas and malignant lesions (25,32). this technique is considered useful in conjunction with chemical shift imaging and provides excellent morphologic assessment of adrenal lesions. Images are obtained in the coronal plain prior to, and repeatedly up to 15 minutes after bolus injection of a gadolinium compound (0.1 mmol/kg body weight). Fat suppression should be used. Scanning parameters can be chosen as follows: TR 100-150 ms/ TE minimal (2-5 ms)/ flip angle 60-90°. Using one excitation, 6-8 mm thick slices and a 20% gap, up to 20 slices can be obtained in one breath hold of about 24 seconds. Beside the above-described MR sequences a multitude of other sequences have been suggested including those using other contrast agents like Mn-DPDP (33). Presently, however, these other sequences do not seem to improve accuracy for distinguishing benign from malignant adrenal masses.

Imaging strategies

Cushing's syndrome

Cushing's syndrome is caused by excessive amounts of circulating cortisol. This can either be caused by an increase in pituitary (in Cushing's disease), or extra-pituitary ACTH production resulting in bilateral adrenal hyperplasia or the increased cortisol levels can be produced in an adrenal tumor. Prolonged administration of high doses of corticosteroids can also cause iatrogenic Cushing's syndrome. Increased ACTH production in the pituitary gland is responsible for about 70% of the cases of hypercortisolism. In about 10% an ectopic ACTH source is responsible for the syndrome. Ectopic ACTH production occurs mostly in small cell bronchogenic carcinoma, or less commonly in medullary thyroid carcinomas, gastrointestinal neuroendocrine cancers, thymic carcinoids and pheochromocytomas. Primary cortisol-producing adrenal tumors are responsible for about 10-20% of all cases of Cushing's syndrome.

Imaging in case of Cushing's syndrome follows clinical and laboratory testing. In case of suspicion of a cortisol-producing adrenal tumor, either CT or MRI can be used to assess this tumor. It is important to realize that in about one third of the cases an adrenocortical carcinoma rather than an adenoma is responsible for the primary hypercortisolism.

The appearance of an adenoma on CT is usually sharp and round with a low density, often near that of water. Cortisol-producing adenomas usually enhance vividly after intravenous contrast administration (34). It is difficult to differentiate an adenoma from a carcinoma or metastasis. If an adrenal tumor is larger than 3 cm, malignancy should be considered. On MRI the signal intensities of an adrenal adenoma resembles normal adrenal tissue (isointense on T1-weighted and hyperintense on T2-weighted sequences).

Adrenocortical scintigraphy is a powerful tool to distinguish cortisol-producing adenoma from ACTH-independent bilateral adrenal hyperplasia (35). However, adrenal scintigraphy is costly and is a time consuming investigation with repeated imaging procedures 3–6 days after the administration of the radiolabeled cholesterol analogue. Therefore, scintigraphy is often omitted in the pre-operative work-up of adrenal endocrinopathy.

Conn's syndrome

Primary hyperaldosteronism or Conn's syndrome is caused by excess excretion of aldosterone. This results in hypokalemia, hypernatremia, hypertension, magnesium depletion and metabolic alkalosis. There are two causes of hyperaldosteronism: in about 80% of the cases a benign adrenocortical adenoma is responsible and in about 20% of the cases bilateral hyperplasia is the cause. In less than 1% of the cases of Conn's syndrome an adrenocortical carcinoma is found. It is essential to distinguish between the two main causes of Conn's syndrome since an adenoma can be treated by adrenalectomy whereas bilateral hyperplasia should be treated medically. Since aldosterone-producing adenomas are usually small (5-35 mm) and hyperplastic nodules in bilateral hyperplasia measure usually less than 10 mm, it is important to choose a small slice thickness in CT or MRI (Figure 4). If CT scanning is unable to locate an adenoma, selective venous sampling can be used to identify very small adenomas (36).

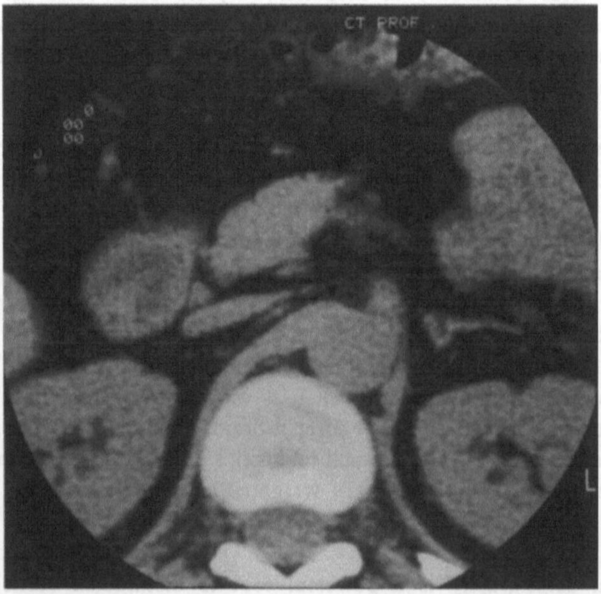

Figure 4. CT scan without intravenous contrast of an aldosterone producing adenoma of the left adrenal gland

Adrenal scintigraphy can distinguish an adenoma from bilateral hyperplasia and sometimes can detect small adenomas missed by CT (35).

The appearance of aldosterone-producing adenomas on non-contrast CT or MRI is similar to that of cortisol-producing adenomas. After intravenous contrast administration producing-producing adenomas usually display no or only little enhancement, whereas cortisol-producing adenomas usually enhance clearly.

Adrenal virilization

The most common cause for adrenal virilization is congenital adrenocortical hyperplasia. An inborn error in the enzyme 22- or 11-beta hydroxylase results in an impaired cortisol and aldosterone synthesis. As a result ACTH stimulation is strongly increased, resulting in an increased androgen production. These symptoms present in early childhood with virilization and pseudohermaphroditism in girls and precocious puberty in boys. In case of virilization later in live, an androgen-producing tumor can be the cause. These tumors are generally malignant (37).

Spiral CT scanning with narrow collimation and thin section reconstructions is probably the best imaging modality for tumor detection. Androgen-secreting adenomas show similar appearance as other adrenal adenomas on CT but the density is somewhat higher ranging from 30-50 Hounsefield Units. The appearance on MRI is indistinguishable from other adenomas.

Pheochromocytoma

Hyperfunctioning tumors of the adrenal medulla include pheochromocytoma and neuroblastoma. Neuroblastoma is a tumor exclusively encountered in young children and, therefore, this subject will not be covered in this chapter. Pheochromocytoma arises as other paragangliomas from the paraganglion cells of the sympatic nervous system. In 90% of cases, paragangliomas are located in the adrenal glands (= pheochromocytomas), in 10% elsewhere in the body (37). Pheochromocytomas are usually hormonally active. The overproduction of catecholamines causes the sometimes life-threatening symptoms like hypertension as well as palpitations, anxiety and excessive perspiration. Other hormones that can be produced by pheochromocytomas are parathyroid hormone (PTH), gastrin, calcitonin, serotonin and corticotrophin (ACTH). In about 10% of cases, pheochromocytomas occur in association with inherited disorders like MEN II syndrome, neurofibromatosis, and Von Hippel-Lindau disease (36).

Imaging of pheochromocytomas can be performed with CT, MRI or Radioiodinated metaiodobenzylguanidine (MIBG) scintigraphy. Although MRI is probably the most sensitive technique and MIBG scintigraphy the most specific technique (38), CT usually will visualize most pheochromocytomas adequately. Optimal CT imaging consists of pre- and post-contrast thin collimation spiral scanning. Small pheochromocytomas usually present as homogenous structures, isodense to renal tissue. Larger pheochromocytomas can show areas of bleeding, necrosis and cystic degeneration. Intravenous contrast administration results in a clear enhancement of the tumor, especially in the periphery (Figure 5). Necrotic areas are accentuated by the contrast enhancement around them.

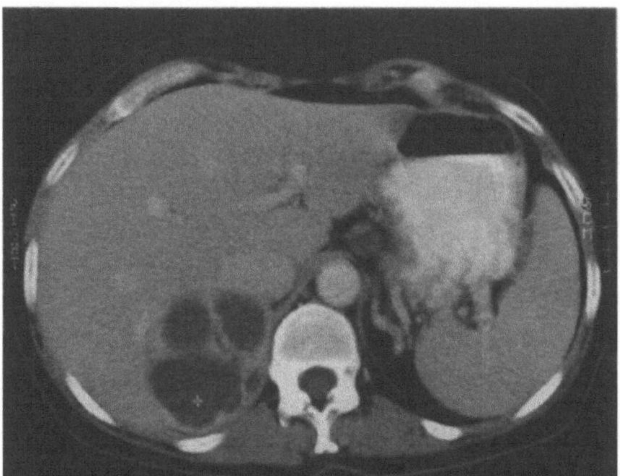

Figure 5. CT scan with intravenous contrast of a large right-sided cystic pheochromocytoma.

On MRI small pheochromocytomas present as an iso- or hypointense structure compared to liver on pre-contrast T1-weighted images while they appear on T2-weighted images markedly intense (23,37,39,40). Larger pheochromocytomas are commonly inhomogeneous due to cystic degeneration, necrosis and/or intratumoral hemorrhage (Figure 6).

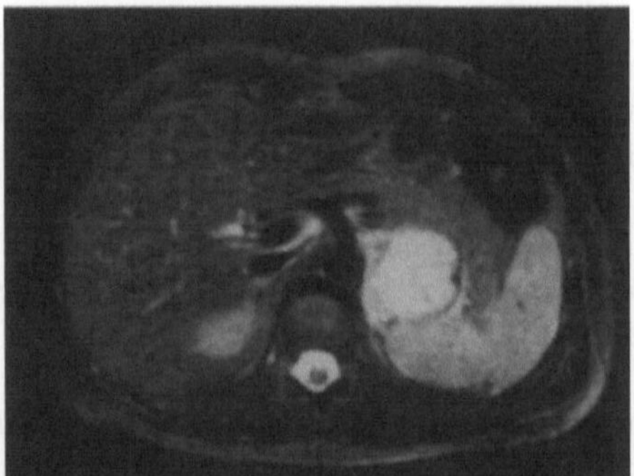

Figure 6. T2-weighted turbo spin echo with fat suppression of a large cystic pheochromocytoma of the left adrenal gland.

Dynamic contrast enhanced T1-weighted gradient echo sequences show rapid enhancement with slow washout, resembling to primary or secondary adrenal malignancies (21,22,30). Chemical shift imaging usually shows lack of signal decrease on the opposed phase images (27,28,41) However, anecdotal reports describe pheochromocytomas with signal decrease due to lipid degeneration or due to the fact that they sometimes contain normal lipid rich adrenocortical cells (42).

Both CT and MRI cannot reliably differentiate pheochromocytomas from metastasis or primary adrenal malignancies. The clinical symptoms will however usually clearly point to pheochromocytoma. For extra-adrenal localization and detection and evaluation of recurrent or metastatic lesions, MIBG scanning is the imaging method of choice (43)

Non-hyperfunctioning adrenal masses

Adenoma

Most adrenal masses are non-hyperfunctioning adrenocortical adenomas. Even in oncology patients, non-hyperfunctioning adenomas are the most common cause of adrenal enlargement (3). Obviously a reliable method for distinguishing adenomas from other not hormonally active adrenal tumors is essential. CT scanning, especially non-contrast enhanced CT allows to some extent to rule out malignancy based on density measurements (Figure 7).

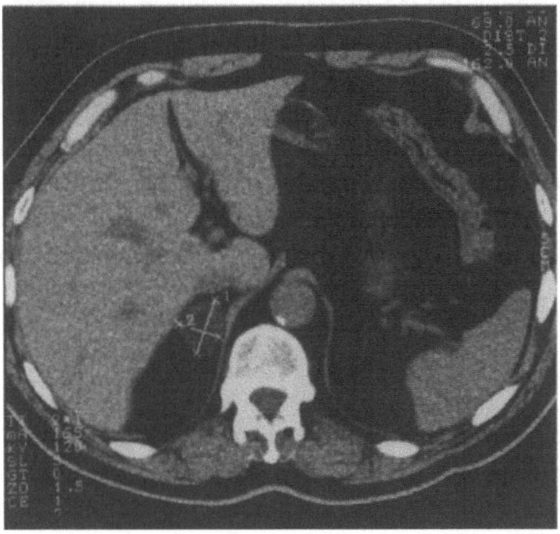

Figure 7. Non-enhanced CT-scan of an adrenal adenoma on the right.

On T1-weighted MR images, adenomas are usually hypo- or isointense compared to liver tissue, and iso-or slightly hyperintense on T2-weighted images (Figure 8).

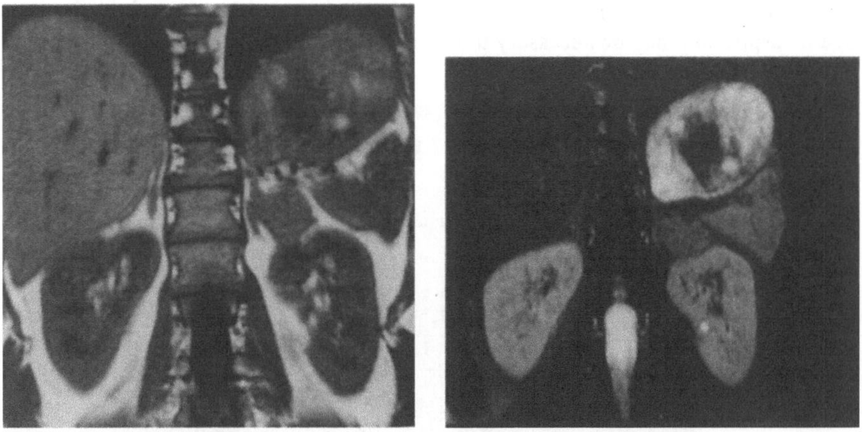

Figure 8. Left: T1-weighted and right: T2-weighted (fat suppressed) coronal images of a left sided adrenal adenoma.

Contrast enhancement is only mild to moderate, i.e. the signal increase is less than 100% followed by a quick washout on dynamic contrast enhanced gradient echo sequences. This contrast enhancement pattern usually allows distinguishing adenomas from metastases and pheochromocytomas (22,30,32,44). However atypical adenomas with avid prolonged contrast enhancement and hyperintense signal compared to liver parenchyma on T2-weighted images have been described (23,30,45).

Currently MRI, especially Chemical Shift Imaging (CSI) is considered to be one of the most reliable methods for the distinction between adenomas and non-adenomas (29,32). Accuracy of this method has been reported to be as high as 100%. However, as this method relies on the lipid content of the adrenal mass, other lipid containing tumors also result in decreased signal intensity on the opposed phase images. Rarely metastases of hepatocellular carcinomas, renal cell carcinomas, liposarcomas and (primary) adrenocortical carcinomas may show areas of signal decrease on opposed phase images (46). On the other hand presumably some benign adenomas may contain insufficient lipids to show a significant signal decrease on the opposed phase images (47).

Myelolipoma

These rare benign adrenal tumors are composed of variable amounts of fat and bone marrow tissue. Myelolipomas are typically asymptomatic and discovered incidentally during CT or MRI scanning (Figure 9). CT scanning is usually sufficient to diagnose this lesion with its characteristic appearance of predominantly fat attenuation. MRI is superior compared to CT in larger tumors, since different imaging planes are helpful to distinguish adrenal myelolipoma from other extra-adrenal retroperitoneal fat containing tumors (malignant retroperitoneal lipoma or liposarcoma, or large renal angiomyolipoma) (48).

The fatty content of myelolipomas can be proved by MRI with fat suppression techniques (23,24,49,50). If a myelolipoma mainly consists of myeloid tissue fine needle aspiration may be necessary to obtain the correct diagnosis (48).

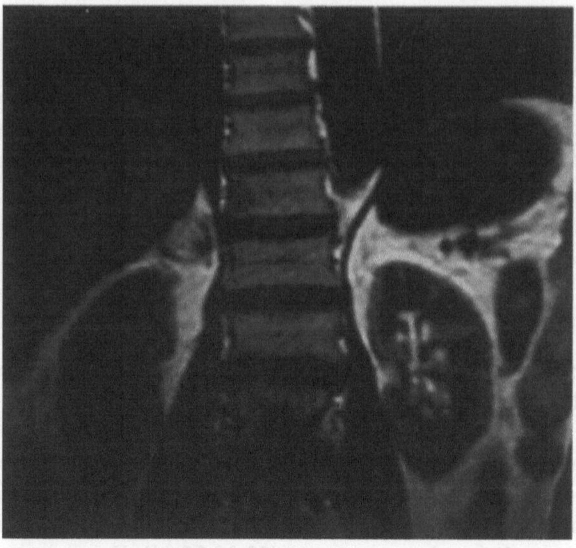

Figure 9. T1-weighted image illustrating the high signal intensity of the fatty content of a myelolipoma of the right adrenal gland.

Adrenal metastasis

Post-mortem studies show that adrenal gland metastases are present in up to 26% of patients with an extra-adrenal malignant disease. Ultrasound can detect most metastases larger than 2 cm. However, especially on the left side even large tumors can be missed, therefore ultrasound is considered insufficient for screening for adrenal metastases. CT is able to detect small adrenal metastases, but the problem is to differentiate metastases from non-hyperfunctioning benign adenomas (Figure 10).

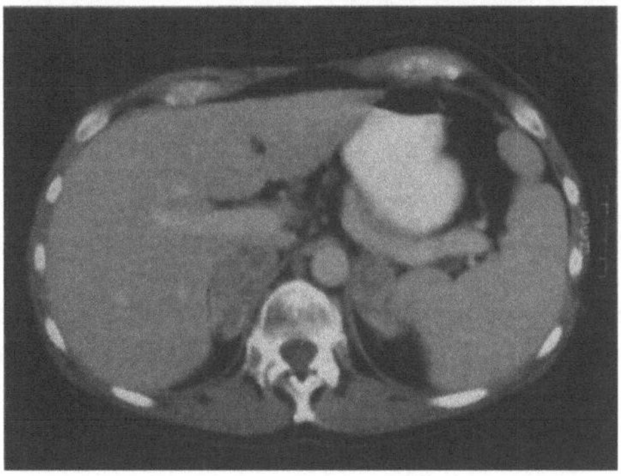

Figure 10. Contrast-enhanced CT scan of bilateral adrenal metastases. Primary tumor: melanoma.

CT appearance strongly suggestive for metastatic lesions are diameter > 5 cm, irregular contours, invasion of neighboring structures and increase in size during follow-up. In equivocal cases fine needle aspiration or biopsy has to be performed. Although the sensitivity of CT for detection of adrenal masses is high, the sensitivity for detection of small adrenal metastases may be rather low (Figure 11). Using biopsy, Pagani found adrenal metastases in patients with small cell lung cancer and normal adrenal glands on CT in 17% (51).

As described earlier, MRI is currently possibly the most reliable technique to distinguish adenomas from malignancies. Criteria suggestive for metastasis are hypo- to isointensity compared to liver on T1-weighted and hyperintensity on T2-weighted sequences (Figure 11) (23,40). On opposed phase Chemical Shift Images, metastases usually demonstrate no signal decrease (27). Some metastases however, like those of renal cell carcinoma, hepatocellular carcinoma and liposarcoma, may contain intracellular lipids and therefore may mimic normal adrenal (41). Metastasis typically show rapid contrast enhancement with a signal increase higher than 150% and a persistent high signal intensity after 10 minutes (>75%)(30,44,52). When Chemical Shift Imaging and dynamic contrast-enhanced MR sequences are combined, accuracy for the distinction between benign from malignant lesions can be increased to approximately 90% (30).

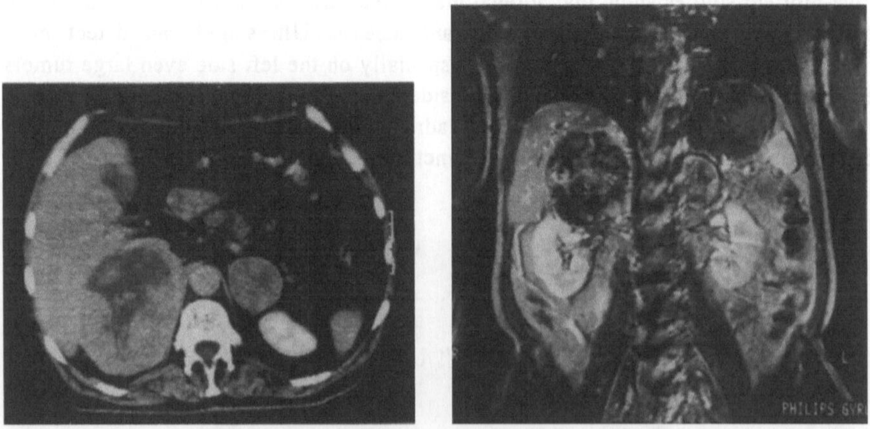

Figure 11. Left: Contrast-enhanced CT scan and right: T1-weighted gradient echo MRI after intravenous gadolinium of large adrenal metastases. Primary tumor: thyroid carcinoma.

Adrenal carcinoma

Primary carcinoma of the adrenal cortex is an uncommon tumor with an annual incidence of approximately one case per million (42). CT and MRI findings do not significantly differ from metastasis (Figure 12). Adrenal carcinomas are usually asymptomatic and therefore often large at time of detection.

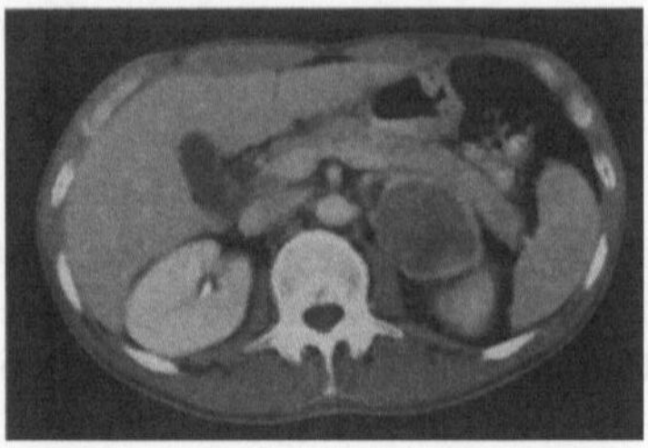

Figure 12. CT scan with intravenous contrast of a large left sided adrenal carcinoma with areas of central necrosis.

In about 15-50% of cases adrenocortical carcinomas are hormonally active. The majority of patients with hormonally active adenocarcinomas present with Cushing's syndrome. The size of the tumor is often larger than 6 cm. Invasion of adjacent organs and the inferior vena cava is possible. Calcifications and large necrotic areas are commonly seen (23,37). MRI is probably the best imaging modality for the evaluation of spread to adjacent organs (23).

Lymphoma

Non-Hodgkin's lymphoma of the adrenal gland is usually not an isolated disease: retroperitoneal lymphomatous involvement is present in most cases. Primary adrenal lymphoma is extremely rare. Adrenal involvement in systemic malignant lymphoma has been documented with CT in only 4% of the cases (53). Lymphomatous involvement of the adrenal glands is more often the case with non-Hodgkin's than with Hodgkin's lymphoma. Like other malignant diseases of the adrenal glands, adrenal lymphomas show on MRI low to isointense signal intensity on T1- and high signal on T2-weighted sequences when compared to liver tissue (54). Contrast enhancement is usually marked and prolonged (55). Chemical Shift sequences show no decreased signal on the opposed phase images, as lymphomatous tissue does not contain lipids (27,32).

Hemorrhage

Adrenal hemorrhage can occur as a result of trauma, anticoagulation, with septicemia, hypertension, thrombocytopenia, disseminated intravascular coagulation (DIC) or spontaneously. Small adrenal hemorrhages are particularly common in infants in the prenatal period. In children and adults meningococcal sepsis is a notorious cause of adrenal hemorrhage (Waterhouse Friderichsen syndrome).

Unenhanced CT images are well suited to image hemorrhages. In cases of chronic adrenal hemorrhage CT can show calcifications, which are not easily appreciated on MRI (56). Depending on the age of the hemorrhage MRI reflects the different stages of hemoglobin oxidation products (57). Methemoglobin with its paramagnetic behavior results in high signal on both T1- and T2-weighted images. Hematomas do not show contrast enhancement.

General conclusion

Both modern CT and MRI scanners are capable of imaging most morphologic adrenal disorders. In case of a patient with endocrinopathy, localization of the suspected hormonally active adrenal tumor is the most important issue. Because of its high resolution and relative simplicity and general availability, CT scanning, especially spiral CT can be considered as the method of choice. In case of a non-functioning adrenal mass, however, MRI can often accurately distinguish benign from malignant lesions. The best results are obtained with a combination of imaging sequences, including chemical shift imaging and dynamic contrast enhanced MRI.

References

1. ME, Walther MM, Phillips VM, et al. CT-guided adrenal biopsies: accuracy, safety, and indications. AJR 1985;144: 67.
2. Oliver TW jr, Bernardino ME, Miller JI, Mansour K, Greene D, Davis WA. Isolated adrenal masses in nonsmall-cell brochogenic carcinoma. Radiology 1984;153:217.
3. Modder U. Röntgendiagnostik der Nebennierenerkrankungen. Internist 1982 23:99.
4. Doppman JL, Gill JR Jr. Hyperaldosteronism: Sampling the Adrenal Veins. Radiology 1996;198:309.
5. Abrams HL, Siegelman SS, Adams DF, Sanders R, Finberg HJ, Hessel SJ, McNeil BJ. Computed Tomography versus Ultrasound of the adrenal gland: a prospective study. Radiology 1982;143:121.
6. Paivansalo M, Lahde S, Merikanto J, Kallionen M. Computed tomography in primary and secondary adrenal tumors. Acta Radiol 1988;29:519.
7. Miyake H, Maeda H, Tashiro M, et al. CT of adrenal tumors: frequency and clinical significance of low-attenuation lesions. AJR 1989;152:1005.
8. Lee MJ, Hahn PF, Papanicolaou N, et al. Benign and malignant adrenal masses: CT distinction with attenuation coefficients, size, and observer analysis. Radiology 1991;179:415.
9. Van Erkel AR, van Gils APG, Lequin M, Kruitwagen C, Bloem JL, Falke THM. CT and MR distinction of adenomas and nonadenomas of the adrenal gland. J Comput Assist Tomogr 1994;18:432.
10. Miyake H, Takaki H, Matsumoto S, Yoshida S, Maeda T, Mori H. Adrenal nonhyperfunctioning and nonadenoma: CT attenuation value as a discriminative index. Abdom Imaging 1995;20:559.
11. McNicholas MMJ, Lee MJ, Mayo-Smith WW, Hahn PF, Boland GW, Mueller PR. An imaging algorithm for the differential diagnosis of adrenal adenomas and metastases. AJR 1995;165:1453.
12. Korobkin M, Brodeur FJ, Yutzy GG, et al. Differentiation of adrenal adenomas from nonadenomas using CT attenuation values. AJR 1996;166:531.
13. Outwater EK, Siegelman ES, Huang AB, Birnbaum BA. Adrenal masses: correlation between CT attenuation value and chemical shift ratio at MR imaging with in-phase and opposed-phased sequences. Radiology 1996;200:749.
14. Szolar DH, Kammerhuber F. Quantitative CT evaluation of adrenal gland masses: a step forward in the differentiation between adenomas and nonadenomas. Radiology 1997;202:517.
15. Boland GW, Hahn PF, Pena C, Mueller PR. Adrenal masses: characterization with delayed contrast-enhanced CT. Radiology 1997;202:693.
16. Boland GW, Lee MJ, Scott Gazelle G, Halpern EF, McNicholas MMJ, Mueller PR. Characterization of adrenal masses using unenhanced CT: An analysis of the CT literature. AJR 1998;171:201.
17. Korobkin M, Brodeur FJ, Francis IR, Quint LE, Reed Dunnick N, Goodsitt M. Delayed enhanced CT for differentiation of benign from malignant adrenal masses. Radiology 1996;200:737.
18. Szolar DH, Kammerhuber FH. Adrenal adenomas and nonadenomas: assessment of washout at delayed contrast-enhanced CT. Radiology 1998;207:369.
19. Korobkin M, Brodeur FJ, Francis IR, Quint LE, Reed Dunnick N, Londy F. CT Time-Attenuation washout curves of adrenal adenomas and nonadenomas. AJR 1998;170:747.

20. Reinig JW, Doppman JL, Dwyer AJ, Frank J. MRI of indeterminate adrenal masses. AJR 1986;147:493.
21. Krestin GP, Steinbrich W, Friedmann G. Adrenal masses: evaluation with fast gradient-echo MR imaging and Gd-DTPA-enhanced dynamic studies. Radiology 1989;171:675.
22. Lee MJ, Mayo-Smith WW, Hahn PF, Goldberg MA, Boland GW, Saini S, Papanicolaou N. State-of-the-art MR imaging of the adrenal gland. RadioGraphics 1994;14:1015.
23. Korobkin M, Giordano TJ, Brodeur FJ, Francis IR, Siegelman ES, Quint LE, Reed Dunnick N, Heiken JP, Wang HH. Adrenal adenomas: relationship between histologic lipid and CT and MR findings. Radiology 1996;200:743.
24. Korobkin M, Lombardi TJ, Aisen AM, Francis IR, Quint LE, Dunnick NR, Londy F, Shapiro B, Gross MD, Thompson NW. Characterization of adrenal masses with chemical shift and gadolinium-enhanced MR imaging. Radiology 1995;197:411.
25. Bilbey JH, McLoughlin RF, Kurkjian PS, Wilkins GEL, Chan NHL, Schmidt N, Singer J. MR imaging of adrenal masses: value of chemical-shift imaging for distinguishing adenomas from other tumors. AJR 1995;164:637.
26. Tsushima Y, Ishizaka H, Matsumoto M. Adrenal masses: differentiation with chemical shift, fast low angle shot MR imaging. Radiology 1993;186:705.
27. Mitchell DG, Crovello M, Matteucci T, Petersen RO, Miettinen MM. Benign adrenocortical masses: diagnosis with chemical shift imaging. Radiology 1992;185:345.
28. Schwartz LH, Panicek DM, Koutcher JA, Brown KT, Getrajdman GI, Heelan RT, Burt M. Adrenal masses in patients with malignancy: prospective comparison of echo-planar, fast spin-echo and chemical shift imaging. Radiology 1995;197:421.
29. Krestin GP, Friedman G, Fischbach R, Neufang KFR, Allolio B. Evaluation of adrenal masses in oncologic patients: dynamic contrast-enhanced MR US CT. J Comput Assist Tomogr 1991;15:104.
30. Semelka RC, Shoenut JP, Lawrence PH, Greenberg HM, Maycher B, Madden TP, Kroeker MA. Evaluation of adrenal masses with gadolineum enhancement and fat-suppressed MR imaging. JMRI 1993;3:337.
31. Reinig JW, Stutley JE, Leonhardt CM, Spicer KM, Margolis M, Caldwell CB. Differentiation of adrenal masses with MR imaging: comparison of techniques. Radiology 1994;192:41.
32. Mitchell DG, Outwater EK, Matteucci T, Rubin DL, Chezmar JL, Saini S. Adrennal gland enhancement at MR imaging with Mn-DPDP. Radiology 1995;194:783.
33. Dunnick NR, Korobkin M, Francis I. Adrenal Radiology: Distinguishing benign from malignant adrenal masses. AJR 1996;167:861.
34. Gross MD, Shapiro B. Adrenocortical scintigraphy. From: Nuclear Medicine in Clinical Diagnosis and Treatment. Editors: Murray IPC, Ell PJ, Van der Wall H, Strauss HW. Churchill Livingstone, Edinburgh 1998, chap. 63, p. 805.
35. Geisinger MA, Zelch MG, Bravo EL, Risius BF, O'Donovan PB, Borkowski GP. Primary hyperaldosteronism: comparison of CT, adrenal venography and venous sampling. AJR 1983; 141:299.
36. Reznek RH, Armstrong P. The adrenal gland. Clinical endocrinology 1994;40:561.
37. Van Gils A, Falke T, van Erkel A, Aerndt JW, Sandler MP, van der Mey AGL, Hoogma RPLM.MR imaging and MIBG scintigraphy of pheochromocytomas and extraadrenal functional paragangliomas. RadioGraphics 1991;11:37.
38. Francis IR, Gross MD, Shapiro B, Korobkin M, Quint LE. Integrated imaging of adrenal disease. Radiology 1992;183:1-13.
39. Newhouse JH. MRI of the adrenal gland. Urol Radiol 1990;12:1.
40. Tsushima Y, Ishizaka H, Kato T, Matsumota M. Differential diagnosis of adrenal masses using out-of-phase FLASH imaging: a preliminary report. Acta Radiol 1992;33:262.

41. McLoughlin RF, Biley JH. Tumors of the adrenal gland: findings on CT and MR imaging. AJR 1994;163:1413.
42. Troncone L, Rufini V. Radiolabeled metaiodobenzylguanidine in the diagnosis of neural crest tumors. From: Nuclear Medicine in Clinical Diagnosis and Treatment. Editors: Murray IPC, Ell PJ, Van der Wall H, Strauss HW. Churchill Livingstone, Edinburgh 1998, chap. 66, p. 843.
43. Reinig JW, Doppman JL, Dwyer AJ, Johnson AR, Knop RH. Distinction between adrenal adenomas and adrenal metastases using MR imaging. J Comput Assist Tomogr 1985;9:898.
44. Klose KC, Andreopoulos D, Adam G, Biesterfeld S. Hypervaskularisiertes Nebennierenadenom. Radiologe 1992;32:32.
45. Schlund JF, Kenney PJ, Brown ED, Ascher SM, Brown JJ, Semelka RC. Adrenocortical carcinoma: MR imaging appearance with current techniques. J Magn Reson Imaging 1995;5:171.
46. Tsushima Y. Different lipid contents between aldosterone-producing and non-hyperfunctioning adrenocortical adenomas: in vivo measurement using chemical shift MRI. J Clin Endocrinol Metab 1994;79:179-1762.
47. Casey LR, Cohen AJ, Wilw AG, Dietrich B. Giant adrenal myelolipomas: CT and MRI findings. Abdom Imaging 1994;19:165.
48. Reinig JW, Doppman JL, Dwyer AJ, Johnson AR, Knop RH. Adrenal masses differentiated by MR. Radiology 1986;158:81.
49. Musante F, Derchi LE, Bazzocchi M, Avataneo T, Gandini G, Pozzi Mucelli RS. MR imaging of adrenal myelolipomas. J Comput Assist Tomogr 1991;15:111.
50. Pagani JJ. Normal adrenal glands in small cell lung carcinoma: CT-guided biopsy. AJR 1983;140:949.
51. Ichikawa T, Ohtoma K, Uchiyama GG, Fujimoto H, Nasu K. Contrast-enhanced dynamic MRI of adrenal masses: classification of characteristic enhancement patterns. Clin Radiol 1995;50:295.
52. Paling MR, Williamson BRJ. Adrenal involvement in non-Hodgkin lymphoma. AJR 1983;141:303.
53. Lee FT jr, Thornbury JR, Grist TM, Kelcz F. MR imaging of adrenal lymphoma. Abdom Imaging 1993;18:95.
54. Krestin GP. Adrenal diseases. In Krestin G, ed. Morphologic and functional MR of the kidneys and adrenal glands. New York: Field & Wood Medical Publishers. 1991:P89.
55. Mezrich R, Banner MP, Pollack HM. Magnetic resonance imaging of the adrenal glands. Urol Radiol 1986;8:127.
56. Ikeda DM, Francis IR, Glazer GM, Amendola MA, Gross MD, Aisen AM. The detection of adrenal tumors and hyperplasia in patients with primary aldosterism: comparison of scintigraphy, CT and MR imaging. AJR 1989;153:301.

9
SCINTIGRAPHY OF ADRENAL DISORDERS

Milton D. Gross, M.D.
Brahm Shapiro, M.B., CH.B., Ph.D.
Paul Shreve, M.D.
Barry I. Shulkin, M.D.
University of Michigan
Ann Arbor, MI 48105, USA

INTRODUCTION

Since the introduction of radioactive ^{131}I and the success achieved in imaging of the thyroid there has been great interest in the development of agents for localization of other endocrine glands. The scintigraphic imaging of the adrenal glands spans an almost 4 decade interval during which high resolution computed tomography (CT), magnetic resonance imaging (MRI) and sensitive hormone analyses have been developed and are now often taken for granted in our modern, medical imaging environment. Despite their advancing age and relative lack of high spatial resolution, even the oldest adrenal scintigraphic techniques continue to provide clinically useful information that is often complimentary, unique and not duplicated by other more contemporary, high resolution, imaging techniques.

Scintigraphy of the adrenal glands provides examples of functional imaging based on a number of fundamental physiological principles: 1) uptake, storage and modulation of accumulation by trophic hormones and secretogogues of metabolic precursors (e.g., adrenocortical scintigraphy with radiolabeled cholesterol analogs); 2) specific receptor binding of radiolabeled hormone analogs to cell surface receptors (e.g., adrenomedullary scintigraphy with radiolabeled somatostatin analogs); and 3) exploitation of hormone/neurotransmitter uptake and storage by radiolabeled catecholamine analogs (e.g., adrenomedullary scintigraphy with radiolabeled metaiodobenzylguanidine and related compounds) (Table 1).

In each of these cases the radiopharmaceuticals are designed not only to resist rapid degradation or extensive metabolism after specific uptake, but also to depict a functional aspect of the target tissues or neoplasm each was designed to localize. Furthermore, manipulation of mechanisms of hormone secretion and radiotracer accumulation has provided insight into the physiology and pathophysiology of adrenal gland disorders, and has also allowed efficacious and cost effective localization of neoplasms of adrenal origin.

TABLE 1

Mechanisms of Uptake Adrenocortical and Adrenomedullary Radiopharmaceuticals

Radiopharmaceutical	Uptake Mechanisms	Metabolism
Adrenal Coretx		
Radiolabeled cholesterol analogs eg., ^{131}I-19-Iodocholesterol, ^{131}I-6ß-Iodomethy-norcholesterol, ^{75}SE-6ß-Seldnomethyl-norcholesterol	Binds to low density lipoprotein (LDL) in circulation	No metabolism of cholesterol esters to radiolabeled adrenocortical hormone analogs
	Bound tracer binds to LDL receptor on adrenocortical cells	
	Esterifcation of cholesterol analog	
	Storage of esterfied tracer in cholesterol ester pool (no further metabolism to radiolabeled steroid hormore analogs)	
Adrenal Medulla		
Radiolabeled somatostatin analogs eg., ^{111}In-octreotide, ^{123}I-tyr-octreotide	Binds to cell surface somatostatin receptors	Clearance of tracer from the circulation slowed by creation of proteolysis resistant analogs
	Possible intracellular translocation of tracer-receptor complex	Different analogs have different affinities to binding to various receptor subtypes
Radiolabeled arylguanidines and analogs, eg., ^{131}I metaiodobenzylguanidine, ^{123}I metaiodobenzylguanidine, ^{11}C-hydroxy-ephedrine	Specific uptake via type 1 catecholamine reuptake mechanisms in cell membrane (tricyclic antidepressent sensitive)	Tracer does not bind to post-synaptic or β adrenergic receptors
	Transport from cytoplasm into the intracellular hormone storage granules (tetrabenazine sensitive) Storage within the intracellular storage granules	Tracer resists metabolism by catecholamine degrading enzymes (eg., MAO or COMT)
	Storage within the intracellular hormone granules	

Historical Perspective

In the early 1970's cholesterol labeled with radioiodine was demonstrated to image the adrenal cortex. Primary and secondary etiologies of Cushing's syndrome were evaluated. Biochemical manipulation of adrenocorticotropic hormone (ACTH) and corticotrophic releasing hormone levels affecting substrate uptake (e.g., dexamethasone suppression of ACTH) expanded the use of iodocholesterol to include primary aldosteronism, adrenal and ovarian etiologies of hyperandrogenism and more recently characterization of incidentally discovered, hormonally silent, adrenal masses. The introduction of single photon emission tomography (SPECT) in the mid-1980's provided some improvement in spatial resolution and adrenal localization over planar imaging techniques. Adrenomedullary imaging became possible in the early 1980's with the availability of metaiodobenzylguanidine (MIBG). Pheochromocytoma and other neuroendocrine neoplasms could be depicted scintigraphically. The pharmacokinetics of MIBG allows for the use of ^{123}I and SPECT. The development in the late 1980's of the long acting somatostatin (SMS) receptor binding analog, octreotide, gave great impetus for the development of suitable radiolabeled analogs for imaging the broad spectrum of tissues and neoplasms expressing SMS receptors. Initial success with an ^{123}I labeled tyrosine analog supported development of a DTPA chelate labeled with ^{111}In, pentetreotide. A wide spectrum of endocrine neoplasms to include pheochromocytoma and neuroblastoma have been imaged with this and other radiolabeled somatostatin analogs. More recently the availability of cyclotron-produced radioisotopes of fluorine, carbon, nitrogen and oxygen allow synthesis of radiolabeled metabolic intermediates, hormones, etc., (e.g. ^{11}C-epinephrine, ^{11}C-hydroxyephedrine, ^{11}C-HED, ^{18}F-fluorodeoxyglucose) as imaging agents that can be used to depict metastatic neoplasms, primary neuroendocrine tumors of the adrenals and their metastases.

Adrenocortical Scintigraphy

Radiolabeled cholesterol analogs when administered intravenously are rapidly incorporated into low density lipoproteins (LDL) and accumulated in target tissues by a specific LDL-receptor mediated process. Cholesterol is the substrate for adrenal steroid hormone synthesis and is derived from LDL (1-3). Radiolabeled cholesterol in the adrenal cortex is esterified and stored within the intracellular lipid pool, but is not further metabolized (1-3). Radiocholesterol analogs are also accumulated by the liver and excreted in bile (1,2,4,5). Accumulation of radiolabeled cholesterol analogs by the adrenal cortex is influenced by modulation of the hypothalamic-pituitary-adrenal (CRH-ACTH-cortisol) and the renin-angiotensin-aldosterone axes and alterations in these feedback pathways can be used to advantage in diagnostic imaging (1,2,4,6) (Figure 1). An elegant alternative approach to adrenocortical scintigraphy has been the use of radiolabeled adrenocortical enzyme inhibitors (e.g., metyrapone and analogs) with some success (14).

Radiopharmaceuticals for Adrenocortical Imaging

The first successful radiopharmaceutical for adrenocortical imaging was ^{131}I-19-iodocholesterol (Figure 1). Sometime later ^{131}I-6-ß-iodomethyl-norcholesterol (NP-59) was identified as a contaminant produced in the synthesis of ^{131}I-19-iodocholesterol possessing a five-fold greater adrenocortical uptake than ^{131}I-19-iodocholesterol (2,4). Scintadren®, ^{75}Se-6-ß-selenomethyl-norcholesterol, has properties similar to NP-59. The ^{75}Selenium label provides some advantage of longer shelf-life (up to 6 weeks) and imaging at times (14 days or more post-injection) when background is very low (6,7). Radiobromine labeled compounds have been synthesized but not used clinically (8). An alternative approach has been to label LDL with ^{131}I, ^{111}In or ^{99m}Tc with some success (9-11). More recently, ^{18}F-fluorodeoxyglucose (^{18}F-FDG) has been used to image metastatic disease to the adrenals, while ^{11}C-etiomidate and ^{11}C-metiomidate, inhibitors of adrenal steroid hormone synthesis, have shown uptake in the adrenal cortex and in some adrenal neoplasms (12,13).

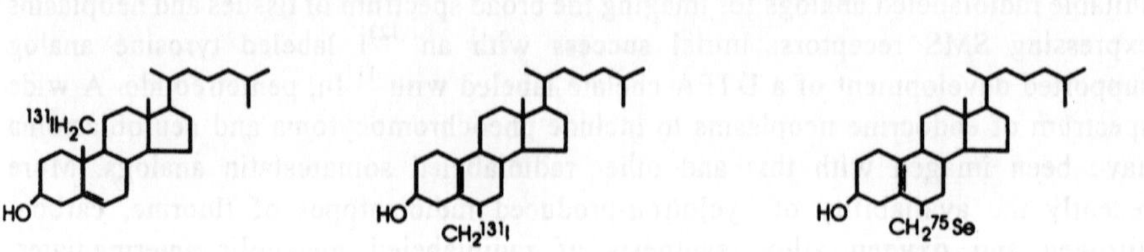

^{131}I-19-Iodocholesterol (*^{131}I-19-Iodocholest-5(6)-en-3β-ol*) — ^{131}I-NP-59 (*6β-^{131}I-Iodomethyl-19-Nor cholest-5(10)-en-3β-ol*) — Scintadren® (*6β-^{75}Se-Seleno Methyl-19-Nor cholest-5(10)-en-3β-ol*)

Figure 1. Radiolabeled cholesterols used for adrenocortical scintigraphy

Procedures for Adrenocortical Imaging

Adrenocortical imaging may be performed under baseline, non-suppressed conditions or performed concomitantly with dexamethasone to suppress ACTH and tracer accumulation in the ACTH-responsive portions of the adrenal cortex, the zona fasiculata and zona reticularis (1,2,4,6,14,15) (Table 2). Pharmacologic manipulation improves detection of small mineralocorticoid and androgen-secreting adrenal adenomas and permits their differentiation from bilateral adrenal hyperplasia. The suppression regimen most frequently employed is 1 mg of dexamethasone administered 4 times daily for seven days before NP-59 injection and continued throughout a 5 day post-NP-59 injection imaging interval (1,14,15). Use of ^{131}I-labeled tracers necessitates thyroid blockade by iodide loading to inhibit uptake of free ^{131}Iodine. The dose of NP-59 and ^{131}I-19-iodocholesterol is 1.0 mCi (or 1 mCi per 1.73 m^2) while for ^{75}Se-selenomethyl-norcholesterol 200-250 μCi is used (1,4,6-9). A mild laxative is usually given, beginning 48 hours prior to imaging, to decrease background gastrointestinal radioactivity. Posterior and lateral images are acquired (occasionally an anterior image is useful) both in analog and digital formats for 50,000-100,000 counts/image. NP-59 studies are performed at baseline (non-suppressed) at five and/or seven days, and at seven and/or 14 days with ^{75}Se-

selenomethyl-norcholesterol (1,4,6,8,9). In dexamethasone suppression studies imaging is performed 3-4 days post injection at a time before the normal adrenal cortex has been observed to image on constant dexamethasone suppression. Later images on day 5 and possibly day 7 may be useful to identify "faint" adrenocortical uptake from background radioactivity. With depth correction and phantom calibration, computer-acquired data can also be used to derive quantitative adrenal uptake measurements (1,2,4).

Biodistribution and Dosimetry of the Radiocholesterols

Normal biodistribution and dosimetry of NP-59 and other radiocholesterols includes prominent liver uptake and biliary excretion (2,4,15) (Table 2). Radiotracer within the gallbladder may at times be confused with the right adrenal, but can be differentiated using anterior and lateral projections. A maneuver to empty the gallbladder with a fatty meal or cholecystokinin (CCK) analogs can also be useful (14). Laxatives are routinely prescribed to eliminate gut radioactivity (16). Normal adrenal glands are visualized as symmetrical foci of ^{131}I accumulation (the right gland is often somewhat more prominent than the left due to liver background and its slightly more superficial posterior location) (1,2,4). Normal left to right asymmetry of adrenal uptake is 0.9 to 1.2. Not surprisingly, baseline adrenal uptake is diminished with dexamethasone suppression ($0.15 \pm 0.04\%$ vs. $0.04 \pm 0.01\%$) (2,4). Earliest normal adrenal visualization on non-suppressed studies is two to three days and five days or later while on dexamethasone suppression (using the 4mg/day x 7 days prior to NP-59 injection regimen). The time to image the adrenal cortex post-injection while on DS appears to be a function of the duration of prior suppression and thus other DS regimens will exhibit different timing of normal gland visualization (1,2,4,14) (Table 2). Usually the visual imaging pattern (interpreted with clinical and biochemical data) is sufficient for diagnostic evaluation, but quantification of uptake may be useful in cases of mild bilateral cortical hyperplasia (1,2,4).

Cushing's Syndrome

All the etiologies of hypercortisolism (Cushing's syndrome-CS) can be studied using adrenocortical scintigraphy (1,2,4,17) (Table 3). In ACTH-dependent CS (Cushing's disease and ectopic ACTH/CRH syndromes) bilateral symmetrical radiopharmaceutical uptake in the adrenal cortex is usually greatest in ectopic ACTH Cushing's syndrome (Figure 2). This is a dramatic scintigraphic depiction of adrenocortical pathophysiology, however the critical clinical problem is identifying the source(s) of ACTH secretion. The greatest clinical value of adrenocortical scintigraphy is in primary adrenal ACTH-independent CS (1,2,4,17).

TABLE 2

Techniques and Dosimetry of Radiopharmaceuticals for Adrenal Scintigraphy

Radiopharmaceuticals	NP-59 *	SMC **	^{131}I-MIBG	^{123}I-MIBG**	^{111}In-pentetreotide
Thyroid blockade† (SSKI 1 drop or Lugol's 2 drops in beverage tid)	start 2 days before injection and continue for 14 days	Not required	start 2 days before injection and continue for 6 days	start 2 days before injection and continue for 4 days	Not required
Adult Dost (i.v.)	37 Mbq	9.25 Mbq	18.5 Mbq-37 Mbq	370 Mbq	222Mbq
Shelf-life	2 weeks frozen	6-8 wks room temp.			
% uptake/adrenal	0.007%-0.26%	0.7%-0.30%	0.01%-0.22%	0.01%-0.22%	-
Dosimetry (cGy/dose)			from package insert	from package insert	
Adrenal	28-88	6.1	0.38 - 0.75	8-28	1.51
Ovaries	8.0	1.9	0.14 - 0.27	0.35	0.98
Liver	2.4	3.5	1.45 - 2.90	0.32	2.43
Kidneys	2.2	-	0.16 - 0.32	-	10.83
Spleen	2.7	-	1.10 - 2.20	-	14.77
Urinary bladder	-	-	1.40 - 2.80	-	6.05
Thyroid	150‡	0.43‡	0.17‡ - 0.33‡	17.7‡	1.49
Whole body	1.2	1.4	-	0.29	-
Effective dose equivalent	-	-	0.35 - 0.70	-	2.61
Beta Emission	Yes	No	Yes	No	No
Laxative (e.g. bisacodyl 5-10 mg p.o. bid)	begin 2 days before & continue during imaging	No	begin post injection	begin post injection	begin post injection
Imaging interval post radiotracer administration (optional additional imaging times)	<u>Non-DS:</u> 1 or more days 5, 6, or 7 post injection <u>DS:</u> 1 or more early: (3), 4 & one or more late: 5, 6, or 7 days post injection	7 (14) days post injection (no large published experience with DS scans)	24, 48 (72) hours post injection	2-6, 24 (48) hours post injection	4-6, 24, (48) hours post injection
Collimator	High-energy, parallel-hole	Medium energy, parallel hole	High-energy, parallel hole	Medium energy, parallel-hole	Medium energy, parallel-hole
Principle photopeak (abundance) window	364 keV (81%) 20% window	137keV (61%), 265 keV (59%), 280 keV (25%) 20% window	364 keV 20% window	159 keV 20% window	172 keV (90%), 245 keV (94%) 20% windows
Imaging time/counts (per view)	20 min/100K	20 min/200K (±SPECT)	20 min/100K	10 min (at 3 hours); 20 min/1M (±SPECT)	head & neck: 10-15 min/300K (at 4-24 hrs) & 15 min/200K (at 48 hrs) chest & abdomen: 10min/500K (±SPECT)

*^{131}I-iodomethylnorcholesterol *75 Se-selenomethylnorcholesterol ***0%-1.4% 125-I contamination †Patients allergic to iodine may be given potassium perchlorate 200 mg every 8 hours after meals or triiodothyronine 20 mg every 8 hours ‡No thyroid blockade (can be reduced to 1%-2% by iodide administration) DS = dexamethasone suppression K = thousand counts M = million counts (Kloos, RT., Khafali, F., Shapiro, B. and Gross, MD.) Chapter 10, Adrenal in Clinical Nuclear Medicine 3rd edition, MN. Maisey, KE. Britton, BD. Collier, 1998 EDS. Chapman and Hall Nuclear Medical London 1998, pp. 359, with permission.

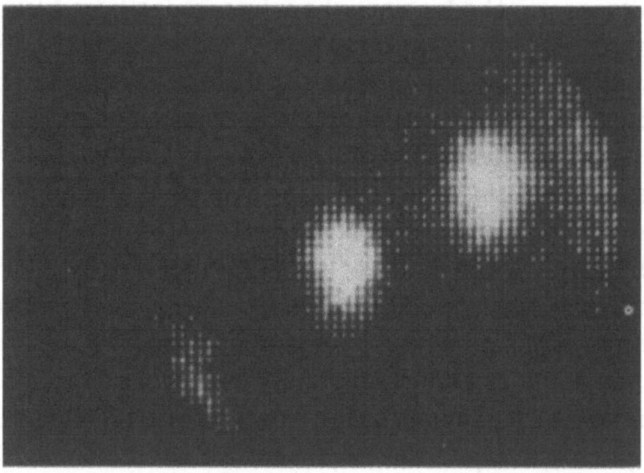

Figure 2. NP-59 scan in ACTH-dependent CS due to pituitary adenoma. Bilaterally symmetric, increased NP-59 uptake by the adrenals depicts adrenocortical hyperplasia from abnormal adrenocorticotrophic hormone secretion.

Table 3

Imaging Patterns in Cushing's Syndrome (without dexamethasone suppression)

Scintigraphic Pattern	Type of Cushing's Syndrome
Bilateral symmetrical imaging	ACTH dependent; hypothalamic; pituitary Cushing's disease; ectopic ACTH syndrome; ectopic CRF syndrome
Bilateral asymmetrical imaging	ACTH independent nodular hyperplasia* (However all causes listed above may rarely cause asymmetrical hyperplasia)
Unilateral imaging	Adrenal adenoma**; adrenal remnants†; ectopic adenocortical tissue†
Bilateral nonvisualization	Adrenal carcinoma **‡; severe hypercholesterolemia††

* Almost always asymmetrical

** Cortisol secreting lesions suppress tracer uptake INTO contralateral gland

† Usually only one focus present, occasionally more than one focus may be present in ectopic locations or metastatic sites

†† A potential cause for interference with the effectiveness of study

‡ Very rarely tumors (and metastases) may accumulate sufficient tracer to image

Hypersecretory adrenocortical adenomas show intense ipsilateral tracer uptake in the adenoma and suppression or absent uptake in the contralateral normal cortex as a result of pituitary ACTH suppression (1,2,4,15,17) (Figure 3). Scintigraphy may be useful in the functional characterization of adrenal masses in ACTH-independent CS due to either carcinoma or adenoma. Adrenalectomy is indicated in either case, and a pre-operative, anatomic imaging procedure may appear helpful to identify local tumor invasion or metastases in the case of carcinoma. However, while CT is very sensitive in identifying adenomas and carcinomas (100%), it often (in up to 40% of cases) fails to identify the bilateral nature of ACTH-independent adrenocortical hyperplasia, where the largest hyperplastic nodule is often misdiagnosed as a unilateral adenoma (1,2,4,15,17,18). Radiocholesterol scintigraphy however, clearly depicts bilateral, frequently asymmetrical, imaging and hence hyperfunction in these cases (1,2,4,6,7,15) (Figure 4). Despite the exquisite resolution afforded by CT and MR, adrenocortical scintigraphy remains the best modality to locate adrenal cortical remnants leading to recurrent Cushing's syndrome after bilateral adrenalectomy (1,2,4,15,17).

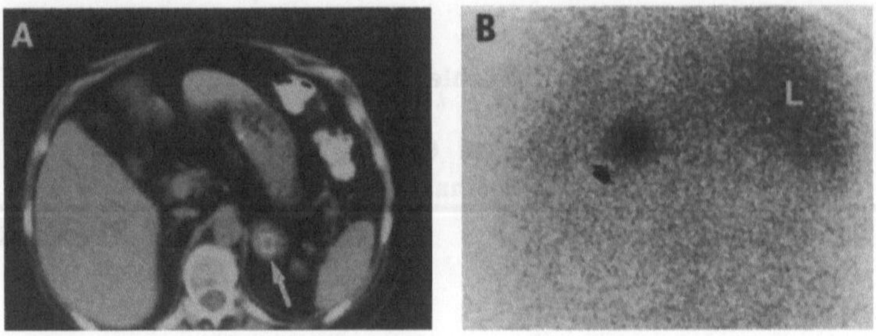

Figure 3. Abdominal CT (A) and posterior abdominal NP-59 scans in ACTH-independent Cushing's syndrome due to an adrenocortical adenoma (arrow). The contralateral right adrenal cortex is not seen as a result of suppression of pituitary adrenocorticotrophic hormone secretion (L=liver). (Fig, LM, et al.: Adrenal localization in the adrenocorticotrophic hormone-independent Cushing's syndrome. Ann.Intern.Med. 1988;109:547-553. with permission).

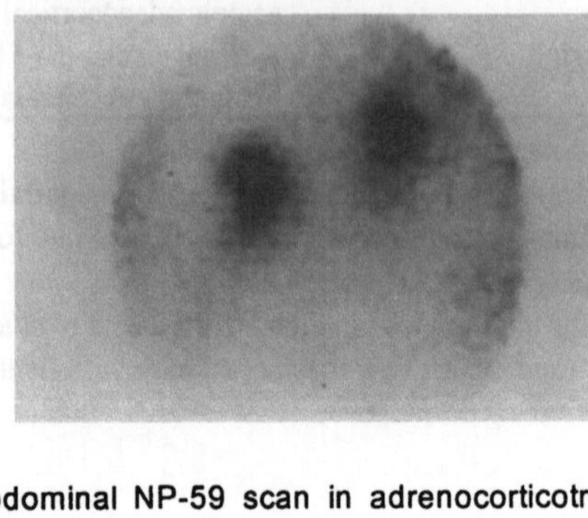

Figure 4. Posterior abdominal NP-59 scan in adrenocorticotrophin-independent CS due to cortical nodular hyperplasia. Bilaterally increased and occasionally asymmetric NP-59 uptake may be seen in this variant of CS.

Primary Aldosteronism

Baseline (non-dexamethasone suppression) adrenocortical scintigraphy in primary aldosteronism (PA) depicts patterns of asymmetrical uptake in adenoma (Conn's tumor) and symmetrically increased iodocholesterol uptake in bilateral hyperplasia (1,4,18,19,20) (Table 4). Differences from normal may be subtle, and estimations of uptake may prove useful in PA (2,4,6,7,15). Baseline imaging, however has suboptimal sensitivity in PA due to high background radioactivity in the inner adrenal cortex. Administration of dexamethasone prior to NP-59 will suppress ACTH and thus reduce ACTH-dependent adrenocortical uptake to enhance the sensitivity of imaging. "Early visualization" before the 5th day post-injection is abnormal, and normal adrenal glands are not visualized before this time interval using this DS regimen (2,4,14,19).

Before day 5 post-injection PA due to adenoma and unilateral hyperplasia (albeit an unusual, but previously reported condition in PA) is visualized as a unilateral focus of NP-59 uptake (Figure 5). Bilateral hyperplasia is characterized by bilateral uptake, either symmetrical or asymmetrical in the case of asymmetrical hyperplasia (which may be erroneously interpreted on CT as a unilateral adenoma) (Figure 6).

While CT is generally effective in positively localizing most adenomas in PA, bilateral hyperplasia is often inferred by the "absence" of an adenoma. Small adenomas not readily depicted by CT may be correctly located by NP-59 scintigraphy and this technique thus retains considerable utility in characterization of primary aldosteronism when used in combination with biochemical evaluation which includes aldosterone levels, aldosterone/renin ratios, postural effects on aldosterone and renin and aldosterone precursor and metabolite levels (2,4,19).

Table 4
Imaging Patterns in Aldosteronism
(With Dexamethasone Suppression)

Scintigraphic Pattern	Type of Aldosteronism
Symmetrical bilateral early imaging (before day 5)	Bilateral autonomous hyperplasia; secondary aldosteronism†
Unilateral early imaging (before day 5)	Unilateral adenoma (Conn's tumor) unilateral malignant aldosterone secreting tumor (rare)
Symmetrical late imaging (on or after day 5); nondiagnostic pattern	Normal adrenals; dexamethasone suppressible aldosteronism (rare)

† Should be excluded by measurement of renin and aldosterone levels and should not require imaging

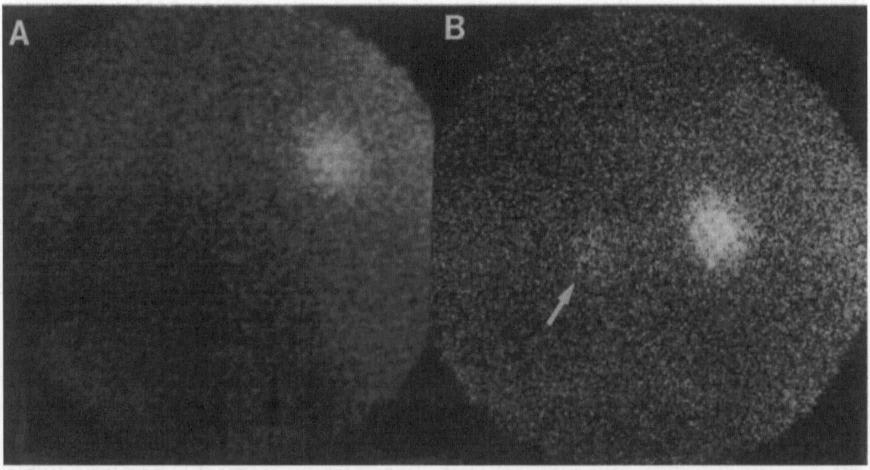

Figure 5. Posterior abdominal scans performed on dexamethasone suppression in primary aldosteronism at 3 days (A) and 5 days (B) post injection of NP-59. Focal uptake is seen in the right adrenal on both studies and faint accumulation of NP-59 is seen in the normal left adrenal cortex (arrow) on the late 5 day post injection image.

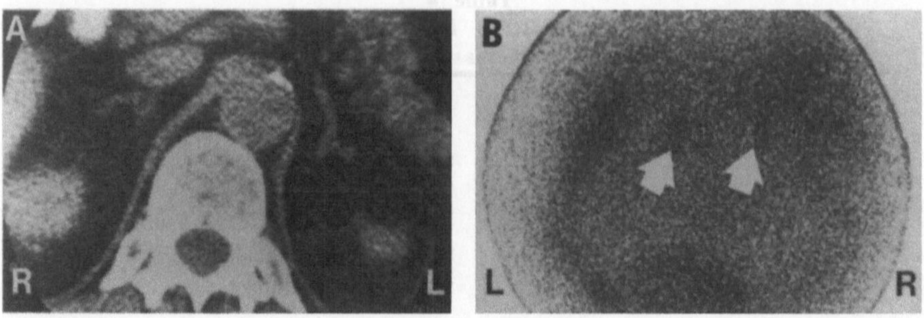

Figure 6. Abdominal CT (A) and posterior abdominal NP-59 scans (B) performed on dexamethasone suppression in primary aldosteronism due to bilateral adrenal hyperplasia. Normal adrenal glands are depicted on the CT scan and abnormal bilateral adrenal NP-59 uptake (arrows) is seen on the day 3 post injection scan. (Gross, MD and Shapiro B. Scintigraphic studies in adrenal hypertension. Semin.Nucl.Med. 1989; 19: 122-143. with permission).

It is critical that a firm biochemical diagnosis of PA be made before any attempts at localization. Secondary hyperaldosteronism has been shown to result in a bilateral pattern of imaging indistinguishable from that seen in primary bilateral hyperplasia (1,2,4,14). Drugs which may alter the renin-angiotensin-aldosterone axis must be omitted prior to biochemical and imaging evaluations. Diuretics, spironolactone, amiloride and other drugs may falsely create a scintigraphic appearance of bilateral hyperplasia in the setting of PA due to an adrenal adenoma (1,4,6,14). Unusual variants of PA such as bilateral nonvisualization of the adrenal glands may occur in PA, due to an adrenal malignancy or DS remediable PA where a return to normal blood pressure while on DS suggests this as a possible diagnosis.

Adrenal Hyperandrogenism

Adrenal hyperandrogenism yields patterns of imaging strikingly similar to those seen in PA. (2,4,14,18). When hyperandrogenism results from impaired cortisol synthesis (e.g., 21-hydroxylase deficiency), baseline imaging depicts the ACTH-dependent bilateral adrenal hyperfunction which may normalize with DS (14).

Adrenal adenomas causing hyperandrogenism image as markedly asymmetric (on baseline) or unilateral (on DS) foci of NP-59 uptake. The adrenal component of the polycystic ovary syndrome can also be depicted by iodocholesterol scintigraphy. In these patients the level of uptake achieved may approach that seen in ACTH dependent CS (21).

Non-hypersecretory, Incidentally Discovered Adrenal Masses

Not unlike the use of radioiodine to distinguish benign from potentially malignant thyroid masses, adrenocortical scintigraphy can be used to depict the function (or lack of function) of adrenocortical tissues in patients with euadrenal, incidentally discovered adrenal masses (1,2,3,18,22,23).

The extensive use of CT scanning discloses adrenal mass lesions ("incidentalomas") in 0.55-5% of patients without clinical evidence of adrenal disease (1-3,18,23). CT scans are most often performed for abdominal pain or in the diagnosis or staging of known or suspected non-adrenal malignancies (4,54). Adrenal metastases usually occur in the presence of wide tumor spread. However, some malignancies of lung and breast may develop early, with isolated adrenal metastases which may radically alter tumor staging and/or subsequent therapy. In a large fraction of patients, if not the majority, the adrenal mass is a benign adenoma. Morphology and size of the mass will often not characterize a lesion. Screening biochemistry must be performed to exclude subclinical CS, PA, adrenal hyperandrogenism, and pheochromocytoma. (2,4,22,23). If adrenal cortical and medullary function is normal, management of patients with incidentally discovered adrenal masses is controversial. Suggested approaches include resection of all masses >3.5-6 cm; serial CT follow-up with resection of masses showing growth; attempts at tissue characterization by MRI or on CT Hounsfield units; and CT-guided needle biopsy (2,3,18,23). The vast majority of incidentalomas are non-hypersecretory, benign adenomas and resection based solely upon size criteria (even for masses ≥5 cm) will lead to many unnecessary adrenalectomies. MRI tissue characterization is often nondiagnostic while needle biopsy is invasive, carries significant risks, and cytology may not distinguish adenoma from well differentiated adrenocortical carcinoma (18,23).

Adrenocortical scintigraphy can be used to characterize adrenal incidentalomas (1,23-27). Three imaging patterns have been described: 1) "Concordant imaging" in which the adrenal mass demonstrates increased NP-59 uptake by a benign, non-hypersecretory adrenal adenoma (Figure 7). The contralateral CT normal gland may show variable degrees of NP-59 suppression. Very rarely these "concordant" lesions may evolve over years towards autonomous cortisol hypersecretion, which is analogous to the natural history of many "warm" or "hot" thyroid nodules. 2) A "discordant pattern" with absent, decreased or distorted NP-59 uptake by the adrenal mass. Discordant lesions are the result of destructive, space occupying, or nonadenomatous lesions (Figure 8).

3) A "non-lateralizing" or normal "symmetrical" pattern of imaging of an adrenal mass on CT. If the mass is ≥2 cm in diameter, the lesion may be a pseudo or peri-adrenal mass arising from stomach, pancreas, kidney or other adjacent abdominal organs. Because of the limited spatial resolution of scintigraphy, some masses ≤2 cm reveal a non-lateralizing imaging pattern (1,3). Thus, for masses >2 cm, NP-59 scintigraphy is an efficacious, non-invasive technique to characterize incidentalomas (1,23-27). Because sensitivity falls modestly for lesions less than 2 cm and specificity is retained, the procedure may still provide important functional insight into the nature of even small adrenal masses (26).

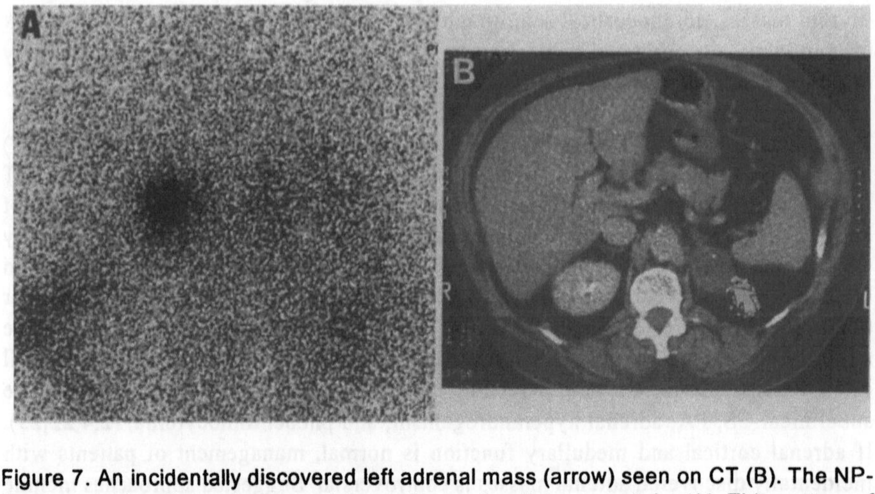

Figure 7. An incidentally discovered left adrenal mass (arrow) seen on CT (B). The NP-59 scan depicts the lesion as an intense focus of radiotracer uptake (A). This pattern of a mass on CT that demonstrates NP-59 uptake that is greater than the contralateral adrenal (in this case note that the right adrenal does not accumulate sufficient NP-59 to be visualized) is a concordant pattern of imaging and functionally characterizes the left adrenal mass as benign.

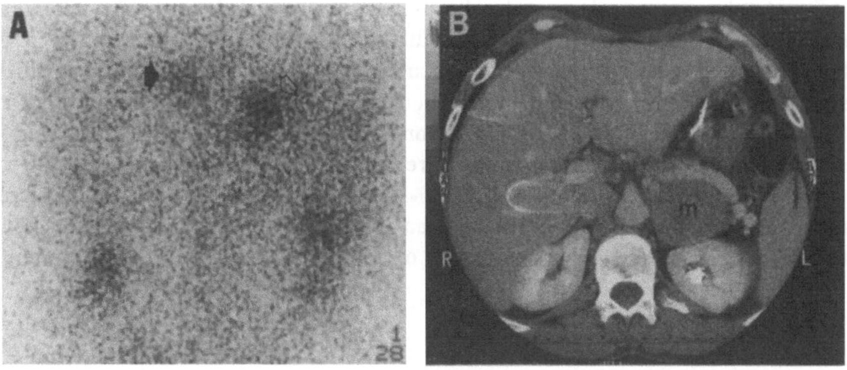

Figure 8. An incidentally discovered left adrenal mass seen on CT (B) done before biochemical investigation was completed. The NP-59 study (A) was performed for evaluation of a non-hypersecretory adrenal mass demonstrates cephalad displacement of the left adrenal (arrow) with less NP-59 uptake than the normal right gland representing a discordant pattern of imaging.

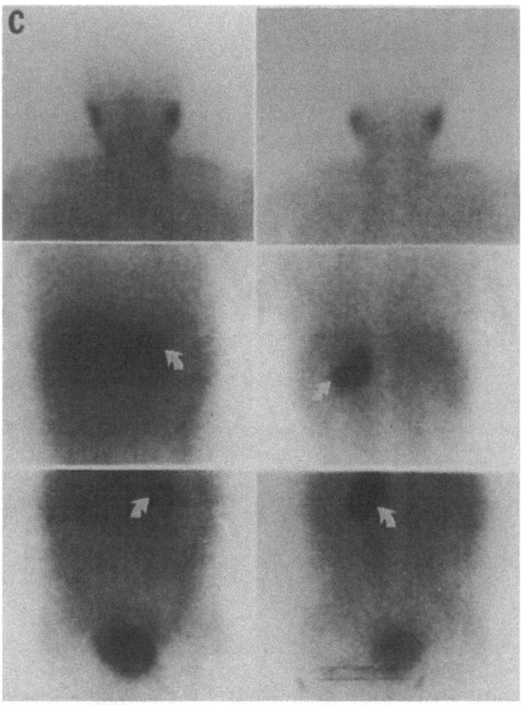

Figure 8. (C) Subsequently mildly abnormal catecholamine metabolites lead to a ^{123}I-MIBG which revealed the mass (arrow) to be a large pheochromocytoma (anterior left vertical column, posterior and right vertical column, scans of the neck and chest and upper and lower abdomen, respectively).

PET radiopharmaceuticals can also be used to distinguish benign from malignant adrenal masses based upon the accumulation of ^{18}F-fluorodeoxyglucose (^{18}F-FDG). The reliance of many malignancies upon anaerobic glycolysis as a primary means of energy production as opposed to more efficient aerobic metabolism can be depicted in vivo using ^{18}F-FDG (Figure 9). An inhibitor of adrenal steroid metabolism, etiomidate and metiomidate labeled with ^{11}C have recently been shown to image the adrenal cortex and adrenal neoplasms. Rapid (20-30 minutes post-injection), PET imaging with these agents may afford not only an insight into the functional status of an adrenal lesion, but allow characterization of adrenal masses as benign vs. malignant (12,23).

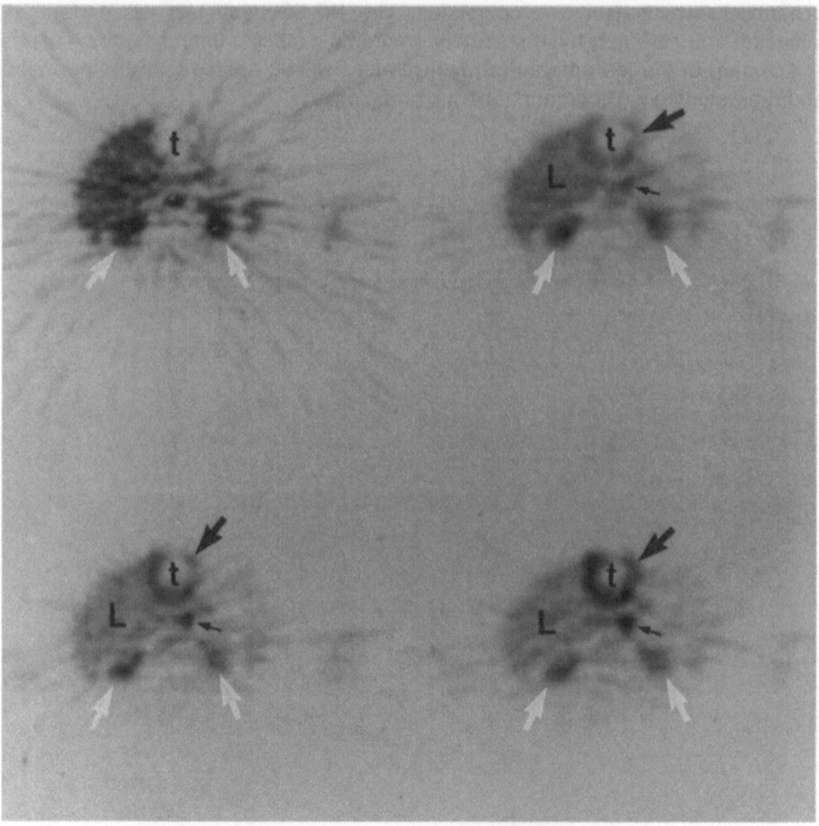

Figure 9. Sequential transverse abdominal ^{18}F-Fluorodeoxyglucose PET scans in metastatic adenocarcinoma of lung to liver and left adrenal. The liver metastasis (t) is depicted as an intrahepatic defect with a necrotic center and a rim of increasing ^{18}F-FDG accumulation (large black arrow). The adrenal metastasis (small black arrow) is also depicted as a focus of increasing ^{18}F-FDG uptake (L=liver, kidneys=white arrows).

Adrenomedullary Scintigraphy

Radiopharmaceuticals for Imaging Adrenomedulla Disease

Radiolabeled catecholamines and analogs were some of the first compounds evaluated as agents to image the adrenal medulla. ^{11}C-labeled dopamine demonstrated significant accumulation in the normal human adrenal medulla, in neuroblastoma and pheochromocytoma (26).

Radiolabeled enzyme inhibitors of catecholamine biosynthesis are another avenue for developing adrenal medullary imaging agents. Inhibitors of phenylethanolamine-N-methyltransferase have been developed and various tyrosine derivatives evaluated, but none has demonstrated sufficient uptake as a clinical adrenal medulla imaging agent (29).

Neuronal blocking agents offered another alternative to the development of clinically useful adrenal medullary imaging agents. Bretylium, demonstrated good adrenal medulla accumulation in the dog, but insufficient uptake in subsequent human studies (30). Guanethidine analogs were then investigated as potential adrenal medulla imaging agents and iodobenzylguanidine radioiodinated in the para and meta positions demonstrated avid adrenal medulla uptake in animal studies (31). The meta isomer demonstrated significantly more rapid uptake and lower background activity with less in vivo deiodination, metaiodobenzylguanidine (MIBG) has been shown to localize the normal adrenal medulla, adrenal medullary tumors and adrenal medullary hyperplasia (32-35) (Figure 10).

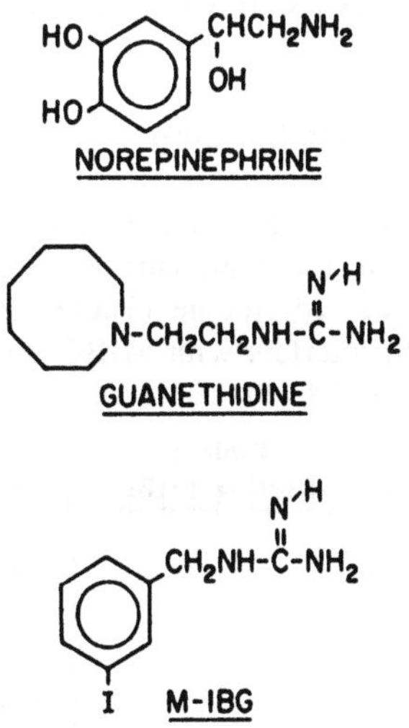

Figure 10. Comparison of structures of the endogenous neurotransmitter hormone norepinephrine, the hypotensive drug guanethidine and the radiopharmaceutical metaiodobenzylguanidine (MIBG). (Gross MD and Shapiro B: Scintigraphic studies in adrenal hypertension. Semin.Nucl.Med. 1989; 19: 122-143. with permission).

Accumulation of metaiodobenzylguanidine (MIBG) is thought to be through the cell membrane type I norepinephrine reuptake mechanism, with subsequent entry of MIBG into catecholamine storage vesicles of neuroendocrine tissues such as adrenergic nerve endings and adrenal medullary cells or tumors derived from them (36). This concept is supported by a series of experiments that indicate MIBG uptake can be reduced or prevented by pretreatment with reserpine, labetalol, a drug which inhibits catecholamine reuptake). The absence of an effect of phenoxybenzamine or propranolol means that clinical studies can be safely performed simultaneously with protective treatment for uncontrolled hypercatecholaminemia (i.e., alpha and beta adrenergic blockade) (33,36,37) (Table 5).

Hydroxyephedrine (HED), a norepinephrine analog has been labeled with ^{11}C for PET and is concentrated by adrenergic nerve terminals by the norepinephrine uptake mechanism (38). This was the first positron-emitting tracer of the adrenergic nervous system suitable for human studies (39). More recently, high specific activity ^{11}C-epinephrine has been synthesized, and early studies suggest that vesicular uptake of epinephrine is greater than that of HED (40). ^{11}C-epinephrine and HED may prove useful for localization of pheochromocytoma and functional characterization of the adrenal medulla and the cardiac sympathetic innervation (40).

Radiation Dosimetry

The clearance of radioiodinated MIBG from blood is rapid with approximately two-thirds of a dose is excreted into the urine in the first 24 hours after administration. The radiation dosimetry for ^{123}I and ^{131}I-MIBG is summarized in Table 2. Thyroid dosimetry is presented with and without iodide administration, and most of the absorbed dose is due to accumulation of radioiodine released by in vivo deiodination of MIBG

Procedures for Adrenomedulla Imaging

Pretreatment with Lugol's iodine or an equivalent preparation beginning 1 day before and continuing for 1 week after the administration of MIBG is important to block thyroidal accumulation of free radioiodine (Table 2). Other than the meticulous exclusion of drugs that might interfere with MIBG uptake no other pretreatment is required for MIBG scintigraphy (33,41) (Table 5).

Table 5
Drugs Affecting MIBG Uptake

Drug	Mechanism
Tricyclic antidepressants	Uptake inhibitor
Cocaine	Uptake inhibitor
Reserpine	Granule depletion Uptake inhibitor
Symphomimitics	Granule depletion
Phenothiazines	Uptake inhibitor
Butyrophenones	Uptake inhibitor
Thioxanthenes	Uptake inhibitor
Adrenergic inhibitors	Granule depletion
Labetalol	Uptake inhibitor Granule depletion
Calcium channel blockers	Unknown

A large-field-of-view gamma-camera equipped with a high-energy, parallel-hole collimator should be employed for ^{131}I-MIBG studies (Table 2). Studies with ^{123}I, require a low energy, high resolution collimator. Simultaneous acquisition of analog and digital images provides the best spectrum of images for MIBG studies. In suspected pheochromocytoma, the entire body is screened in scanning mode or with multiple overlapping anterior and posterior conjugate views to include the skull and the infra-pelvic region. Most pheochromocytomas will be visualized at 48 hours, but some variability in imaging necessitates 24, 48, and 72 hour scans following injection with ^{131}I-MIBG. Each image should contain between 50,000 and 100,000 counts. ^{123}I-MIBG provides excellent images early, 6 hours postinjection and late 24-hour images (Figure 11). Radioactive surface markers can be used for anatomic orientation, and when necessary, additional radiopharmaceuticals can be used to simultaneously image other abdominal organs for more specific anatomic localization. Scintigraphic depiction of the kidneys, liver, spleen, skeleton, cardiac blood pool, and/or left ventricular myocardium have all been used to aid in localization of neoplasms seen on MIBG scans (35,36,41,42).

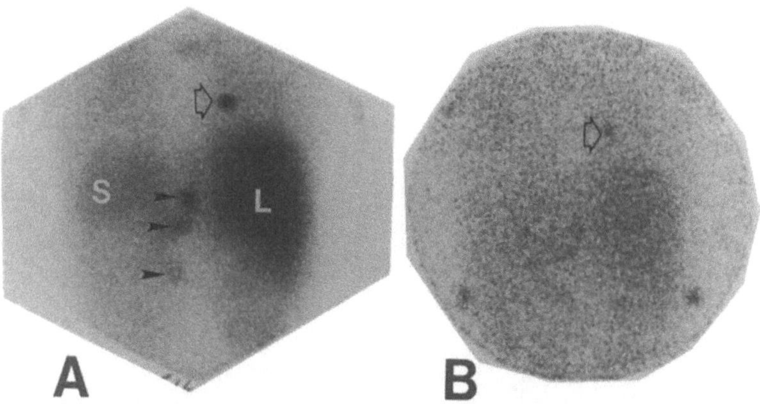

Figure 11. Comparison of posterior chest and abdomen images in malignant, metastatic pheochromocytoma. (A) ^{123}I-MIBG (10 mCi dose) done at 24 hr. post injection; (B) ^{131}I-MIBG (0.5 mCi dose) done at 24 hr. post injection. Improved sensitivity and quality of ^{123}I-MIBG over ^{131}I-MIBG is demonstrated. (Lynn M., et al., Pheochromocytoma and normal adrenal medulla: improved visualization with ^{123}I-MIBG scintigraphy. Radiology. 1985;156:789-792, with permission)

Normal Sympathomedulla Imaging with MIBG

Radioactivity from ^{131}I-MIBG is routinely seen in the salivary glands, liver, spleen, and bladder in normal subjects. Kidney uptake is early but usually transient. Variable amounts of radioactivity are seen in the heart and lungs. Free radioiodine will localize in the thyroid, stomach and in the colon on later images.

The normal adrenal medulla is infrequently and faintly visualized with ^{131}I-MIBG (less than 20% of cases at 48 hours) (35). In contrast to ^{131}I-MIBG the normal adrenal medulla is frequently seen on ^{123}I-MIBG studies, it is not however imaged on ^{11}C-HED-PET studies (39). Salivary gland, heart, liver, kidney, and bladder activity are seen in normal subjects (39).

Localization of Sympathomedulla Tumors

The majority of pheochromocytomas are sporadic and located within the adrenal gland(s) (41). When greater than 1.5 cm in diameter, pheochromocytomas are readily depicted by CT and MRI (43). As a "hot spot" imaging technique, MIBG scintigraphy detects both large and small pheochromocytomas and has the additional advantage of whole body screening that may locate multifocal (10% of cases) or metastatic (10% or more of cases) disease (33,35,41) (Figures 11,12,13).

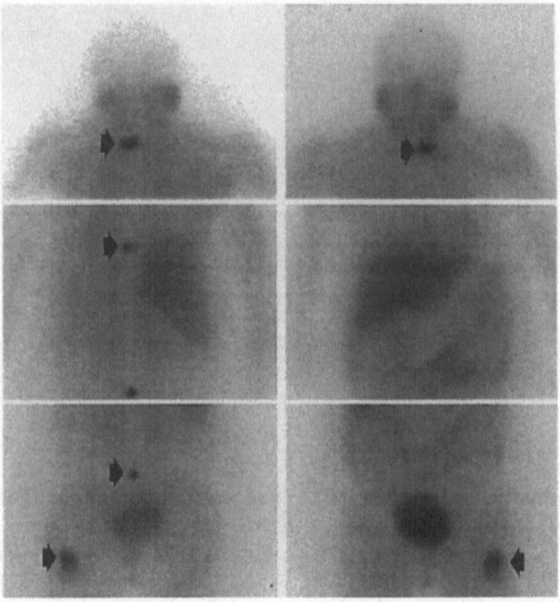

Figure 12. ^{123}I-MIBG body scan in widely metastatic malignant pheochromocytoma left vertical column-anterior and right vertical column-posterior head, neck, chest, abdomen and pelvis; arrows identify metastatic pheochromocytoma.

Metaiodobenzylguanidine scintigraphy is of particular value in the localization of extra-adrenal pheochromocytomas. These lesions occur at many locations from the base of the skull to the pelvis and are frequently not detected by CT because of size and close relationship to other structures (44) (Figure 14). Venous catecholamine sampling may suggest the level of a given lesion, but this is invasive and not a practical means of surveying the entire body (45).

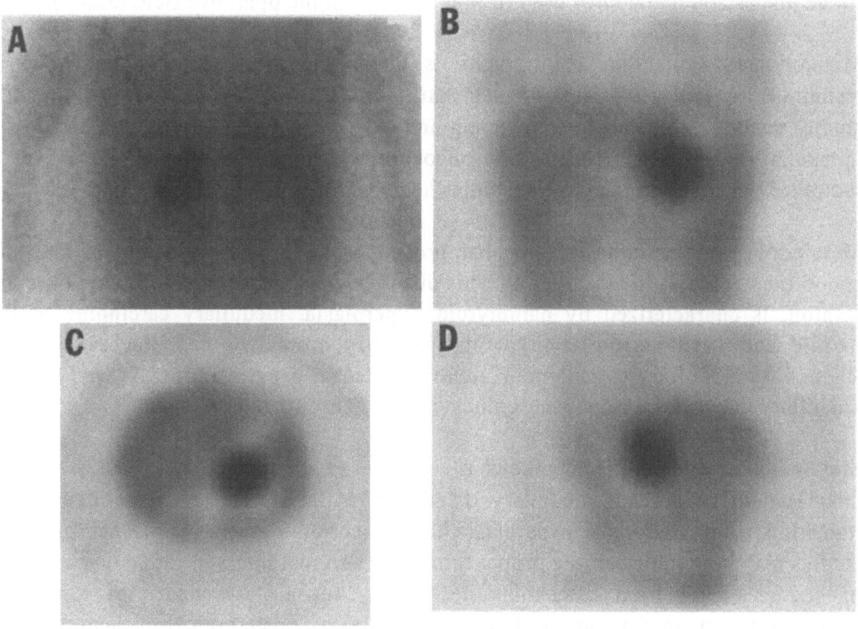

Figure 13. A large left adrenal pheochromocytoma is depicted on ^{123}I-MIBG scintigraphy. (A) Posterior chest and abdomen planar image; (B) coronal, (C) transaxial and (D) parasaggital projection SPECT images.

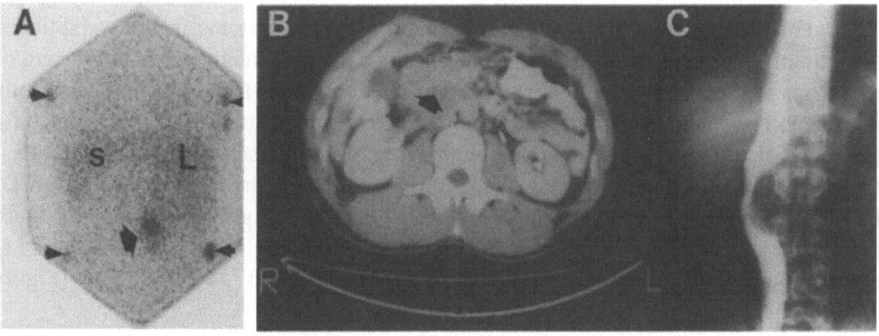

Figure 14. Familial extra-adrenal pheochromocytoma. (A) ^{131}I-MIGB scan of the posterior chest and abdomen (S=spleen, L=liver, arrowheads=surface markers, large arrow=right para-renal pheochromocytoma; (B) abdominal CT scan (arrow=right para-renal pheochromocytoma; (C) inferior venocavogram shows tumor indenting the vena cava. (Glowniak J., et al., Familial extra-adrenal pheochromocytoma: a new syndrome. Arch.Int.Med. 1985;145:257-261, with permission)

Both CT and MRI may fail to identify recurrence because of distorted anatomy and tissue planes and metal clips used for homeostasis in the operative field (33,41).

Metaiodobenzylguanidine scintigraphy is the single most sensitive and specific technique for evaluating sites of metastatic disease compared to other radionuclide studies such as bone and liver scanning and CT (36,46). The intense and prolonged uptake of ^{131}I-MIBG by metastatic pheochromocytoma has allowed its use as a radiotherapeutic agent, and initial studies have been promising in this regard (47).

Metaiodobenzylguanidine imaging has proven useful in the evaluation of multiple endocrine neoplasia (MEN) type II. This disorder, transmitted in autosomal dominant fashion, is characterized by parathyroid hyperplasia, medullary carcinoma of the thyroid, and adrenal medullary hyperplasia or pheochromocytoma in the case of MEN IIa, and by medullary carcinoma of thyroid, mucosal ganglioneuromata, and adrenal medullary hyperplasia or pheochromocytoma in MEN IIb.

Metaiodobenzylguanidine uptake has been used to depict the course of the development of adrenal medullary disease in MEN II, and may distinguish the transition from medullary hyperplasia to pheochromocytoma. Serial scintigraphic studies may help in discerning proper timing for surgical intervention to decrease risk of sudden death from catecholamine excess, but aid by means of functional characterization, in delaying as long as possible the post-surgical consequences of definitive bilateral adrenalectomy therapy, for the adrenal disease of MEN II. (34).

Patients with neurofibromatosis and Von Hippel Lindau disease have also been studied with MIBG scintigraphy. These patients have a somewhat increased incidence of pheochromocytoma and because of the difficulty of differentiation of pheochromocytoma from retroperitoneal neurofibromas and other tumors, functional imaging with MIBG has great utility and efficacy (48).

The role of MIBG imaging in the management of neuroblastoma is well-established (49). Scintigraphy has been shown useful for the detection, staging and monitoring of responses to therapy and in the distinction of residual tumor from scar. The technique is especially sensitive for detection of bone marrow metastases and highly specific (more so than bone scans anatomical imaging or other scintigraphic techniques) (Figure 15). In addition to locating pheochromocytomas ^{11}C-hydroxyephedrine (HED) has also been used for neuroblastoma (50). High quality PET images of these neoplasms can be obtained as early as 10 minutes following injection and images are comparable to SPECT images obtained after 24 hours with ^{123}I-MIBG (50) (Figure 16).

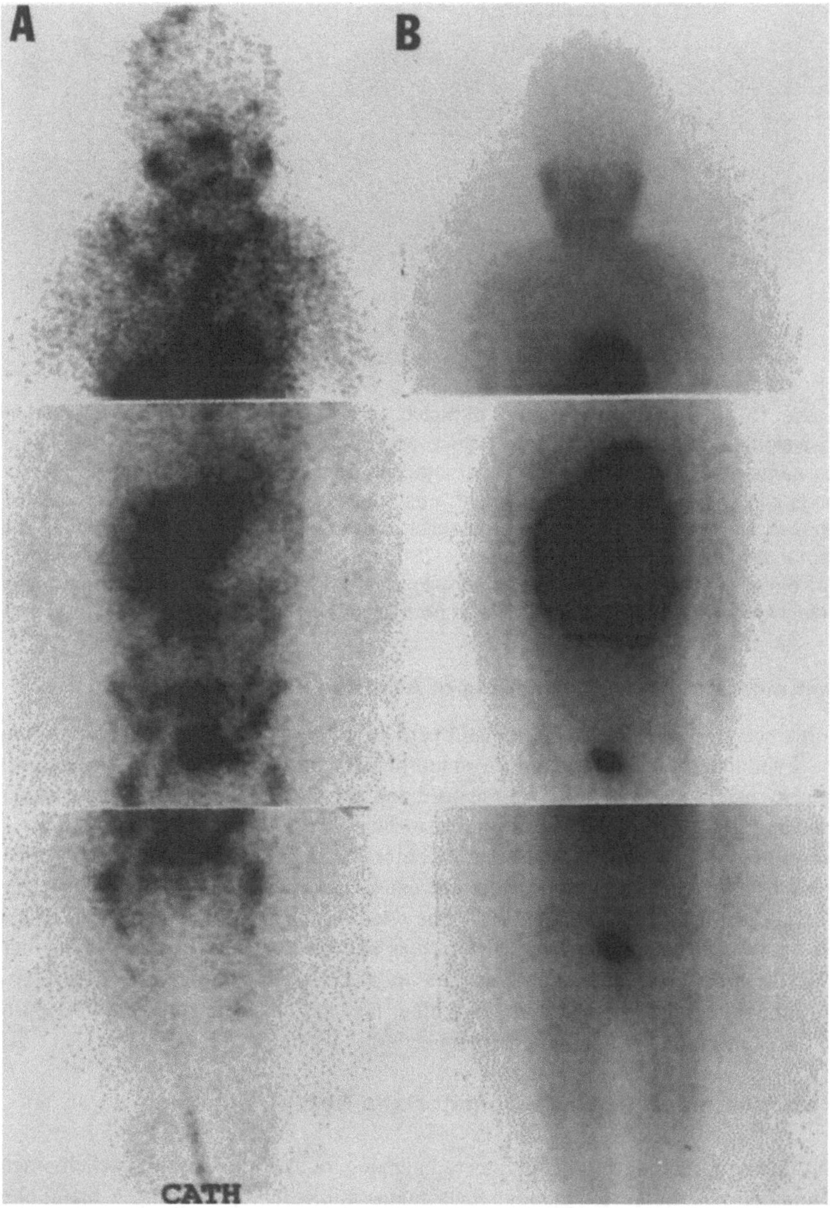

Figure 15. Whole body ^{123}I-MIBG scans done to monitor the response to chemotherapy in a patient with advanced neuroblastoma. (A) Pretherapy anterior images from head to mid-calf level demonstrate widespread tumor involvement. (B) Post therapy anterior images demonstrate excellent response as documented on this series of images.

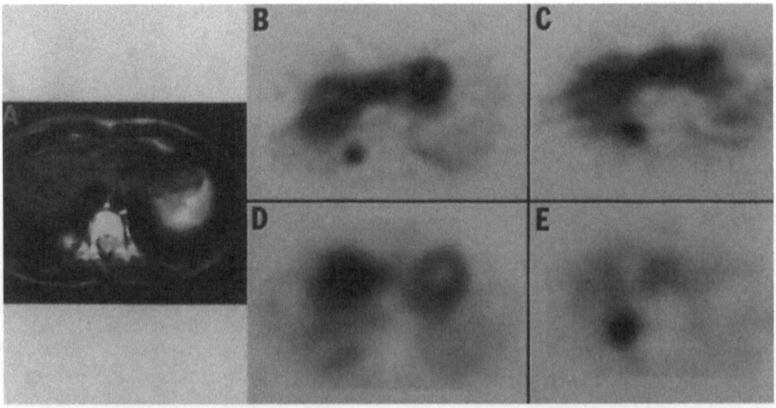

Figure 16. (A) A neuroblastoma is depicted as a mass with high signal intensity on a T2-weighted MRI scan of the lower chest and upper abdomen. (B) A ^{11}C-HED scan at the same level acquired 10 min. post injection demonstrates the tumor as a discrete focus of ^{11}C-HED uptake and (C) 1 hr. post injection. (D) No discernable ^{123}I-MIBG is seen in the mass at 10 min. post injection, but (E) at 24 hrs there is a focal uptake demonstrated by SPECT imaging. (Shulkin B., et al., PET scanning with hydroxyephedrine: a new approach to the localization of pheochromocytoma. J.Nucl.Med. 1992; 33: 1125-1131, with permission).

Somatostatin Receptor Imaging of Adrenal Disorders

Somatostatin is a 14 or 28 amino acid peptide with multiple functions; a hormone in the hypothalamic pituitary portal, enterohepatic portal and general circulations; a neurotransmitter in the brain, spinal cord and peripheral nervous system; a paracrine transmitter in the stomach, gut and elsewhere; an autocrine modulator of its own secretion; and a lymphocyte immune modulator. There are 5 subcategories of somatostatin receptor subtypes that are expressed on various tissues. The receptor-ligand complex may be internalized. The wide distribution of somatostatin receptors on many neuroendocrine and other tissues and tumors derived from them include pheochromocytoma and neuroblastoma in addition to a long list of benign and malignant neuroendocrine tumors and other lesions. This offers yet another approach to the scintigraphy of adrenal disorders.

Radiopharmaceuticals for Somatostatin Receptor Imaging

Synthesis of the long acting somatostatin analog, octreotide led to the development of a number of radiolabeled analogs for somatostatin receptor imaging. A metal chelate compound, DTPA-D-phe^1-octreotide, labeled with ^{111}In (^{111}In-pentetreotide) has been shown to scintigraphically localize a wide spectrum of neuroendocrine and non-neuroendocrine neoplasms and tissues which express somatostatin receptors to include pheochromocytoma and neuroblastoma (51). This tracer binds with greatest affinity for the type 2 and 5 subtypes of receptor (51,52).

Procedures for Somatostatin Receptor Imaging

With the exception of octreotide therapy, which should be stopped at least 24 hours before ^{111}In-pentetreotide scanning, other drugs do not generally affect uptake of the radiotracer. Good hydration and a mild laxative are recommended for a 24 to 48 hour imaging interval. Three to 6 mCi of ^{111}In-pentetreotide is administered intravenously. A gamma camera equipped with a medium energy collimator interfaced to a computer and set to detect the 2 primary photo peaks, 171 KEV and 245 KEV of ^{111}In is used to obtain the planar and SPECT images from the abdomen and other suspected affected sites (Table 2) (51,52).

Somatostatin Receptor Adrenal Imaging

The normal biodistribution of ^{111}In-pentetreotide is complex and includes; the kidneys, liver, gall bladder, bladder and gut. At times the thyroid can be visualized and , this finding has been ascribed to high concentration of somatostatin receptors on cells within the gland. Pheochromocytoma and neuroblastoma are depicted as foci of ^{111}In-pentetreotide uptake (Figures 17,18). SPECT is important in distinguishing neoplasms from background, especially in the upper abdomen, chest and in metastatic involvement of the liver (51,52) (Figure 17).

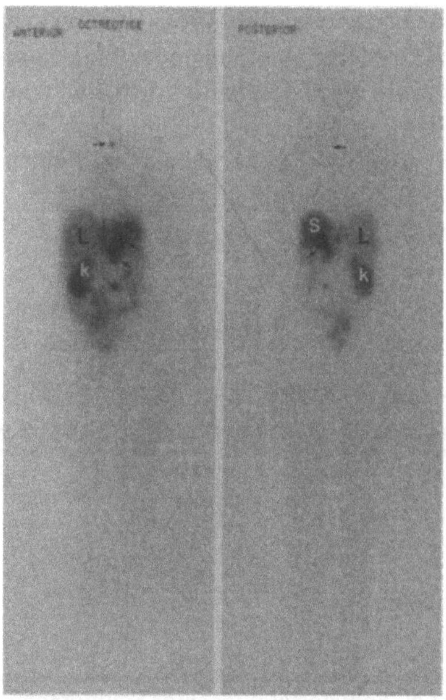

Figure 17. Metastatic pheochromocytoma is depicted on whole body ^{111}In-octreotide scans. Multiple retroperitoneal and liver metastases in addition to solitary supraclavicular lymph node metastases are identified (arrow). The left kidney is surgically absent. (L=liver, S=spleen, K=kidney).

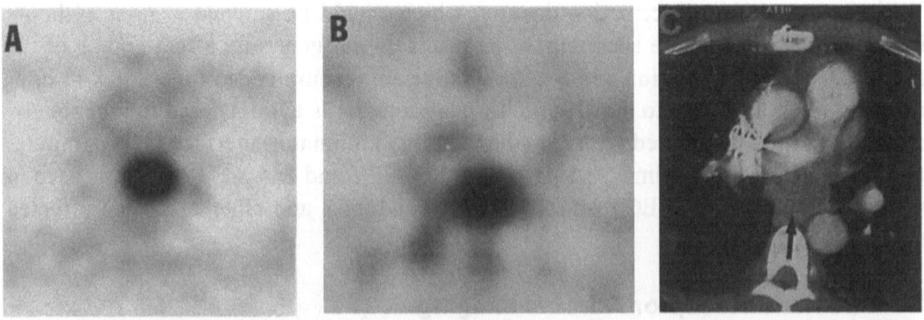

Figure 18. Comparative imaging in pheochromocytoma. (A) ^{18}F-FDG PET scan depicts a recurrent pericardiac pheochromocytoma as an intense focus of uptake in the chest. (B) ^{111}In-octreotide SPECT scan confirms the presence of this intrathorasic pheochromocytoma. (C) Transverse CT scan of the chest depicts a retrocardiac mass (arrow).

Comparative studies indicate that ^{111}In-pentetreotide and MIBG are comparable in the localization of intra-adrenal pheochromocytoma and neuroblastoma (Table 6). MIBG localizes metastatic pheochromocytoma and neuroblastoma somewhat better and with greater specificity than ^{111}In-pentetreotide (51). However, localization of carcinoid, medullary carcinoma of the thyroid, chemodectoma, paragangliomas and other neuroendocrine neoplasms are more frequently identified with ^{111}In-pentetreotide than MIBG (52). Very high doses (150 mCi on multiple occasions) of ^{111}In-DTPA-pentetreotide has been used for experimental radiopharmaceutical therapy of neuroendocrine tumors (53). The pure ß emitter ^{90}Y-DOTA-octreotide has also been developed for this purpose.

Table 6

Comparison of MIBG and In-111-pentetreotide Imaging of Neuroendocrine Neoplasms

Neoplasms	MIBG	Pentetreotide
Pheochromocytoma	86%	88%
Neuroblastoma	91%	89%
Paraganglioma	52%	100%
Medullary thyroid carcinoma	35%	71%
Carcinoid	70%	96%
Pancreatic Tumors	25%	80%

(From Krenning, EP, et al. Somatostatin receptor Scintigraphy with [^{111}In-DTPA-D-Phe^{1}] and [^{123}I-Tyr^{3}]-octreotide: The Rotterdam experience with more than 1000 patients. Eur. J. Nucl. Med. 20:716-731, 1993, with permission).

REFERENCES

1. Shapiro B, Gross MD. Adrenocortical Scintigraphy. (Chapter 64) In: Murray PS, Ell ICP (editors), Nuclear Medicine in clinical diagnosis and treatment (Volume 2), Churchill Livingston, Edinburgh UK, 1994, p. 737.
2. Gross MD, Falke THM, Shapiro B, Sandler MD. Adrenal glands. In: Sandler MD, Patton JA, Gross MD, Shapiro B, Falke THM, (editors), Endocrine Imaging, Appleton and Lange, Connecticut, 1992, p. 271.
3. Gross MD, Shapiro B, Bouffard JA, et al. Distinguishing benign from malignant euadrenal masses. Ann Int Med. 1988;109:613.
4. Shapiro B, Fig LM, Gross MD,, Khafagi F. Radiochemical diagnosis of adrenal disease. Crit Rev Clin Lab Sci. 1989;27:265.
5. Lynn MD, Gross MD, Shapiro B. Entero-hepatic circulation and distribution of I-131-6-iodomethyl-19-norcholesterol (NP-59). Nucl Med Comm. 1986;7:625.
6. Hawkins LA, Britton KE, Shapiro B. Selenium 75 selenomethyl cholesterol: A new agent for quantitative functional scintigraphy of the adrenals: Physical aspects. Brit J Radiol. 1980;53:833.
7. Shapiro B, Britton KE, Hawkins LA, Edwards CE. Clinical experience with 75 Se-selenomethyl-cholesterol adrenal imaging. Clin Endocrinol. 1981;15:19.
8. Liu B-L, Jin Y-T, Pan Z-Y, Minora M, Masaharu K. Radiobromine labeled cholesterol analogs; synthesis and tissue distribution of Bromine 82 labeled 6 Bromocholesterol. J Labl Comp Radiopharm. 1982;19:1089.
9. Hay RV, Flemming RM, Ryan JW, et al. Nuclear Imaging analysis of human low density lipoprotein biodistribution in rabbits and monkeys. J Nucl Med. 1991;32:1239.
10. Hay RV, Ryan JW, Williams KA, et al. Biodistribution parameters and radiation absorbed close estimates for radiolabeled human low density lipoprotein. In: Watson, EE, Schlafke-Stelson, AT (editors), Fifth International Radiopharmaceutical Dosimetry Symposium Proceedings of Oak Ridge Tennessee Conference May 7-10, 1991, US Department of Energy, 1992, p. 256.
11. Isaacsohn JL, Lees AM, Lees RS, Strauss HW, Barlai-Kovach M, Moore TJ. Adrenal Imaging with Technetium-99m-labeled low density lipoproteins. Metabolism 1986;35:364.
12. Boland GN, Goldberg MA, Lee MJ, et al. Intermediate adrenal mass in patients with cancer: evaluation at PET with 2[F-18]-fluoro-2-dioxy-D-glucose. Radiology 1995;194:131.
13. Bergstrom M,Bonasera TA, Bergstrom E, Backlin C, Juhlin C, Langstrom B. *In vivo* and *in vitro* primate evaluation of carbon 11-etiomidate and carbon-11-metomidate as potential tracers for PET imaging of the adrenal cortex and its tumors. J Nucl Med. 1998;39:982.
14. Gross MD, Walk TW, Swanson DP, et al. The role of pharmacologic manipulation in adrenal cortical scintigraphy. Semin Nucl Med. 1981;9:128.
15. Gross MD, Shapiro B, Beierwaltes WH. Functional characterization of the adrenal gland by quantitative scintigraphy. In: Winshell S, Lawrence J (editors), Recent Adv Nucl Med. Academic Press, 1983;6:83.
16. Shapiro B, Nakajo M, Gross MD, Freitas JE, Copp JE, Beierwaltes WH. Value of bowel preparation in adrenocortical scintigraphy with NP-59. J Nucl Med. 1983;24:732.
17. Fig LM, Gross MD, Shapiro B, et al. Adrenal localization in ACTH-independent Cushing's syndrome. Ann Intern Med. 1988;109:547.
18. Francis IR, Korobkin M, Quint L, Gross MD, Shapiro B. Integrated imaging of adrenal disease. Radiology 1992;182:1.

19. Gross MD, Thompson NW, Beierwaltes WH: Scintigraphic approach to the localization of adrenal lesions causing hypertension. Urologic Radiology 1982;3:241.
20. Gross MD, Shapiro B, Grekin RJ, et al. The scintigraphic localization of the adrenal lesion in primary aldosteronism. Am J Med. 1984;77:839.
21. Mountz EM, Gross MD, Shapiro B, et al. Scintigraphic localization of ovarian dysfunction I-131-6-ß-iodomethyl-norcholesterol (NP-59). J Nucl Med. 1988;29:1644.
22. Shapiro B, Gross MD. Functional imaging of the adrenal cortex. In: Bhatt HR, James VHT, Besser GM, Bottazzo GF, Keen H (editors). Advances in Thomas Addison's Diseases: Clinical developments in adrenal cortical disease and vitamin B12 deficiency (Volume 1), The Society for Endocrinology and the Thomas Addison Society, Page Brothers, Norwich, UK, 1994, p. 143.
23. Kloos RT, Gross MD, Francis IR, Korobkin M, Shapiro B. Incidentally discovered adrenal masses. Endocr Rev. 1995;16:460.
24. Gross MD, Shapiro B, Francis IR, Glazer GM, et al. Scintigraphic evaluation of clinically silent adrenal masses. J Nucl Med. 1994;35:1145.
25. Gross MD, Shapiro B, Francis IR, Bree RI, et al. Incidentally discovered bilateral adrenal masses. Eur J Nucl Med. 1995;22:315.
26. Kloos RT, Gross MD, Shapiro B, Francis IR, et al. The diagnostic dilemma of small incidentally discovered adrenal masses: a role for ^{131}I-6ß-Iodomethyl-norcholesterol (NP-59) scintigraphy. World J Surgery. 1997;21:36.
27. Dwamena B, Kloos RT, Fendrick AM, Gross MD, et al. Diagnostic evaluation of the adrenal incidentaloma decision and cost effectiveness analyses. J Nucl Med. 1998;39:707.
28. Lieberman LM, Beierwaltes WH, Varma VM, Weinhold P, Ling R. Labeled dopamine concentration in human adrenal medulla and in neuroblastoma. J Nucl Med. 1969;10:93.
29. Yu T, Wieland DM, Brown LE, Beierwaltes WH. Synthesis of radiolabeled inhibitors of phenylethanol-amine-N-methyltransferase. J Labeled Compd. 1979;16:173.
30. Korn N, Buswink A, Yu T, Carr EA, Carroll M, Counsell RE. A radioiodinated bretylium analog as a potential agent for scanning the adrenal medulla. J Nucl Med. 1977;18:87.
31. Wieland DM, Wu JL, Brown LE, Mangner TJ, Swanson DP, Beierwaltes WH. Radiolabeled adrenergic neuron blocking agents: Adrenal medulla imaging with (^{131}I) iodobenzylguanidine. J Nucl Med. 1980;21:349.
32. Wieland DM, Brown LE, Tobes MD, et al. Imaging the primate adrenal medulla with ^{123}I and ^{131}I metaiodobenzylguanidine. J Nucl Med. 1981;22:358.
33. Sisson JD, Frager MS, Valk TW, et al. Scintigraphic localization of pheochromocytoma. N Engl J Med. 1981;305:12.
34. Valk TW, Frager MS, Gross MD, et al. Spectrum of pheochromocytoma in multiple endocrine neoplasia: A scintigraphic portrayal using ^{131}-I-metaiodobenzylguanidine. Ann Intern Med. 1981;94:762.
35. Nakajo M, Shapiro B, Copp J, et al: The normal and abnormal distribution of the adrenomedullary imaging agent I-131-metaiodobenzylguanidine (^{131}I-MIBG) in man: Evaluation by scintigraphy. J Nucl Med. 1983;24:672.
36. Shapiro B, Wieland DM, Brown, LE, Nakajo M, Sisson JC, Beierwaltes WH. ^{131}I-meta-iodobenzylguanidine. (MIBG) adrenal medullary scintigraphy: interventional studies. In: Spencer RP, ed. Interventional Nuclear Medicine. New York: Grune, Stratton, p. 451, 1983.
37. Khafagi FA, Shapiro B, Fig LM, Mallette S, Sisson JC. Labetalol reduces iodine-131 MIBG uptake by pheochromocytoma and normal tissues. J Nucl Med. 1989;30:481.
38. Schwaiger M, Kalff V, Rosenspire KC, et al. The noninvasive evaluation of the sympathetic nervous system in the human heart by PET. Circulation 1990;82:457.

39. Shulkin BL, Wieland DM, Schwaiger M, et al. PET scanning with hydroxyepinephrine: An approach to the localization of pheochromocytoma. J Nucl Med. 1992;33:1125.
40. Chakraborty PK, Gildersleeve DL, Jewett DM., et al. High yield synthesis of high specific activity R-(-) {11C}16 epinephrine for routine PET studies in humans. Nucl Med Biol. 1993;20:939.
41. Shapiro B, Sisson JC, Beierwaltes WH. Experience with the use of 131-I-metaiodobenzylguanidine for locating pheochromocytomas. In: Raynaud C, ed. Nuclear Medicine and Biology. Vol. II. Paris: Pergamon Press, 1982: p. 1265.
42. Lynn MD, Shapiro B, Sisson JC, et al. Portrayal of pheochromocytoma and normal human adrenal medulla by ^{123}I-metaiodobenzylguanidine ^{123}I-MIBG. J Nucl Med. 1984;25:436.
43. Manger W, Gifford RW Current concepts of pheochromocytoma. Cardiovasc Med. 1978;12:289.
44. Shapiro B, Sisson JC, Kalff V, et al. The location of middle mediastinal pheochromocytomas. J Thorac Cardiovasc Surg. 1984;87:814.
45. Shapiro B, Sisson JC, Lloyd RV, et al. A newly described type of familial pheochromocytoma: Fulfilling the possibilities. Clin Res. 1982;30:721A.
46. Shapiro B, Sisson JC, Lloyd R, Satterlee W, Beierwaltes WH. Malignant pheochromocytoma: Clinical, biochemical and scintigraphic characterization. Clin Endocrinol.1984;20:189.
47. Sisson JD, Shapiro B, Beierwaltes WH et al. Radiopharmaceutical treatment of malignant pheochromocytoma. J Nucl Med. 1984;25:197.
48. Kalff V, Shapiro B, Lloyd R, et al. The spectrum of pheochromocytoma in hypertensive patients with neurofibromatosis. Arch Intern Med. 1982;142:2092.
49. Shulkin BL, Shapiro B, Radioiodinated metaiodobenzylguanidine in the management of neuroblastoma. In: Pochedly C, ed. Neuroblastoma. Boca Raton, FL: CRC Press, 1990: p. 171.
50. Shulkin Bl, Wieland DM, Baro ME, et al. PET studies of neuroblastoma with carbon 11-hydroxyephedrine. J Nucl Med. 1993;33:220.
51. Krenning EP, Kwekkeboom DJ, Bakker WH, Breeman WAP, et al. Somatostatin receptor scintigraphy with [^{111}In-DTPA-d-Phe^{1}] and ^{123}-I-Tyr^{3}} - octreotide: The Rotterdam experience with more than 1,000 patients. Eur J Nucl Med. 1994;21:545.
52. Hoefnagel CA Metaiodobenzylguanidine and somatostatin in oncology: Role in the management of neural crest tumors. Eur J Nucl Med. 1994;21:561.
53. Stolz B, Weckbecker G, Smith-Jones PM, Albert R, Raulf F, Bruns, C.The somatostatin receptor-targeted radiotherapeutic [^{90}Y-DOTA-d-Phe1,Tyr^{3}] octreotide (^{90}Y-SMT 487) eradicates experimental rat pancreatic tumors. Eur J Nucl Med. 1998;25:668.

10
ADRENAL INCIDENTALOMAS

Massimo Terzolo, M.D.
Giangiacomo Osella, M.D.
Anna Alì, M.D.
Alberto Angeli, M.D.
Università di Torino,
Turin, Italy.

INTRODUCTION

In the heyday of high-tech medicine, routine use of sophisticated radiological techniques frequently results in the incidental discovery of an adrenal mass. The unexpected finding of an adrenal mass offers the possibility of presymptomatic diagnosis and, therefore, early treatment of a potentially dangerous disease. However, the quintessence of the problem is whether or when an incidental adrenal mass puts the patient at increased risk for an unfavorable outcome (1). From the estimated prevalence of clinically significant adrenal tumors in the general population, it can be predicted that the excess morbidity and mortality resulting from an unexpected adrenal mass will be actually low (2). However, this estimate could not be entirely accurate and possibly underrated, because a number of assumptions were based on autopsy or population series, which were both geographically and demographically limited (2-5). The other important question is whether early diagnosis and treatment is more effective in presymptomatic patients and whether the beneficial effects justify the costs. Studies on this issue are subject to lead-time bias, which refers to fictitious extension of life due to an anticipated time of diagnosis and not to true prolongation of survival (1). The financial aspects of this problem have to be carefully weighted since the detection of adrenal masses, as incidental findings, will be progressively increasing with further radiological advancements.

The optimal use of radiological and laboratory procedures requires a reasonable estimate of the disease prevalence and high power of available diagnostic tests. In a study population presenting with non-specific signs, such as patients with an incidentally discovered adrenal mass, the predictive values of various screening tests can be considerably different from those obtained in a population with a high pre-test probability of disease, like patients presenting with typical clinical features (6).

Despite the abundance of recently published specific literature, the above-mentioned considerations highlight the many uncertainties associated with the diagnosis and management of adrenal incidentalomas. Adrenal incidentalomas were indeed considered as “very rare” in a paper of Lewinsky and collegues in 1974 (7), but in the last years this view has completely changed to the point that they were even regarded as a new endocrine epidemic (8).

The purpose of this chapter is to address some "hot" topics on adrenal incidentalomas. For a more comprehensive overview, the reader is referred to a number of excellent reviews (1,9-11).

Epidemiology

Current prevalence of unsuspected adrenal masses is approximately 3-4% in abdominal computed tomography (CT) scan series (12,13). This rate is likely to be underestimated because adrenal adenomas were found in approximately 10% of autopsies of subjects not suspected of having adrenal disease during life (9,11). However, inconsistent tumor classification systems have significant impact on the description of small lesions. Consequently, there is wide variation in the reported prevalence in autopsy series (9,14). Adrenal incidentaloma is an "umbrella" definition applying to many different pathologies sharing the same modality of discovery. The great heterogeneity of adrenal incidentalomas represents a problem for useful comparison of different series and explains why epidemiological data, often obtained using meta-analyses, have resulted in wide ranges of prevalence for any tumor type (9). Such variability in the reported estimates can be explained by the small sample size of the studies in which they were obtained.

Most of the epidemiological data that will be herewith presented are derived from a multi-institutional survey performed in Italy, which collected 1004 cases between 1980 and 1995 (15). The limit of the retrospective, multicenter design did not restrain us from drawing some interesting conclusions. In agreement with previous studies, the prevalence of adrenal incidentalomas was highest between 50 and 60 years of age (9,16). This pattern merely reflects a higher number of diagnostic procedures in these age decades or is the consequence of the aging process of the adrenal glands, which may be characterized by increased formation of adrenocortical nodules secondary to vascular changes (17). The higher prevalence in women could be explained by referral bias (i.e. more imaging studies in women due to higher prevalence of biliary disease) as in autopsy series non-functioning adrenal adenomas occurred as frequent in males as in females (18,19). Taking into account the possibility of selection bias, the prevalence of hypertension (41%), obesity (28%) and diabetes (10%) in this cohort of adrenal incidentalomas did not seem significantly higher than that found in the general Italian population matched for age (15). The possible association of silent adrenal masses and hypertension, diabetes or obesity is a debated issue that should be clarified by prospective evaluation of large series (9,10,14,20). The size of the adrenal masses estimated by CT ranged from 0.5 to 25 cm (median 3.0 cm) although most lesions were less than 4.0 cm (15). Among the 1004 patients, 380 underwent adrenalectomy and the most frequent histological diagnoses are given in Figure 1. Obviously, the frequency of adrenal carcinoma and pheochromocytoma was overestimated, because this cohort of patients was selected from the overall series of patients . In the literature, the frequency of adrenal carcinoma among incidentalomas ranged between 0-25%, that of pheochromocytoma between 0-11% and that of secondary malignancy from extra-adrenal primary neoplasms between 0-21% in non-oncological series and between 32-73% in oncological patients (9).

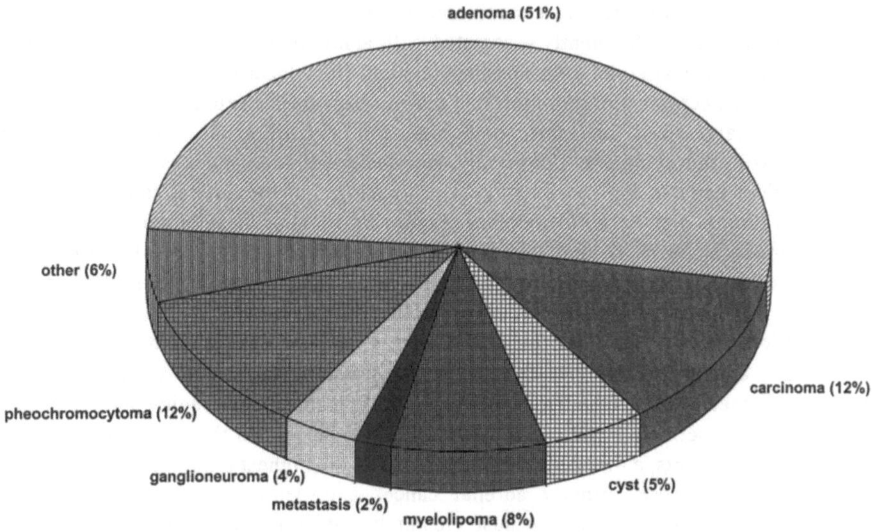

Figure 1. Italian survey on adrenal incidentaloma: histological diagnoses in the 380 patients who underwent adrenalectomy.

Incidental detection of an adrenal malignancy

The first consideration in a patient presenting with an adrenal incidentaloma is to exclude malignancy, although primary or secondary malignant adrenal tumors occur very infrequently. Primary adrenal carcinoma is an aggressive tumor, which prognosis is far better in early stages (21,22). Therefore, this tumor has to be actively searched for. The unexpected discovery of an adrenal metastasis may be less appealing in terms of possible benefit for the patient as it usually heralds advanced neoplastic disease. The primary tumors are most commonly carcinomas arising from breast, lung, or kidney; melanoma or lymphoma represent other possibilities (23,24). These tumors usually do not escape detection by routine diagnostic work-up. A subtler problem is to assess the secondary nature of an adrenal mass in patients with a known extra-adrenal tumor but no other evidence of metastatic disease, as this will result in a different tumor management. In our opinion, however, an adrenal mass detected in the course of tumor staging should not be considered as incidental and many of the relevant diagnostic considerations for adrenal incidentalomas do not fully apply to these tumors.

In the Italian survey, primary adrenocortical carcinoma was not rare. However, the majority of incidentalomas were benign (15). The low rate of adrenal metastases largely depended on the exclusion of patients with known extra-adrenal neoplasms. The outcome of this study has lead to the assumption that primary adrenocortical carcinoma is the most common incidental adrenal malignancy in non-oncological patients. Even assuming that all non-operated lesions were benign, the overall frequency of adrenal carcinoma was approximately 4%. This figure fits well with a recent meta-analysis reporting 26 primary adrenal malignancies over 630 incidentalomas (median 4%, range 0-25%) (25). In the Italian experience, adrenocortical carcinoma occurred at younger age without gender predominance and was frequently associated with abdominal pain at presentation, either as dull pain or typical colic. Pain possibly resulted from local infiltration, intratumoral hemorrhage or necrosis. Large tumor size did not necessarily explain all complaints of pain, since large-sized pheochromocytomas and myelolipomas were not closely associated with this symptom. Conversely, adrenocortical adenoma was more frequently found in older patients and in women (15). On average, adrenocortical carcinomas were the largest tumors among incidentalomas (Figure 2). Most of these tumors were already in MacFarlane stage II-III, and this finding dampens the enthusiasm of a precocious diagnosis of adrenal carcinoma through the incidental detection of an adrenal mass. The probability for an adrenal incidentaloma of being a primary adrenal malignancy increases as a function of tumor size, but this correlation is far from perfect, as different adrenal lesions may appear as large masses (26). In the literature, there is no consensus on the threshold diameter below which a lesion may be safely considered benign and the critical cut-off has been set between 2.5 and 6.0 cm (2,12,16,26-30). In the cohort of surgically treated Italian patients, a threshold of 4.0 cm showed the highest sensitivity (93%) for the discrimination between primary adrenal cancer and benign lesions. However, the specificity of this value was low because the number of benign lesions still exceeded that of malignant ones at this threshold value (15).

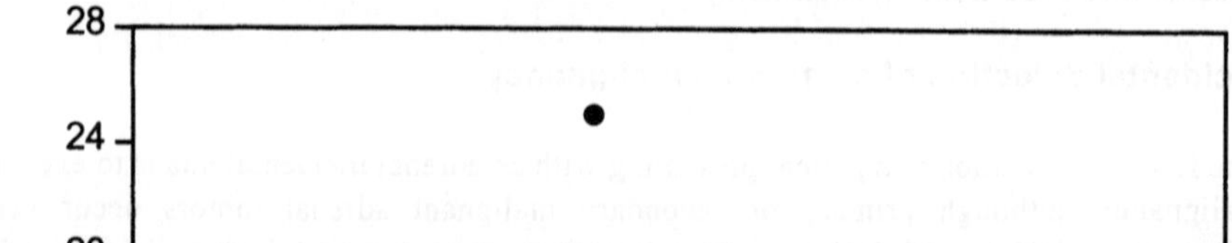

Figure 2. Italian survey on adrenal incidentaloma: distribution of mass size (CT estimate) by histology.

Small-sized adrenocortical carcinomas occur infrequently but it is obvious that at an early stage of development they are still tiny. The smallest cancer in the Italian group was of 2.6 cm (15). It is therefore advisable to follow-up any incidentaloma, even when the optimal frequency for serial scanning and appropriate duration of follow-up are presently unknown (14,25,28,31). From the available follow-up studies, it can be shown that clinically significant mass growth has been infrequently observed. Usually, a benign tumor has been found in those cases (32,33).

Considering mass size only, complete separation between benign and malignant incidentalomas is impossible. However, other imaging features have gained importance as a result of an impressive technical evolution of radiology. In recent years, several studies have demonstrated high sensitivity and specificity for unenhanced CT scan and opposed-phase chemical-shift magnetic resonance imaging (MRI) in differentiating benign adrenal adenomas from other non-adenomatous lesions. These techniques use differences in fat content among adrenal masses, as demonstrated by the close correlation observed between lipid content in histological sections and either CT attenuation values or signal intensity loss on chemical shift MRI (34). Generally, adrenal adenomas are lipid-rich tumors, while adrenal carcinomas, metastases and other non-adenomatous lesions (except myelolipomas) are typically devoid of lipids (35). Lipid-rich adenomas show reduced attenuation values on unenhanced CT scan and a decrease in relative signal intensity using chemical shift MR.

There is considerable debate in the literature on the threshold of attenuation value on unenhanced CT scan for the diagnosis of a benign adenoma (9,14). Having compared data from historical series with their own, Korobkin and collegues concluded that an attenuation threshold value of 10 Hounsfield units, or less has an overall specificity of 96% and sensitivity of 73% for the diagnosis of adenoma (36). However, incidentalomas are usually found by CT scans performed with intravenous contrast enhancement not specifically tailored to evaluate adrenal glands. Regretfully, attenuation values on enhanced CT scan are less reliable. Nevertheless, it was demonstrated that a threshold of 30 Hounsfield units, or less on a delayed CT scan obtained one hour after routine enhanced CT had 100% specificity and 95% sensitivity for the correct diagnosis of an adrenocortical adenoma (37). The sensitivity and specificity of opposed-phase chemical-shift MRI in differentiating adenoma from other lesions were 94% and 100%, respectively (38). For the identification of an adenoma, the diagnostic accuracy for unenhanced CT and chemical-shift MRI in the same patients was very comparable (39). The small number of primary adrenal carcinomas evaluated in these radiological series makes additional studies necessary before more definite conclusions can be drawn on their clinical utility (9). In particular, early adrenocortical cancers smaller than 4.0 cm have not been studied into details. Hypothetically, a small, well-differentiated adrenal cancer may contain sufficient lipid to resemble an adenoma.

Iodocholesterol adrenal scintigraphy, usually employing $[^{131}I]$-6β-iodomethyl-norcholesterol (NP-59) as radiopharmaceutical, is another useful imaging technique for the characterization of adrenal incidentalomas. Benign adrenocortical tissue accumulates the tracer showing a "concordant" imaging pattern characterized by an increased NP-59 uptake on the side of the mass as compared to the contra-lateral adrenal gland. Thus, scintigraphic visualization of an adrenal tumor predicts its benign nature (40,41). Conversely, primary and metastatic malignancies, or space-occupying and destructive adrenal lesions (cysts or hemorrhages), typically show decreased or absent NP-59 uptake by the relevant side in comparison with the contra-lateral adrenal gland. This imaging pattern has been called "discordant" uptake (40-42). Characteristically, adrenocortical carcinomas are not capable of taking up sufficient amounts of tracer to be visualized by NP-59 scintigraphy. This is generally the result of inefficient cholesterol uptake and hormone synthesis. However, a number of well-differentiated adrenocortical carcinomas showing NP-59 uptake have been reported (43). Almost all of these exceptional tumors were associated with overt Cushing's syndrome or mineralocorticoid excess (43). NP-59 adrenal scintigraphy was reported to have 100% specificity and approximately 75% sensitivity in distinguishing benign from malignant incidentalomas (41). Due to the limited resolution of scintigraphy, concordant and discordant patterns of uptake may not be observed when adrenal tumors are less than 2.0 cm in diameter (41,44). However, scintigraphy has been recently put forward also in the evaluation of these smaller incidentalomas (45,46). It has also to be considered that some benign adrenal tumors of extra-adrenocortical origin, i.e. myelolipoma, do produce a discordant pattern of uptake (suggestive of malignancy). Overall, insufficient spatial resolution, lack of widespread expertise, and length of the procedure, needing serial scanning over a 5- to 7-day span, are the main inconveniences of this technique (44).

Some authors advocate employ fine needle aspiration (FNA) biopsy to differentiate primary from metastatic tumors in the adrenal glands (11,12,44,47). According to this strategy, when FNA biopsy reveals a metastatic lesion, a search for the primary tumor has to be initiated, whereas when it reveals adrenal tissue the tumor should be removed in case its radiological characteristics look suspicious for primary adrenal cancer (11). FNA is not accurate in differentiating benign from malignant primary adrenal tumors. Performing FNA biopsy carries a small but definitive risk of morbidity and mortality from pneumothorax, bleeding and pancreatitis with an overall rate of complications ranging from 8 to 12% (9). For these reasons, this procedure should be restricted to selected cases since the use of non-invasive imaging techniques allows correct classification of most incidentalomas. When primary adrenal cancer is suspected we advocate to proceed directly to surgery. The most accepted indication for FNA biopsy is to establish a definitive diagnosis of adrenal metastasis in patients with a known primary extra-adrenal tumor and no evidence of other metastatic disease.

Hormonal data could aid to distinguish primary adrenal carcinoma because great elevations of adrenal androgens, and in particular of dehydroepiandrosterone sulfate (DHEA-S) give a clue for the presence of this tumor (48). However, DHEA-S had insufficient sensitivity to be proposed as a screening test (49). We have recently pursued a different way of interpreting results of DHEA-S measurement considering that reduced DHEA-S levels represent a marker of benignity while normal results are not discriminating, and elevated levels seem very suspect for primary adrenal malignancy. In our experience, evaluation of DHEA-S levels was a useful supplementary test in the differential diagnosis of an incidental adrenal mass (50). Since other authors have not replicated these results (51, 52), the role of DHEA-S still remains investigational.

Silent pheochromocytoma

As for adrenal carcinoma, there is little doubt that a precocious diagnosis of pheochromocytoma is beneficial for the patient. Early recognition of the tumor allows prevention of potentially lethal hypertensive crises that could occur either spontaneously, or can be induced by anesthesia and surgical procedures (3,53). The discovery of an unsuspected adrenal mass carries a risk for pheochromocytoma comparable to that of the classic symptom triad (headache, palpitation, diaphoresis) in a hypertensive patient (9). The frequency of pheochromocytoma among adrenal incidentalomas was roughly comparable to that of adrenal carcinoma in the Italian survey (approximately 4%) (15). An equivalent figure can be obtained from calculating a weighted mean from the different estimations reported in the literature (9,11).

In the Italian survey, about half of patients with incidental pheochromocytoma were normotensive (15). At the reverse side of the problem, approximately 10% of the benign sporadic adrenal pheochromocytomas diagnosed at the Mayo Clinic from 1978 to 1995 presented as incidentalomas. About 90% of these cases were hypertensive and had diagnostic values of urinary catecholamines or metanephrines (54). Both these findings confirm that the tumor may present with mild or little symptomatology (3,55,56). In fact, several authors have reported that pheochromocytoma may only be unexpectedly discovered by autopsy in a relevant number of cases (3,53,57). Incidental pheochromocytomas are generally larger than 4 cm (15,55). Large pheochromocytomas can extensively metabolize catecholamines prior to secretion and therefore may cause less clinical symptoms than small tumors (58).

The sensitivity of unenhanced CT for the detection of adrenal pheochromocytoma ranges from 93 to 100% (59). Intravenous contrast enhancement is not generally needed even if most tumors markedly enhance after intravenous contrast medium (42). MRI may have higher specificity than CT in diagnosing adrenal pheochromocytomas and is also more accurate in detecting the less frequently occurring extra-adrenal pheochromocytomas (60,61). T2 weighted MRI may be particularly helpful, as this tumor usually shows a high signal intensity (higher than primary carcinoma or metastasis) (9,62).

Adrenal scintigraphy with [^{131}I] metaiodobenzylguanidine (MIBG) provides anatomical localization and functional characterization of the tumor. This technique has lower sensitivity (78%) as compared with CT or MRI but superior specificity (100%). MIBG scintigraphy may be useful in patients with equivocal imaging and biochemical data, or when a malignant or multifocal pheochromocytoma is suspected (63).

It can be debated which test has to be considered as the gold standard for biochemical screening of (incidental) pheochromocytoma. There are currently two different approaches, one advocating measurement of plasma catecholamines (64), the other relying on urinary biochemistry (65). Plasma catecholamines are more subject to spurious elevation and more frequently are in the normal range between hypertensive paroxysms than urinary catecholamines and their metabolites. Pharmacological stimulation or suppression of plasma catecholamines may occasionally be helpful (66). Most experts recommend measurement of urinary catecholamines as the first step, also because of its large availability and low costs. These levels should be at least two times above the upper limit of normal to exclude false positives (65). Urinary metanephrines may be the most sensitive screening test (67) while urinary vanillylmandelic acid is less sensitive but just as specific (68). However, assuming that the samples were complete and properly collected while the patient was not receiving interfering medications, the three major urinary determinations had comparable operating characteristics (9,66). It should be noted that some patients with incidental pheochromocytoma may show a completely negative biochemical work-up (69). Serum chromogranin A is markedly elevated in many patients with pheochromocytoma and thus has potential diagnostic value (70) but its specificity has been questioned. It has not been widely used and further experience is required. It should be locally determined which diagnostic test is the best on the basis of personal experience. It is our practice to screen patients with adrenal incidentalomas using urinary measurements of catecholamines and vanillylmandelic acid. We are also currently evaluating the diagnostic utility of plasma chromogranin A determinations and preliminary results look promising.

Subclinical Cushing's syndrome

Subclinical Cushing's syndrome is possibly the most intriguing issue concerning adrenal incidentalomas since it raises many questions and uncertainties. The first one concerns the terminology used to describe this condition characterized by autonomous and unregulated cortisol secretion, not fully restrained by pituitary feed-back. In this context, the terms "preclinical Cushing's syndrome" (71-74) or "subclinical Cushing's syndrome" (6,75) have sometimes been interchangeably used. As proposed by Ross (6), the term subclinical Cushing's syndrome is probably more accurate not implying any assumption on the possible development of the clinical syndrome. The diagnostic criteria of subclinical Cushing's syndrome and the management strategy of the patients who qualify for this condition are again very controversial.

By definition, patients with incidentally discovered adrenal masses do not present with overt physical stigmata of Cushing's syndrome. Therefore, only subtle states of cortisol excess should be discovered in these patients. The study of subclinical cortisol excess is difficult to pursue as standard biochemical tests for the existence of Cushing's syndrome are generally ill-suited for the assessment of patients who have no, or very mild signs of cortisol excess only (1,6). In the absence of reliable clinical clues, it is difficult to distinguish between true- and false-positivity. Moreover, the frequency of subclinical Cushing's syndrome among patients with adrenal incidentaloma is roughly comparable to the false-positive rate of the tests used for endocrine screening.

In the literature, the prevalence of subclinical Cushing's syndrome ranged from 5 to 12% (74-80). This discrepancy may be explained by the following considerations: a) the different series were heterogeneous with regard to sample size and inclusion of non-adenomatous lesions, b) various endocrine protocols were applied, c) disparate criteria were employed to define a mild degree of cortisol excess (Table I). Moreover, it should be considered that there may be a continuous spectrum from a non-secretory adenoma to subclinical Cushing's syndrome (80). Therefore, variability in methodological approach has precluded the definition of an uniform entity. Overall, when the HPA axis was studied in detail, mixed endocrine findings were produced using a number of possible combinations of abnormal tests (74,75,79,81). However, considering the largest screening studies some general conclusions can be drawn. Loss of the normal circadian rhythm of cortisol, with blunted nyctohemeral variation, frequently occurred despite normal baseline cortisol levels (74,75,77,81). Moreover, adrenal incidentalomas infrequently caused elevation of urinary free cortisol excretion (10,74,75,79-82). However, the cortisol excess might be relatively mild but sufficient to suppress ACTH secretion, as low to undetectable ACTH levels have been repeatedly reported in silent adrenal tumors (74,75,77-80). The response of ACTH and cortisol to CRH may also be blunted in these patients but in our experience CRH stimulation tests do not add significant information to baseline ACTH levels (74,75,79,81). The interpretation of CRH test is confounded by the wide range of ACTH and cortisol responses and by their divergent patterns in patients as well as in healthy controls. The discrepancy between the ACTH and cortisol response to CRH stimulation in patients with an adrenal adenoma (74,75,83) may be due to the capability of the tumor to respond to minimal ACTH increments. It has also been shown that adrenocortical adenomas may express functional ACTH receptors (84).

Dexamethasone suppression tests were extensively employed to screen for autonomous cortisol secretion. However, protocols differed with regard to the dexamethasone dose used and the threshold value for adequate cortisol suppression. Most endocrinologists either used an overnight 1 mg or a standard low-dose suppression test (85,86). The classical test may be more accurate than the overnight test (87) but is also more difficult to apply in everyday practice. Some authors have advocated to reduce the threshold of the post-test cortisol value in order to improve the sensitivity of the test, since in healthy subjects cortisol is usually hardly detectable following 1 mg dexamethasone (10,88). Conversely, other authors have suggested a high-dose dexamethasone test (3 or even 8 mg) to minimize false positive results, because the diagnosis of pituitary Cushing's syndrome is not under consideration (1,74). At present, there are insufficient data to solve this controversy. We believe that overnight 1 mg suppression test should be used for screening purposes, since this test is specifically tailored for diagnosing hypercortisolism, while the high-dose tests were designed for the differential diagnosis of Cushing's syndrome (89). Moreover, there is less experience with the use of high-dose tests in the general, unselected population and a 8 mg dexamethasone dose may produce discomfort during the hours following administration.

TABLE I. Study of the hypothalamic-pituitary-adrenal axis in patients with adrenal incidentaloma: review of the literature.

Author	Patients	UFC	Baseline ACTH	Cortisol after DST	ACTH after CRH
Rizza et al. (1973)	4	normal*	-	suppression 1/1 (8 mg)	-
Charbonnel et al. (1981)	1	normal*	decreased	>5 μg/dl (8mg)	-
Bertagna & Orth (1981)	3	increased 2/3*	decreased 1/3	>5 μg/dl 2/3 (8mg)	-
Bogner et al. (1986)	1	increased	-	>5 μg/dl (8 mg)	-
Gross et al. (1987)	7	increased 1/7	-	Suppression 7/7	-
Huiras et al. (1989)	2	normal 2/2	decreased 1/1	>5 μg/dl 1/1	-
Mcleod et al. (1990)	6	increased 2/5	decreased 5/6	>5 μg/dl 3/3	-
Hensen et al. (1990)	13	normal 13/13	decreased 2/13	>5 μg/dl 3/13	normal
Rosen & Swartz (1992)	1	normal	-	>5 μg/dl	normal
Jockenhövel et al. (1992)	18	increased 1/18	decreased 1/18	>5 μg/dl 9/18 (2 mg)	-
Reincke et al. (1992)	66	increased 1/66	decreased 5/66	>5 μg/dl 8/66 (8 mg)	reduced 5/66
Kobayashi et al. (1993)	14	increased 5/10*	-	> 5 μg/dl 7/14 (2 mg)	-
Osella et al. (1994)	45	increased 1/26	-	>5 μg/dl 7/45	reduced 8/23
Flecchia et al. (1994)	22	increased 5/24	decreased 6/24	>5 μg/dl 4/24	-
Fernandez-Real et al. (1994)	3	increased 1/3	decreased 2/3	>5 μg/dl 3/3 (2 mg)	normal 1/1
Lavoie & Lacroix (1995)	3	normal 3/3	decreased 1/3	>5 μg/dl 1/3	-
Ambrosi et al. (1995)	32	increased 4/32	decreased 1/32	>5 μg/dl 4/29	reduced 6/18
Bardet et al. (1996)	35	increased 4/35	decreased 3/14	>5 μg/dl 2/15 (2 mg)	-
Terzolo et al. (1998)	53	increased 4/53	decreased 5/53	>5μg/dl 9/53	reduced 6/53

UFC = urinary free cortisol excretion, DST = dexamethasone suppression test (1 mg if not differently specified), *urinary 17-hydroxycorticosteroid excretion.

Reduced DHEA-S concentrations were frequently found in patients with adrenal incidentalomas and this is probably the most frequent hormonal alteration (51,52,79,81,90,91). Low DHEA-S levels were thought to reflect suppression of the HPA axis by autonomous cortisol secretion (51,81). However, these studies failed to demonstrate a significant correlation between DHEA-S and basal ACTH levels (51,81) and further studies showed that reduced DHEA-S concentrations were not restricted to patients with silent hypercortisolism (92). Therefore, it was concluded that low DHEA-S levels were not a reliable marker of subclinical Cushing's syndrome (52). A recent study challenges this conclusion, because high post-dexamethasone cortisol concentrations were associated with low DHEA-S levels (91). At present, we believe that the cause of this DHEA-S reduction remains to be clarified.

Iodocholesterol adrenal scintigraphy was also extensively used to assess functional autonomy of adrenal incidentalomas (adenomas) and to differentiate functioning from non-functioning tumors (93). Some adrenal adenomas can progressively grow until they can produce sufficient amounts of cortisol to suppress ACTH secretion and iodocholestrol uptake of the contralateral gland, but not sufficient to cause clinically overt signs (41,45,90,91,93). Bardet and colleagues (90) reported that patients with concordant unilateral uptake showed overall lower baseline ACTH levels and higher cortisol after an overnight dexamethasone suppression test than patients with bilateral uptake. The relationship between scintigraphic uptake and the degree of functional autonomy was challenged by Rizza and colleagues who argued that increased uptake simply reflects the presence of enlarged adrenal tissue (94). In our experience, NP-59 uptake on the side of the mass with non-visualization of the contra-lateral adrenal gland (concordant uptake) may occur despite overall normal endocrine tests (75,81). Scintigraphic uptake may represent a very early sign of functional autonomy, allowing the detection of adrenocortical adenomas which do accumulate LDL cholesterol (and therefore NP-59) but do not secrete cortisol in significant excess, in analogy with hot, pre-toxic, thyroid nodules (41).

If there is no doubt that many incidentally discovered adrenal adenomas are able to secrete cortisol autonomously, exhaustive endocrine evaluation may provide a spectrum of results so variable that it is difficult to define the amount of cortisol excess which is truly relevant to cause subclinical Cushing's syndrome. Reincke and colleagues (74) have proposed a hypothetical model of development from non-functioning to autonomous adrenal adenomas, but other studies (75,79-81) do not support such a multi-step approach. Conversely, different hormonal patterns may be observed as a consequence of a variable degree and, possibly, duration of cortisol hypersecretion. It is also conceivable that a larger tumor size increases the probability that cortisol may be secreted in excess (95). Therefore, when comparing different series this variable should also be adjusted for.

We have recently developed a categorization of subclinical Cushing's syndrome resulting in different levels of probability according to the extent of endocrine alterations. The association of two abnormal tests is required to reduce the possibility that a patient qualifies for subclinical Cushing's syndrome as a result of false positive tests. In the presence of an increased urinary free cortisol excretion and failure of cortisol to suppress after overnight 1 mg dexamethasone subclinical Cushing's syndrome has the highest degree of probability. These alterations were considered as major criteria since they represent the most reliable markers of hypercortisolism (89) and negative test results have the highest negative predictive value (6). Lower degrees of probability for subclinical Cushing's syndrome were defined by the presence of other combinations of hormonal alterations (Table II).

TABLE II. Classification of subclinical Cushing's syndrome in patients with adrenal incidentaloma.

Definitive subclinical Cushing's syndrome
Presence of both major criteria
Probable subclinical Cushing's syndrome
Presence of a major criterion and at least one minor criterion
Possible subclinical Cushing's syndrome
Presence of at least two minor criteria

Major criteria: i) Elevated urinary free cortisol.
ii) Inadequate cortisol suppressibility after 1 mg dexamethasone.

Minor criteria: i) Low baseline ACTH, or blunted ACTH response to CRH.
ii) Disturbed cortisol rhythm: elevated serum levels, or reduced day/night amplitude.

The present definition is possibly too rigid and not fully adequate to fit in with a heterogeneous and ill-defined clinical condition characterized by continuous variability. Moreover, silent hypercortisolism may be more frequently characterized by qualitative rather than quantitative alterations of cortisol secretion (81). However, this classification is a somewhat provocative attempt to demonstrate that subclinical Cushing's syndrome is a complex condition and that a general definition is needed to compare data from different series.

The natural history of patients with silent hypercortisolism is presently unknown. In the literature, controversy exists on the risk of progression from subclinical to full-blown hypercortisolism (71-75,83,96). The rare occurrence of Cushing's syndrome in the general population strongly suggests that the vast majority of patients with subclinical Cushing's syndrome will never progress to clinically significant disease (6). Our follow-up data suggest that endocrine alterations were non-progressive, at least in the mid-term, and even self-limiting in some patients. This raises the possibility of intermittent hypersecretion with intervening phases of quiescence (75,81). As reported in the literature, only few patients have progressed to overt Cushing's syndrome (72,74,83,96).

The key question with regard to subclinical Cushing's syndrome is whether this state has any impact on the clinical condition of patients with adrenal incidentalomas (95). At present, there are insufficient data to estimate the morbidity and potential long-term complications of subclinical Cushing's syndrome. In this respect, it is critical to exclude any patient with very mild, or cyclical Cushing's syndrome, or patients with pseudo-Cushing's states. The appropriate management of patients with subclinical Cushing's syndrome remains controversial unless detrimental effects of silent hypercortisolism will be clearly proven (9,74,79,81). At present, there is no evidence that this subset of patients would always benefit from adrenalectomy but post-operative weight loss, improvement of hypertension and glycemic control have been reported in some patients (9,74,81,85). Conversely, the possibility of post-operative adrenal insufficiency, resulting from suppression of the contra-lateral adrenal gland, should be considered as a cause of morbidity (9,74,76-81). It is difficult to predict the occurrence of post-operative adrenal insufficiency on the basis of endocrinological and scintigraphic data. Thus a peri-operative steroid cover is recommended to avoid a potential Addisonian crisis after adrenalectomy. It is likely that other factors, such as the duration of silent hypercortisolism, may be important for the determination of the degree of suppression of the HPA axis and the subsequent risk of post-operative hypocortisolism.

Unsuspected Conn's syndrome

In comparison to the HPA axis, the renin-angiotensin-aldosterone (RAA) axis has attracted considerably less interest in the evaluation of adrenal incidentalomas. Until very recently, primary hyperaldosteronism was considered to occur only infrequently when hypokalemia was absent. In keeping with this view, it was stated that in a hypertensive patient with an adrenal incidentaloma screening for spontaneous hypokalemia was all that was required (2). Hormonal evaluation of the RAA axis was considered to be cost-effective only in patients with both hypertension and hypokalemia. This view has been recently challenged by the demonstration that more than half of the patients with primary hyperaldosteronism is normokalemic (97). Screening studies have shown that primary aldosteronism occurs in approximately 10% of hypertensive patients (98). As a result, it should be considered as the most frequent cause of endocrine hypertension. Calculating the aldosterone to plasma renin activity (PRA) ratio is the most effective screening method for primary aldosteronism (99-101). However, awareness of interfering medication is required for appropriate interpretation of the results. Still, primary aldosteronism can be excluded in the majority of patients even when anti-hypertensive medication is continued (100). A ratio of plasma aldosterone to PRA of 30 or greater would require confirmatory testing usually by means of a fludrocortisone test (102). According to recent epidemiological evidence, it is recommended to obtain a paired upright plasma aldosterone concentration and PRA in patients with an adrenal incidentaloma who are hypertensive (9). This is also our current practice because primary hyperaldosteronism is a curable form of hypertension. It is essential to remember at this point that when there is strong suspicion of secondary hypertension, an adrenal mass should generally not be considered as incidental.

A model for the evolution of primary hyperaldosteronism from an early preclinical stage, only recognizable biochemically, to a florid and clinically obvious stage has been proposed (97,103). It is, therefore, possible that an incidentally discovered adrenal adenoma may secrete aldosterone autonomously in a normotensive and normokalemic patient. Preliminary data by Gordon and coworkers seem to support this model (104), This condition, therefore, resembles subclinical Cushing's syndrome.

Suggested management of adrenal incidentalomas

The potential mortality because of adrenal carcinoma implicates that it is mandatory to recognize and remove these lesions early in their course thereby attempting to improve the prognosis of these patients. Notwithstanding the substantial controversy over the value of mass size as a predictor of malignancy and on the optimal cut-off size, most authors agree that tumors larger than 4.0 cm should be surgically resected. We also support these recommendations. Following these indications, the majority of pheochromocytomas will be removed as well.

Whatever the mass size, adrenalectomy should be recommended if imaging criteria look suspicious for malignancy. CT scan is the pivotal imaging technique; we only use MRI or adrenal scintigraphy, or both, in equivocal cases. Other factors contributing to the risk of malignancy are patient's age, abdominal pain at presentation, and high DHEA-S concentrations. FNA biopsy should be only used if a definitive diagnosis of metastatic disease is crucial to patient management (9).

The second objective is to rule out pheochromocytoma since this tumor is usually benign and curable, but potentially lethal. Surgical removal, or even FNA biopsy, of an adrenal mass should never be done until a pheochromocytoma is excluded. Specific biochemical screening should not be limited to hypertensive subjects because some patients may be asymptomatic (15,69). The biochemical screening procedures are determined by local settings. We currently use measurement of urinary catecholamines and VMA and plasma chromogranin A.

The demonstration of autonomous cortisol secretion by an adrenal incidentaloma, defining the so-called "subclinical Cushing's syndrome", is still a subject to many controversies. This uncertainty arises from the definition of incidentaloma (mass discovered serendipitously in the absence of overt signs or symptoms of adrenal disease) which makes any definition of subclinical Cushing's syndrome based only on endocrine data somewhat arbitrary. Adrenal incidentalomas represent a heterogeneous group of lesions, perhaps with distinct patterns of cortisol secretion (92). Overall, it is possible to demonstrate some degree of glucocorticoid autonomy in many adrenal incidentalomas by means of an extensive endocrine work-up. However, it remains to be established which tests should be performed in clinical practice (95). We suggest that the cortisol secretory status has to be investigated using an overnight 1 mg dexamethasone suppression test and measurement of urinary free cortisol excretion. Determination of cortisol rhythm, even with paired 0800 and midnight cortisol levels, in association with measurement of basal ACTH concentrations only should also be considered. The clinical utility of DHEA-S measurement has not been established.

In some patients, where clustering of several abnormalities in the HPA axis occurs, subclinical Cushing's syndrome could be assumed. This denomination should be preferred to that of pre-clinical Cushing's syndrome since the biochemical abnormalities do not seem to become clinically manifest in most patients. Although patients with Cushing's syndrome generally present with clinically evident complications, the morbidity of patients with subclinical disease is less established even when recent evidence suggests a link with increased risk for hypertension, diabetes, obesity and dyslipidemia (20,74,79,81,91,105,106). Our strategy is conservative and consists of yearly follow-up with CT scan and measurement of urinary free cortisol excretion and serum cortisol after 1 mg dexamethasone. However, the optimal duration of follow-up is undetermined and observation involves both monetary and psychological costs (1). Surgery should be employed in case of progression from subclinical to overt Cushing's syndrome. Factors such as young age, coexistence of hypertension, diabetes, or osteoporosis might influence the decision in favor of surgery (10,74). The significant decrease in surgical morbidity and economic costs using a laparoscopic approach to adrenalectomy is actually widening indications to surgery (107,108).

Recent epidemiological evidence outlines that normokalemic primary aldosteronism is much more common than previously suspected (97). The ratio between plasma renin activity to aldosterone levels should be used for screening hypertensive patients with adrenal incidentaloma.

References

1. Chidiac RM, Aron DC. Incidentalomas. A disease of modern technology. Endocrinol Metab Clin North Am 1997;26:233.
2. Ross NS, Aron DC. Hormonal evaluation of the patient with an incidentally discovered adrenal mass. N Engl J Med 1990;323:1401.
3. Sutton MG, Sheps SG, Lie JT. Prevalence of clinically unsuspected pheochromocytoma: review of a 50-year autopsy series. Mayo Clin Proc 1981;56:354.
4. Iimura O, Shimamoto K, Nakahashi Y, Nakamura Y. Actual incidence of adrenal tumors in Hokkaido. In: Takeda R, Miyamori (eds) Controversies in disorders of adrenal hormones: proceedings of the Open Symposium of Adrenal Hormones p. 37. New York: Elseviers Sciences 1988.
5. Melby JC. Diagnosis and treatment of primary aldosteronism and isolated hypoaldosteronism. J Clin Endocrinol Metab 1985;14:977.
6. Ross NS. Epidemiology of Cushing's syndrome and subclinical disease. Endocrinol Clin North Am 1994;23:539.
7. Lewinsky BS, Grigor KM, Symington T, Neville AM. The clinical and pathologic features of "non-hormonal" adrenocortical tumors. Report of twenty new cases and review of the literature. Cancer 1974;33:778.
8. Griffing G. A-I-D-S: The new endocrine epidemic. J Clin Endocrinol Metab 1994;79:1530.
9. Kloos RT, Gross MD, Francis IR, Korobkin M, Shapiro B. Incidentally discovered adrenal masses. End Rev 1995;16:460.
10. Lavoie H, Lacroix A .Partially autonomous cortisol secretion by incidentally discovered adrenal adenomas. Trends Endocrinol Metab 1995;6:191.
11. Cook DM, Loriaux DL. The incidental adrenal mass. Am J Med 1996;101:88.
12. Glazer HS, Weyman PJ, Sagel SS, Levitt RG, McClennan BL. Nonfunctioning adrenal masses: incidental discovery on computed tomography. Am J Roengtenol 1982;139:81.
13. Peppercorn PD, Grossman AB, Rezneck RH. Imaging of incidentally discovered adrenal masses. Clin. Endocrinol 1998;48:379.
14. Turner HE, Moore NR, Byrne JV, Wass JAH. Pituitary, adrenal and thyroid incidentalomas. Endocrine-Related Cancer 1998;5:131.
15. Terzolo M, Ali A, Osella G, Angeli A. Adrenal incidentaloma (1):epidemiological and clinical data from the national Italian Study Group. Proceedings of the 79 annual meeting of the Endocrine Society. June 11-14, 1997, Minneapolis (Abstract).
16. Herrera MF, Grant CS, Van Heerden JA, Sheedy PF, Ilstrup DM. Incidentally discovered adrenal tumors: an institutional perspective. Surgery 1991;110:1014.
17. Dobbie JW Adrenocortical nodular hyperplasias: the ageing adrenal. J Pathol 1969;99:1.
18. Russi S, Blumenthal HT, Gray SH. Small adenomas of the adrenal cortex in hypertension and diabetes. Arch Intern Med 1945;76:284.
19. Commons RR, Callaway CP. Adenomas of the adrenal cortex. Arch Intern Med 1948;81:37.
20. Leibowitz G, Tsur A, Chayen SD, et al. Pre-clinical Cushing's syndrome. An unexpected frequent cause of poor glycaemic control in obese diabetic patients. Clin Endocrinol 1996;44:717.
21. Luton JP, Cerdas S, Billaud L, et al. Clinical features of adrenocortical carcinoma, prognostic factors, and the effect of mitotane therapy. N Engl J Med 1990;322:1195.
22. Crucitti F, Bellantone R, Ferrante A, et al. The Italian registry for adrenal cortical carcinoma: analysis of a multiinstitutional series of 129 patients. Surgery 1996;119:161.

23. Glomset DA. The incidence of metastasis of malignant tumors to the adrenals. Am J Cancer 1938;32:57.
24. de la Monte SM, Hutchinns GM, Moore GW. Endocrine organ metastases from breast carcinoma. Am J Pathol 1984;114:131.
25. Siren JE, Haapiainen RK, Huikuri KT, Sivula AH. Incidentalomas of the adrenal gland:36 operated patients and review of literature. World J Surg 1993;17:634.
26. Copeland PM. The incidentally discovered adrenal mass. Ann Int Med 1983;98:940.
27. Mitnick JS, Bosniak MH, Megibow AJ, Naidich DP. Nonfunctioning adrenal adenomas discovered incidentally on computed tomography. Radiology 1983;148:495.
28. Abecassis M, McLoughin MJ, Langer B, Kudlow JE. Serendipitous adrenal masses: prevalence significance and management. Am J Surg 1985;149:783.
29. Belldegrun A, Hussain S, Seltzer SE, Loughlin KR , Gittes RF, Richie JP. Incidentally discovered mass of the adrenal gland. Surg Gynecol Obstet 1986;163:203.
30. Bernardino ME. Management of the asymptomatic patient with a unilateral adrenal mass. Radiology 1988;166:121.
31. Staren ED, Prinz RA. Selection of patients with adrenal incidentalomas for operation. Surg Clin North Am 1995;75:499.
32. Courtade A, Cornaille B, Ernst O, Renan CA, L'Herminé C, Proye C. Outcome of incidentally discovered adrenal masses not operated on: 44 cases over 7 years. Eur J Surg 1997;163:315.
33. Barry MK, van Heerden JA, Farley DR, Grant CS, Thompson GB, Ilstrup DM. Can adrenal incidentaloma be safely observed? World J Surg 1998;22:599.
34. Korobkin M, Giordano TJ, Brodeur FJ et al. Adrenal adenomas: relationship between histologic lipid and CT and MR findings. Radiology 1996;200:743.
35. Amberson JB, Gray GF. Adrenal pathology. In: Vaughan ED, Carey RM (eds.) Adrenal disorders p. 18. New York: Thieme Medical 1989.
36. Korobkin M, Brodeur FJ, Yutzy GG, et al. Differentiation of adrenal adenomas from nonadenomas using CT attenuation values Am J Roengtenol 1996;166:531.
37. Korobkin M, Brodeur FJ, Francis IR, Quint LE, Dunnick NR, Goodsitt M. Delayed enhanced CT for differentiation of benign from malignant adrenal masses. Radiology 1996;200:737.
38. Schwartz LH, Panicek DM, Doyle MV, et al. Comparison of two algorithms and their associated charges when evaluating adrenal masses in patients with malignancies Am J Roentgenol 1997;168:1575.
39. Outwater EK, Siegelman ES, Huang AB, Birnbaum BA Adrenal masses: correlation between CT attenuation value and chemical shift ratio at MR imaging with in-phase and opposed-phase sequences. Radiology 1996;200:749.
40. Gross MD, Shapiro B, Bouffard AJ, et al. Distinguishing benign from malignant euadrenal masses. Ann Intern Med 1988;109:613.
41. Gross MD, Shapiro B, Francis IR, et al. Scintigraphic evaluation of clinically silent adrenal masses. J Nucl Med 1994;35:1145.
42. Korobkin M, Francis IR. Imaging of adrenal masses. Urol Clin North Am 1997;24:603.
43. Pasieka JL, McLeod MK, Thompson NW, Gross MD, Schteingart DE. Adrenal scintigraphy of well-differentiated (functioning) adrenocortical carcinomas: potential surgical pitfalls. Surgery 1992;112:884.
44. Falke THM, Sandler MP. Classification of silent adrenal masses: time to get practical. J Nucl Med 1994;35:1152.
45. Barzon L, Scaroni C, Sonino N, et al. Incidentally discovered adrenal tumors: endocrine and scintigraphic correlates. J Clin Endocrinol Metab 1988;83:55.
46. Kloos RT, Gross MD, Shapiro B, Francis IR, Korobkin M, Thompson NW. Diagnostic dilemma of small incidentally discovered adrenal masses: role for 131-I6-β-iodomethyl-norcholesterol scintigraphy. World J Surg 1997;21:36.

47. Katz RL, Shirkhonda E. Diagnostic approach to incidental adrenal nodules in the cancer patient. Results of a clinical, radiologic, and fine-needle aspiration study. Cancer 1985;55:1995.
48. Margioris AN, Chrousos GP. Cushing's syndrome: diagnostic evaluation. In: Biglieri EG, Melby JC (eds) Endocrine Hypertension pp 99-111. New York: Raven Press. 1990.
49. Mantero F, Masini AM, Arnaldi G, Giovagnetti M, Mancini V, Opocher G. Adrenal incidentaloma (2): an overview of hormonal data from the national Italian Study Group. Proceedings of the 79 annual meeting of the Endocrine Society. June 11-14, 1997, Minneapolis (Abstract).
50. Terzolo M, Ali A, Osella G, et al. DHEAS measurement in the differential diagnosis between benign and malignant adrenal masses. J Endocrinol Invest 1998;21:33 (Abstract).
51. Flecchia D, Mazza E, Carlini M, et al. Reduced serum levels of dehydroepiandrosterone sulphate in adrenal incidentalomas: a marker of adrenocortical tumour. Clin Endocrinol 1995;42:129.
52. Bencsik, Z., Szabolcs, I., Kovacs, Z., et al. Low dehydroepiandrosterone sulfate (DHEA-S) level is not a good predictor of hormonal activity in nonselected patients with incidentally detected adrenal tumors. J Clin Endocrinol Metab 1996;81:1726.
53. Hartley L, Perry-Keene D. Phaeochromocytoma in Queensland-1970-83. Aust N Z J Surg 1985;55:471.
54. Kudva YC, Young WF. Pheochromocytomas presenting as incidentalomas. Proceedings of the International Conference on the Management of "Non-Functioning" Adrenal Tumors. September 14-16, 1997, Athens.
55. Krane NK. Clinically unsuspected pheochromocytoma: experience at Henry Ford Hospital and a review of the literature. Arch Intern Med 1986;146:54.
56. Manger WM, Gifford RW, Hoffman BB. Pheochromocytoma: a clinical and experimental overview. Curr Probl Cancer 1985;9:1.
57. Modlin IM, Farndon JR, Sheperd A, et al. Phaeochromocytomas in 72 patients: clinical and diagnostic features, treatment and long term results. Br J Surg 1979;66:456.
58. Bravo EL. Pheochromocytoma: new concepts and future trends. Kidney Int 1991;40:544.
59. Quint LE, Glazer GM, Francis IR, Shapiro B, Chenevert TC. Pheochromocytoma and paraganglioma. Comparison of MR imaging with CT and I^{131} MIBG scintigraphy. Radiology 1987;165:89.
60. Lee MJ, Hahn PF, Papanicolau N, et al. Benign and malignant adrenal masses CT distinction with attenuation co-efficients, size and observer analysis. Radiology 1991;179:771.
61. Falke THM, te Strake L, Sandler MP, et al. Magnetic resonance imaging of the adrenal glands. Radiographics 1987;7:343.
62. Doppman JL, Reinig JW, Dwyer AJ, et al. Differentiation of adrenal masses by magnetic resonance imaging. Surgery 1987;102:1018.
63. Bravo EL. Evolving concepts in the pathophysiology, diagnosis and treatment of pheochromocytoma. End Rev 1994;15:356.
64. Bravo EL, Gifford RW. Pheochromocytoma: diagnosis, localization and management. N Engl J Med 1984;311:1298.
65. Landsberg L, Young JB. Catecholamines and the adrenal medulla. In: Foster DW, Wilson JD (eds) William Textbook of Endocrinology p. 891. Philadelphia: WB Saunders. 1985
66. Daly PA, Landsberg L. Phaeochromocytoma: diagnosis and management. Baillières Clin Endocrinol Metab 1992;6:143.

67. Kudva YC, Young WF. Specificity and positive predictive value of 24-hour urine metanephrines and fractionated catecholamines in pheochromocytoma. Proceedings of the 80th annual meeting of the Endocrine Society. June 24-27, 1998, New Orleans.
68. Gifford RW, Manger MD, Bravo EL. Pheochromocytoma. Endocrinol Metab Clin North Am 1994;23:387.
69. Mannelli M, Pupilli C, Lanzillotti R, et al. nonsecreting phaeochromocytoma presenting as an incidental adrenal mass. Report of a case. J Endocrinol Invest 1993;16:817.
70. O'Connor DT, Bernstein KN. Radioimmunoassay of chromogranin A in plasma as a measure of exocytotic sympathicoadrenal activity in normal subjects and patients with pheochromocytoma. N Engl J Med 1984;311:764.
71. Bertagna C, Orth DN. Clinical and laboratory findings and results of therapy in 58 patients with adrenocortical tumours admitted to a single medical center (1951 to 1978). Am J Med 1981;71:855.
72. Charbonnel B, Chatal JF, Ozanne P. Does the corticoadrenal adenoma with pre-Cushing syndrome exist? J Nucl Med 1981;22:1059.
73. Bogner U, Eggens U, Hensen J, Oelkers W. Incidentally discovered ACTH-dependent adrenal adenoma presenting as "pre-Cushing's syndrome". Acta Endocrinol 1986;111:89.
74. Reincke M, Nieke J, Krestin GP, Saeger W, Allolio B, Winkelman W. Preclinical Cushing's syndrome in adrenal "incidentalomas": comparison with adrenal Cushing's syndrome. J Clin Endocrinol Metab 1992;75:826.
75. Terzolo M, All A, Osella G, Cesario F, Paccotti P, Angeli A. Subclinical Cushing's syndrome in adrenal incidentaloma. Clin Endocrinol 1998;48:89.
76. Huiras CM, Pehlig GB, Caplan RH. Adrenal insufficiency after operative removal of apparently nonfunctioning adrenal adenomas. J A M A 1989;261:894.
77. McLeod M, Thompson N, Gross M, Bondeson A, Bondeson L. Sub-clinical Cushing's syndrome in patients with adrenal gland incidentalomas. Pitfalls in diagnosis and management. Am Surgeon 1990;56:398.
78. Caplan RH, Strutt PJ, Wickus GG. Subclinical hormone secretion by incidentally discovered adrenal masses. Arch Surg 1994;129:291.
79. Ambrosi B, Peverelli S, Passini E, et al. Abnormalities of endocrine function in patients with clinically "silent" adrenal masses. Eur J Endocrinol 1995;132:422.
80. Fernandez-Real JM, Ricart-Engel, W, Simò R. Pre-clinical Cushing's syndrome: report of three cases and literature review. Horm Res 1994;41:230.
81. Osella G, Terzolo M, Borretta G, et al. Endocrine evaluation of incidentally discovered adrenal masses (incidentalomas). J Clin Endocrinol Metab 1994;79:1532.
82. Jockenhövel F, Kuck W, Hauffa B, et al. Conservative and surgical management of incidentally discovered adrenal tumours (incidentalomas). J Endocrinol Invest 1992;15:331.
83. Hensen J, Buhl M, Bahr V, Oelkers W. Endocrine activity of the "silent" adrenocortical adenoma is uncovered by response to corticotropin-releasing hormone. Klin Wochenschr 1990;68:608.
84. Reincke M, Beuschlein F, Latronico AC, Arlt W, Chrousos GP, Allolio B. Expression of adrenocorticotrophic hormone receptor mRNA in human adrenocortical neoplasms: correlation with P450scc expression. Clin Endocrinol 1997;46:619.
85. Kobayashi S, Seki T, Nonomura K, Gotoh T, Togashi M, Koyanagi T. Clinical experience of incidentally discovered adrenal tumor with particular reference to cortical function. J Urol 1993;150:8.
86. Tsagarakis S, Kokkoris P, Roboti C, et al. The low-dose dexamethasone suppression test in patients with adrenal incidentalomas: comparisons with clinically euadrenal subjects and patients with Cushing's syndrome. Clin Endocrinol 1998;48:627.

87. Trainer PJ, Grossman A. The diagnosis and differential diagnosis of Cushing's syndrome. Clin Endocrinol 1991;34:317.
88. Huizenga NATM, Koper JW, De Lange P, et al. A polymorphism in the glucocorticoid receptor gene may be associated with an increased sensitivity to glucocorticoids in vivo. J Clin Endocrinol Metab 1998;83:144.
89. Kaye TB, Crapo L. The Cushing's syndrome: an update on diagnostic tests. Ann Intern Med 1990;112:434.
90. Bardet S, Rohmer V, Murat A, et al. ^{131}I-6-β-iodomethylnorcholesterol scintigraphy: an assessment of its role in the investigation of adrenocortical incidentalomas. Clin Endocrinol 1996;44:587.
91. Tsagarakis S, Roboti C, Kokkoris P, Vasiliou V, Alevizaki C, Thalassinon N. Elevated post-dexamethasone suppression cortisol concentrations correlate with hormonal alterations of the hypothalamo-pituitary-adrenal axis in patients with adrenal incidentalomas. Clin Endocrinol 1998;49:165.
92. Terzolo M, Osella G, Ali A, et al. Different patterns of steroid secretion in patients with adrenal incidentaloma. J Clin Endocrinol Metab 1996;81:740.
93. Gross MD, Wilton G, Shapiro B, et al. Functional and scintigraphic evaluation of the silent adrenal mass. J Nucl Med 1987;28:1401.
94. Rizza RA, Wahner HW, Spelsberg TC, Northcutt RC, Moses HL. Visualization of nonfunctioning adrenal adenomas with iodocholesterol: possible relationship to subcellular distribution of tracer. J Nucl Med 1978;19:458.
95. Aron DC. Adrenal incidentalomas and glucocorticoid autonomy. Clin Endocrinol 1998;49:157.
96. Rosen HN, Swartz SL. Subtle glucocorticoid excess in patients with adrenal incidentaloma. Am J Med 1992;92:213.
97. Gordon RD. Primary aldosteronism. J Endocrinol Invest 1995;18:495.
98. Gordon RD, Ziesak MD, Tunny TJ, Stowasser M, Klemm SA. Evidence that primary aldosteronism may not be uncommon - twelve percent among antihypertensive drug trial volunteers. Clin Exp Pharmacol Physiol 1993;20:296.
99. Hiramatsu K, Yamada T, Yukimura Y, Komiya I, Ichikawa K, Ishihara M A. Screening test to identify aldosterone-producing-adenoma by measuring plasma renin activity. Arch Int Med 1981;141:1589.
100. Weinberger MH, Fineberg NS. The diagnosis of primary aldosteronism and separation of two major subtypes. Arch Intern Med 1993;153:2125.
101. Vallotton MB. Primary aldosteronism. Part I Diagnosis of Primary hyperaldosteronism. Clin Endocrinol 1996;45:47.
102. Gordon RD, Stowasser M, Klemm SA, Tunny TJ. Primary aldosteronism and other forms of mineralocorticoid hypertension. In: Swales JD (ed). Textbook of Hypertension p. 865. London: Blackwell Scientific 1995.
103. Gordon RD. Mineralocorticoid hypertension. Lancet 1994;344:240.
104. Gordon RD, Rutherford JC, Stowasser M, Taylor WL. Adrenal hypertension and the significance of apparently non-functioning neoplasms. Proceedings of the International Conference on the Management of "Non-Functioning" Adrenal Tumors. September 14-16, 1997, Athens.
105. Osella G, Terzolo M, Reimondo G, et al. Serum markers of bone and collagen turnover in patients with Cushing's syndrome and in subject with adrenal incidentalomas. J Clin Endocrinol Metab 1997;82:3303.
106. Sartorio A, Conti A, Ferrero S, et al. Evaluation of markers of bone and collagen turnover in patients with active and preclinical Cushing's syndrome and in patients with adrenal incidentaloma. Eur J Endocrinol 1998;138:146.
107. Gagner M, Lacroix A, Prinz RA, et al. Early experience with laparoscopic approach for adrenalectomy. Surgery 1993;114:1120.

108. Jacobs JK, Goldstein RE, Geer RJ. Laparoscopic adrenalectomy. A new standard of care. Ann Surg 1997;225:495.

PANCREATIC NEUROENDOCRINE TUMORS AND CARCINOIDS

11
ULTRASOUND, CT AND MRI APPEARANCES OF PANCREATIC NEUROENDOCRINE TUMORS AND CARCINOIDS

Melanie P. Hiorns, M.R.C.P., F.R.C.R.
Rodney H. Reznek, F.R.C.P., F.R.C.R.
St Bartholomew's Hospital
London ECIA 7BE, United Kingdom

INTRODUCTION

Cross sectional imaging plays a key role in the management of patients presenting with clinical and biochemical evidence of pancreatic neuroendocrine tumors as accurate localization of these tumors will, in large part, dictate much of the management strategy. For example, spontaneous hypoglycemia in association with a single lesion in the pancreas on imaging will, in general, be treated surgically, with the surgeon relying in large part on the findings of the radiologist. Under such circumstances, surgery has a cure rate of over 90% (1). In contrast, the presence of multifocal disease and/or nodal or liver deposits from a secretory islet cell tumor is more likely to be treated medically, with control of the symptoms arising from hormone secretion the overriding concern. To date, no single imaging technique has proved absolutely reliable in the detection of neuroendocrine tumors, which are often small, multiple and frequently do not distort the pancreatic contour (2,3). However, recent technological advances which have improved the spatial and contrast resolution of all cross-sectional techniques, have undoubtedly also improved their sensitivity for the detection of islet cell tumors. The choice of the appropriate technique for imaging these tumors will depend on several factors other than accuracy; the availability and cost of each investigation, local expertise and local preference will all influence the decision. In many instances, more than one imaging technique will be required, often combined with functional studies (4).

This chapter reviews the features of pancreatic neuroendocrine tumors and carcinoids on cross-sectional imaging techniques and discusses factors influencing the choice of imaging technique for their localization.

IMAGING FEATURES

The radiological appearances of any tumor are, at least in part, governed by the biological behavior of that tumor. For example, at presentation, a non-secretory neuroendocrine tumor arising in the tail of the pancreas is likely to be significantly larger, at the point of imaging, than a pancreatic gastrinoma causing symptoms early in its natural history.

A. Sonography

Identification of islet cell tumors by ultrasound depends largely on the tumor causing a different echo pattern to the surrounding normal pancreas, although distortion of the normal anatomy by large tumors may provide an additional clue. Three techniques of ultrasound are available: transabdominal, endoscopic and intra-operative.

1. Transabdominal ultrasound

This technique is widely available, non-invasive, non-ionizing and relatively inexpensive. Normal pancreatic tissue is of mid-echogenicity: replacement of normal parenchyma by fat (either pathologically or with advancing age) causes increased echogenicity. Most islet cell tumors (insulinomas, gastrinomas and non-functioning tumors) appear as well-defined, round or oval areas of decreased echogenicity compared to the normal surrounding pancreas (Figure 1A). A minority of tumors, notably some gastrinomas, is hyperechoic. A very small number of islet cell tumors are iso-echoic and their detection therefore relies on the distortion of the surrounding pancreatic anatomy. Some larger tumors, particularly non-functioning islet cell tumors (NFITs) may exhibit evidence of necrosis or calcification (5). Rarely, islet cell tumors may be cystic or partially cystic and will then appear anechoic or hypoechoic with through transmission (Figure 2A).

The reported sensitivity of transabdominal ultrasound in the detection of islet cell tumors varies widely, although the size threshold for high detection rates seems to be around 8-10 mm (6,7). This probably accounts for a higher sensitivity for the detection of insulinomas compared to gastrinomas which, typically, are very small (< 1 cm). Reported sensitivities for single insulinomas are as high as 70% (8) compared to 41% for intrapancreatic gastrinomas (9). An additional reason for the relatively poor sensitivity of transabdominal ultrasound at detecting gastrinomas (intra and extra-pancreatic) is that as many as 90% lie in the so-called 'gastrinoma triangle' (10, 11), an area bounded by the junction of the cystic and common bile ducts superiorly, the second and third portions of the duodenum inferiorly and the junction between the neck and body of the pancreas medially. Ultrasound detection of lesions lying within this area may be hampered by overlying bowel gas. Similarly, small masses in the tail of the pancreas, often obscured by stomach gas, may also be difficult to demonstrate.

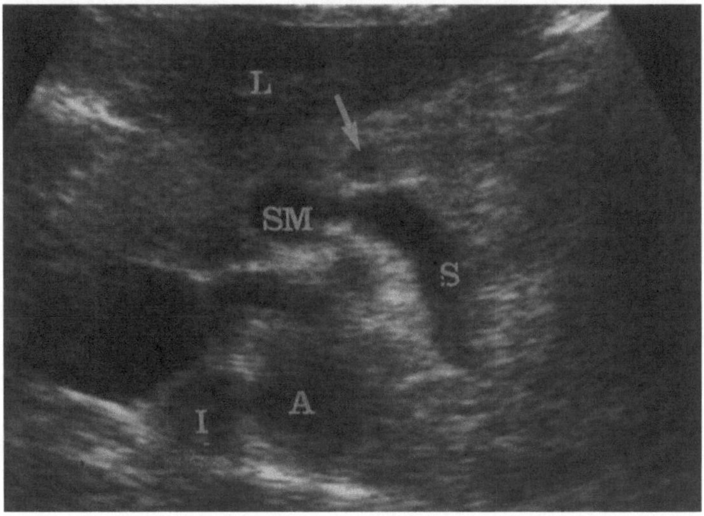
L
SM
S
I
A

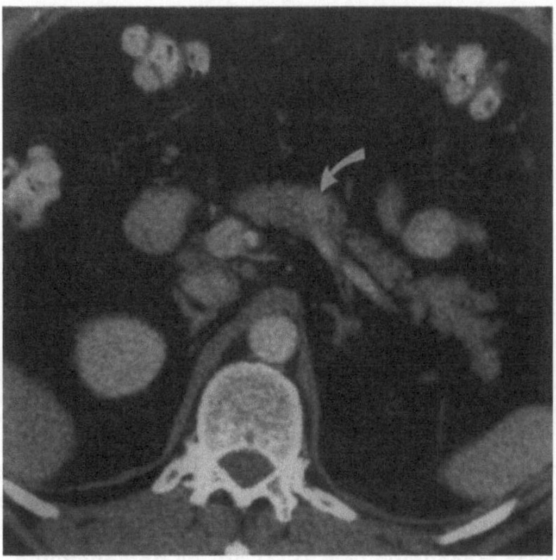

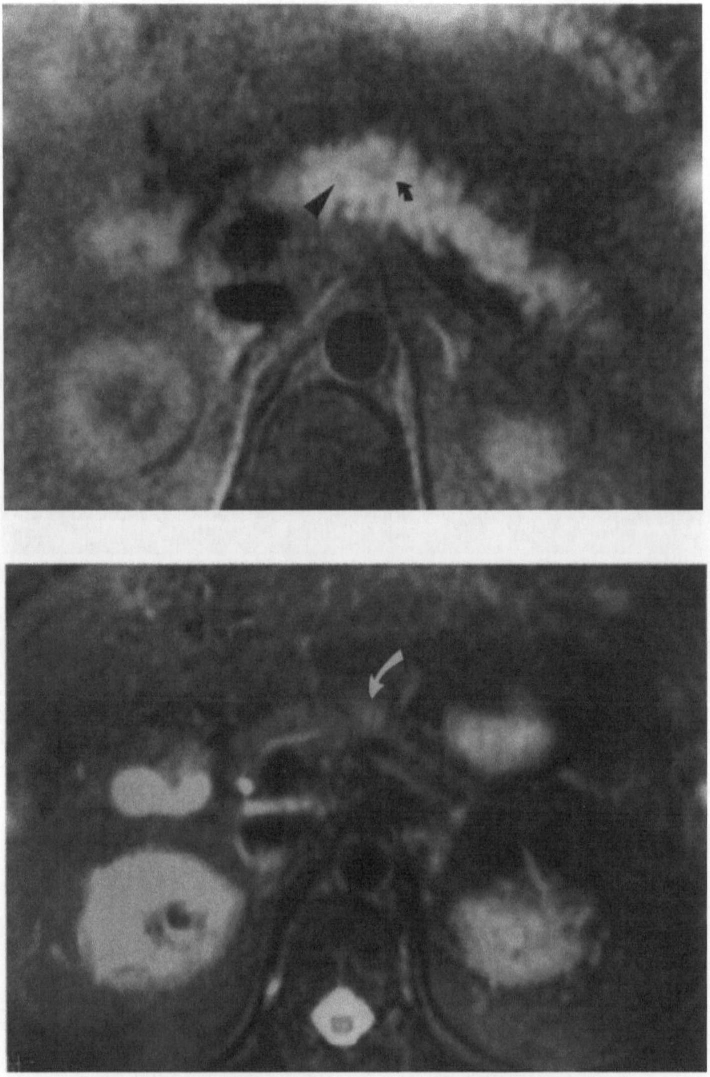

Figure 1. A: Transverse ultrasound through the upper abdomen, showing an 8 mm focal abnormality within the body of the pancreas of decreased echogenicity (white arrow). The left lobe of the liver (L), the aorta (A), the inferior vena cava (I), the splenic vein (S) and superior mesenteric vein (SM) are all demonstrated. B: CT scan in the same patient showing the small lesion in the body of the pancreas (white arrow). The lesion can be seen to extremely vascular. C: Fat suppressed T1 weighted MRI scan in the same patient showing the same small lesion of decreased signal intensity (curved arrow). The fat suppression has resulted in increased signal intensity of the normal pancreas (arrowhead). D: Fat suppressed T2 weighted image in the same patient. This shows the small lesion within the body of the pancreas of increased signal intensity (white arrow).

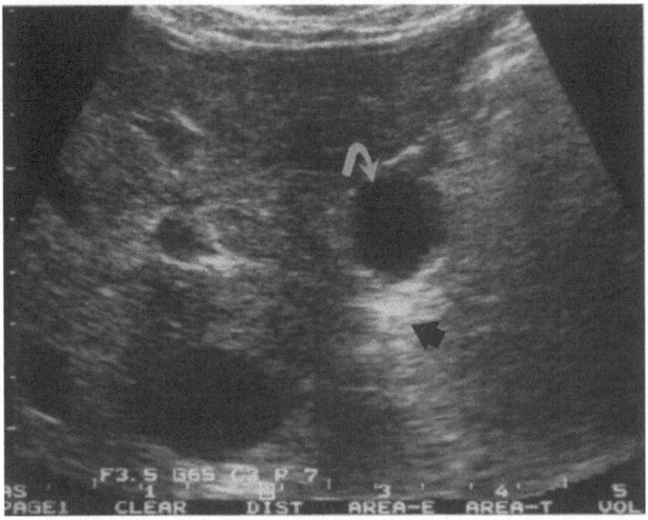
PAGE1 CLEAR DIST AREA-E AREA-T VOL

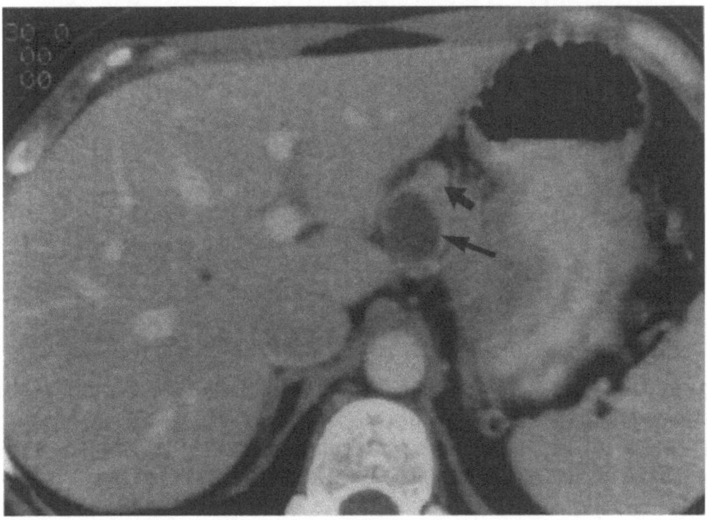

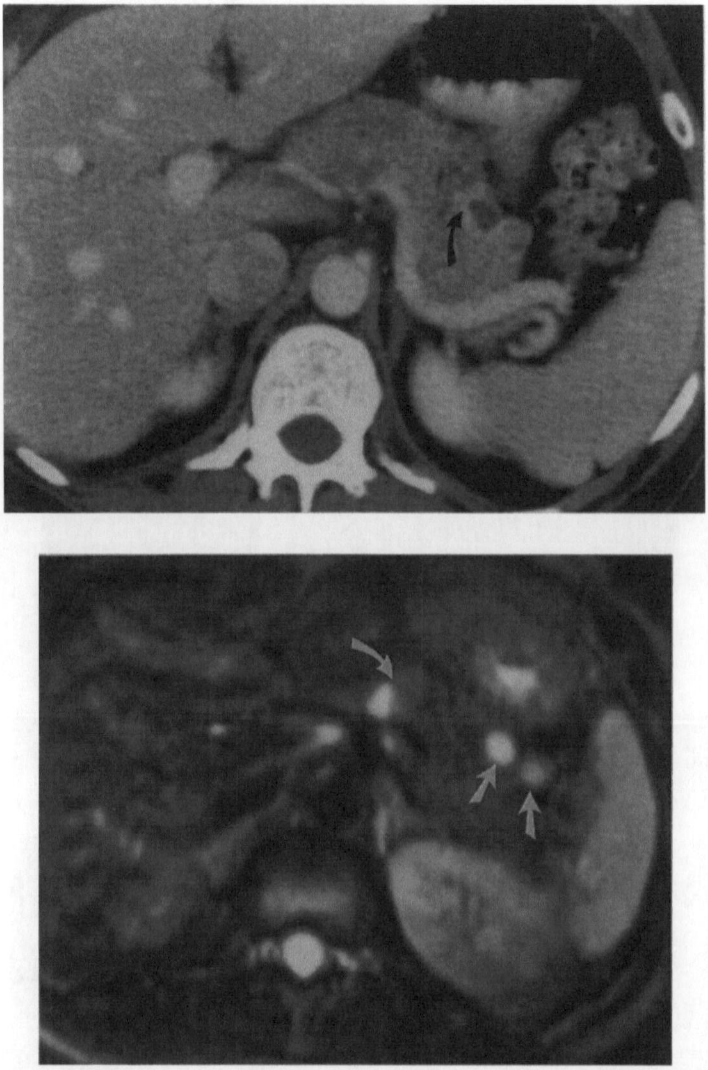

Figure 2. A: Transverse upper abdominal ultrasound examination in a patient with a glucagonoma showing a mass in the body of the pancreas which is predominantly anechoic (white arrow).The increased through transmission (short black arrow) is due to the presence of fluid within the lesion. Note that the soft tissue component is also seen within the mass. B and C: CT scan in the same patient. B shows the same cystic lesion (long arrow) seen on the ultrasound within the body of the pancreas. Note the enhancing portion of the lesion (short arrow). C: Further cystic lesions can be demonstrated in the tail with similar characteristics to those seen in the larger lesion in the head (curved arrow). D. T2 weighted MRI scan showing all three lesions. The large lesion in the head of the pancreas can be seen to have a substantial soft tissue component, although it can also be seen to be cystic. Two further cystic lesions, also demonstrated on the CT scan, are seen in the tail of the pancreas (white arrows).

Transabdominal ultrasound is useful for screening for metastases from pancreatic neuroendocrine tumors. Gastrinoma metastases are almost invariably hyperechoic compared to the surrounding liver (9), unlike the lesions of metastatic pancreatic carcinoma, which usually appear as hypoechoic lesions on ultrasound.

A major disadvantage of ultrasound in the imaging of pancreatic lesions is that visualization of the entire gland may be restricted by overlying bowel gas, particularly in the lateral aspect of the head and in the tail of the pancreas. This inevitably reduces sensitivity so that, although sensitivity rates for the detection of single insulinomas may be as high as 70% if the whole pancreas is imaged (8), overall figures (including cases where visualization may be suboptimal) are significantly lower and vary between 25 and 63% (8,7). Detection rates also fall, possibly to as low as 15% for insulinomas, when multiple islet cell tumors are present (7).

2. Endoscopic ultrasound

In this technique a high-frequency (10 MHz) transducer is passed through an endoscope to lie adjacent to the pancreas either within the duodenum (for visualization of the pancreatic head) or the stomach (for the body and tail). In experienced hands, accurate, high-resolution images of the entire pancreas may be obtained, with the exception of the tip of the pancreatic tail, which does not lie in close proximity to the stomach (12). The higher frequency transducer permits the detection of smaller lesions, with the threshold for detection falling to around 5 mm in some centers (13). As with transabdominal ultrasound, most islet cell tumors appear as hypoechoic areas compared to the surrounding pancreas (Figures 3A, 4A). Endoscopic ultrasound is available at relatively few centers and, being a comparatively new technique, its role in the imaging of pancreatic neuroendocrine tumors and carcinoids is not yet fully established. Early reports, however, are highly encouraging. In one series (13), 82% of tumors not visualized either with transabdominal ultrasound or CT were detected: a figure that compared favorably with the 27% detection rate of angiography in the same patients. Other centers report even greater success with this technique (14).

3. Intraoperative ultrasound

This technique involves the use of a high-frequency transducer placed directly on the pancreas. High-resolution images of the entire gland may be obtained. Mobilization of the pancreatic tail from behind the peritoneum may be required to gain adequate images of this portion of the pancreas, a procedure that may be associated with splenic injury (15). Again, most islet cell Tumors appear as sharply defined hypoechoic masses compared to the surrounding pancreas. IOUS is able to detect around 90% of solitary insulinomas (16) and should be regarded as an adjunct to careful palpation of the gland by an experienced surgeon. These two techniques together have been associated with detection rates of 100% of insulinomas (7). Detection rates of intra-pancreatic gastrinomas with IOUS are also excellent, with 100% reported in one series (15). The reduced detection rate of gastrinomas as a whole with IOUS (15) again reflects the fact that many such tumors are located within the gastrinoma triangle.

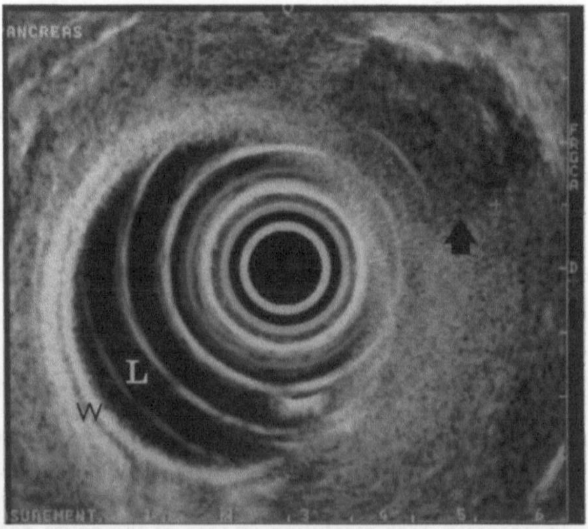

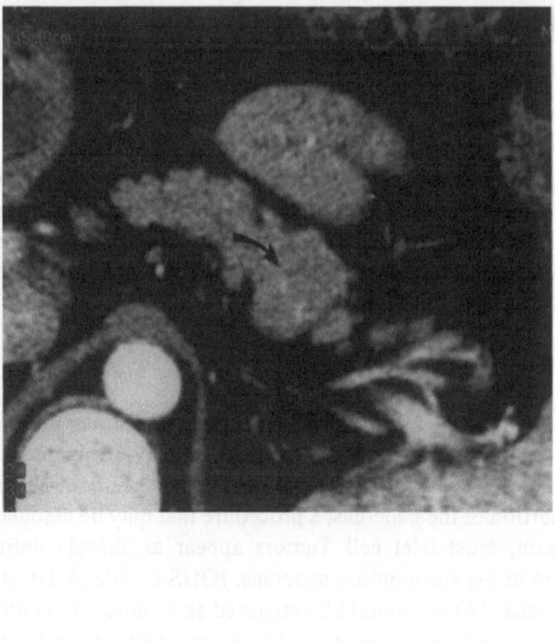

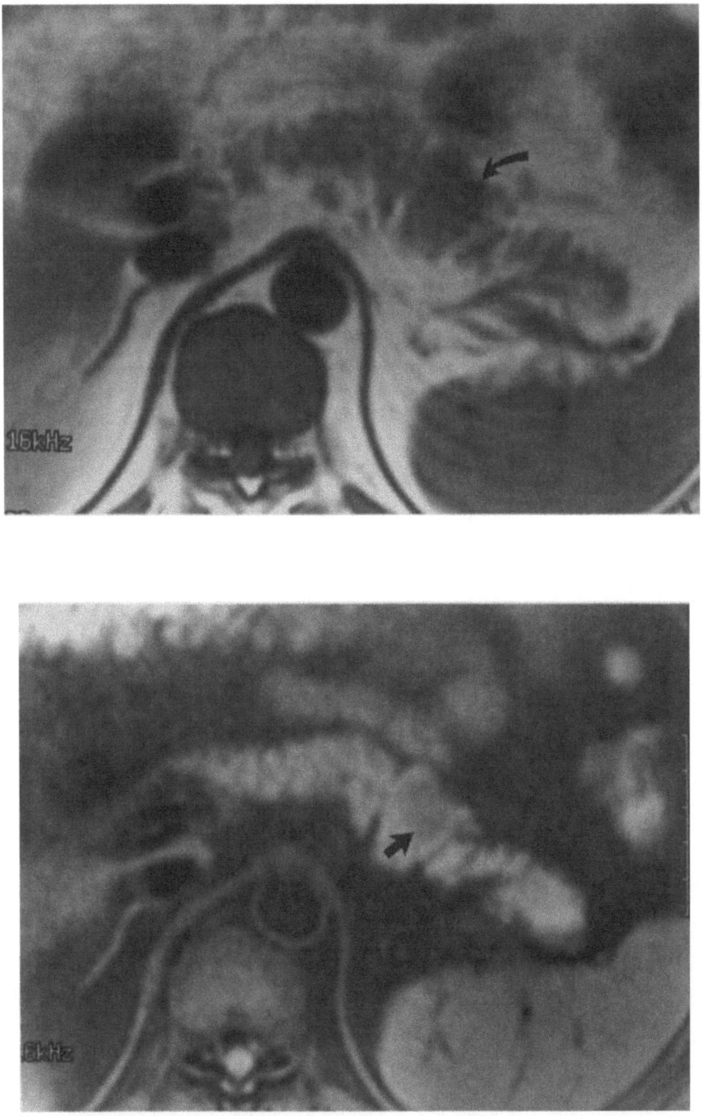

Figure 3. A: Endoscopic ultrasound examination in a patient with a gastrinoma of the pancreas, showing a 1.5 cm mass lesion in the tail of the pancreas (black arrow). The wall of the stomach is demonstrated (W). The circular probe lies within the lumen of the stomach (L). B: CT in the same patient following intravenous injection of contrast medium, showing an enhancing mass within the tail of the pancreas (curved arrow). C: T1 weighted MRI scan in the same patient showing the mass, typically of low signal intensity (curved arrow). D: Fat suppressed T1 weighted MRI scan showing the mass of low signal intensity (arrow). Note that the mass is better seen on the fat suppressed than on the conventional spin-echo sequences.

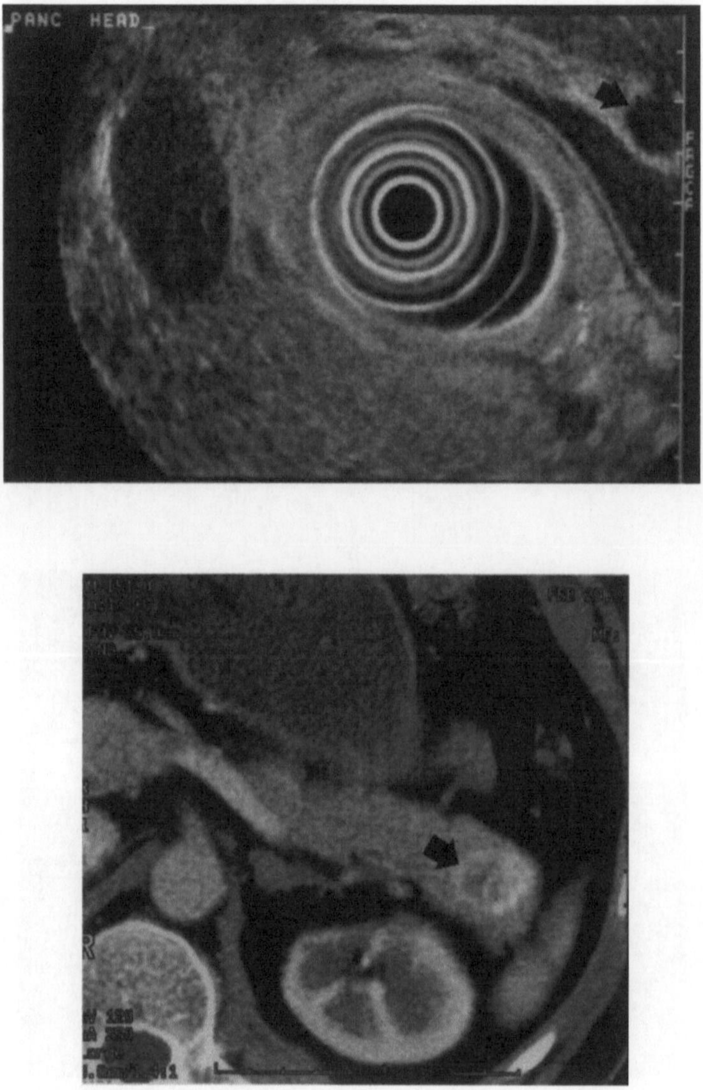
PANC HEAD

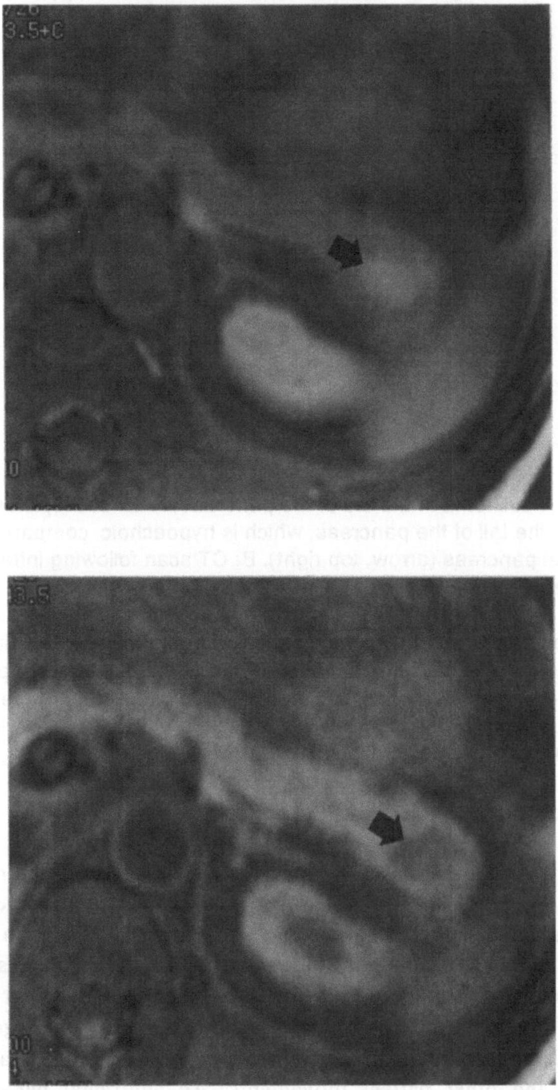

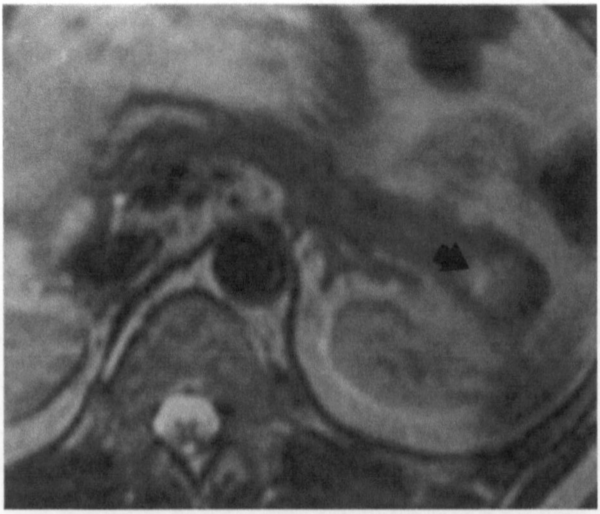

Figure 4. Calcified insulinoma in the tail of the pancreas. A: Endoscopic ultrasound showing a mass in the tail of the pancreas, which is hypoechoic, compared to the surrounding normal pancreas (arrow, top right). B: CT scan following intravenous injection of contrast medium. Note the 1 cm lesion in the tail, which is not distorting the pancreatic outline (arrow). Calcification can clearly be seen within the mass. C: Fat suppressed T1 weighted scan showing the typical appearance of a low signal intensity mass (arrow). Note that the calcium cannot be demonstrated. D: Fat suppressed T1 weighted scan following intravenous injection of gadolinium. Note that the mass lesion (arrow) enhances intensely with contrast. E: T2 weighted MRI scan showing the typical appearance of a mass of high signal intensity (arrow).

B. Computed tomography (CT)

CT is now widely available, minimally invasive and is currently the most frequent mode of imaging for pancreatic endocrine tumors. Despite its extensive use, there is considerable variation in the reported sensitivity of CT for the detection of pancreatic neuroendocrine tumors and carcinoids, a fact that reflects various levels of expertise, age of scanners and the protocols used for dynamic CT in different centers. The advent of 'spiral' or helical scanners allows the entire gland to be imaged in 3-5 mm intervals during a single breath hold, thereby reducing considerably the artifact arising from respiratory and other patient movements. An additional benefit is greater vascular opacification during scans enhanced with contrast medium injected intravenously, as the images can be acquired when the concentration of contrast medium is at its maximum in the arterial phase. This is an important consideration as islet cell tumors are usually very vascular.

Useful diagnostic information may be present on scans obtained both before and after the intravenous injection of contrast medium and the authors recommend that both be performed when imaging the pancreas. The stomach and duodenum should be tilled either with oral contrast medium or water and a muscle relaxant such as hyoscine-Nbutylbromide or glucagon administered. This allows optimal visualization of the bowel wall and pancreas following intravenous administration of contrast medium. Islet cell tumors are generally iso-dense with surrounding pancreas and are only seen after contrast injection. However, helpful features on a pre-contrast scan include distortion of the gland architecture, central necrosis and, in about 10% of cases, well-defined nodular calcification (Figure 4B). Approximately 70% of calcified islet cell tumors are malignant (17) (Figure 5A). A small minority of islet cell tumors are hypodense and, in exceptional circumstances, may arise in the wall of an apparently benign cystic pancreatic lesion (18) (Figures 2B, 2C).

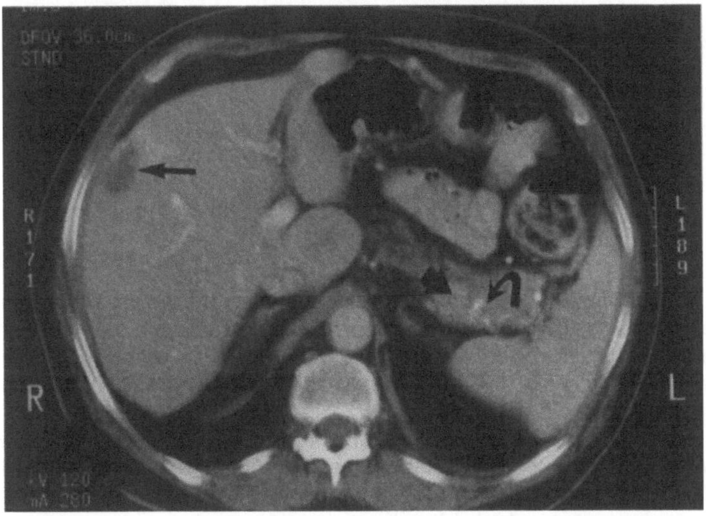

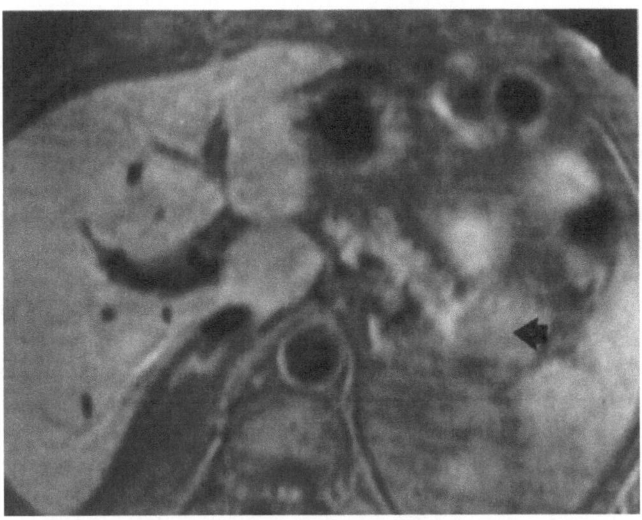

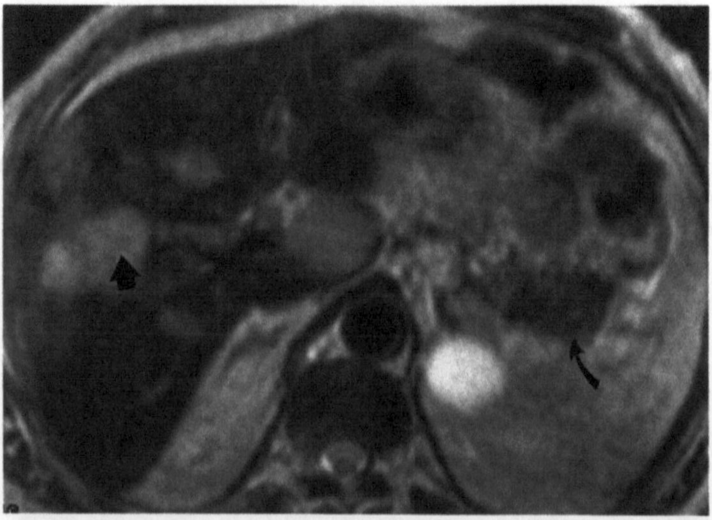

Figure 5. A: This shows an enhancing mass in the tail of the pancreas (straight arrow) of a patient with a malignant carcinoid tumor. It can also be seen that there are flecks of calcium within this lesion (curved arrow). A deposit with an enhancing rim is present within the liver (long arrow). B: Fat suppressed T1 weighted MRI scan in the same patient showing the islet cell tumor of decreased signal intensity in the tail (arrow). Note that the liver deposits cannot be demonstrated on this image. C: T2 weighted MRI scan in the same patient showing the liver deposits of high signal intensity (arrow). Note that the mass in the tail of the pancreas is of low signal intensity – an unusual appearance (curved arrow).

The improved detection rate following intravenous contrast medium is due to the fact that the vascular tumor enhances more readily than the surrounding normal pancreas. In many cases, the difference in attenuation between tumor and normal surrounding pancreas may be extremely subtle and it may be necessary to use narrow window settings to be certain of not missing a small lesion (Figures 6A, 6B).

The wide variation in scanning techniques and the rapidly changing technology of the equipment used makes an assessment of the accuracy of CT scanning in the detection of islet cell tumors difficult. Solitary insulinomas seem to be more elusive than single intrapancreatic gastrinomas (7,19). The size detection limit is certainly smaller than that of TAUS, but probably no better (around 5 mm) than EUS or IOUS. As with ultrasound, detection rates fall considerably in the presence of multiple lesions. Non-functioning islet cell tumors and carcinoids tend to be larger at presentation than either insulinomas or gastrinomas. Detection rates are therefore correspondingly higher.

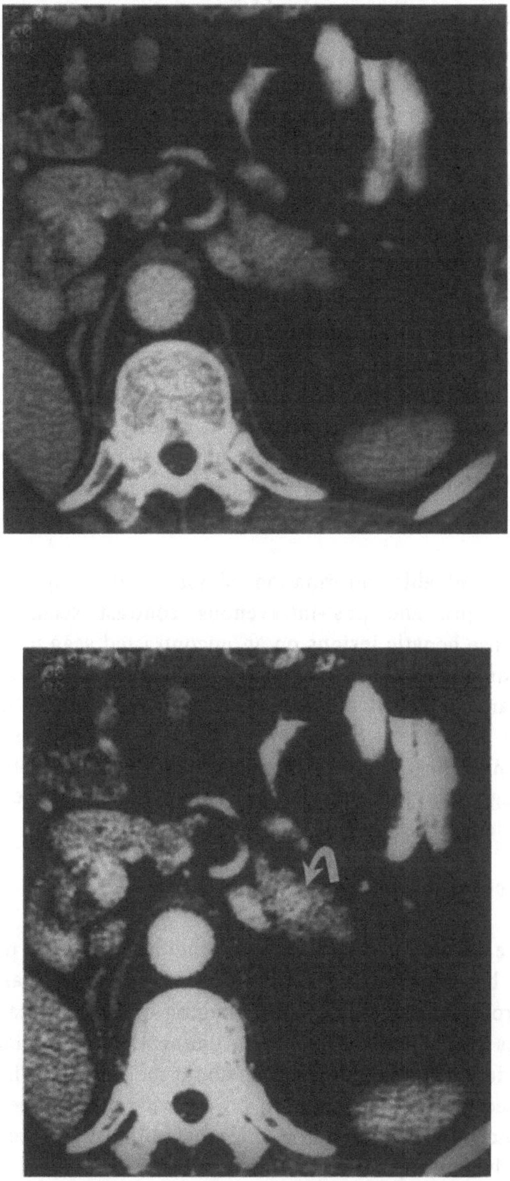

Figure 6. A: CT scan following intravenous injection of contrast medium. An abnormality cannot definitely be demonstrated within the pancreas. B: The same CT scan with post processing. The 'window level' and the window center have been altered to increase the contrast. A lesion can now clearly be seen within the tail of the pancreas showing the typical enhancement following contrast medium (white arrow).

Conventional CT with contrast has a disappointing sensitivity in the detection of islet cell tumors (20). However, the use of dual phase spiral CT (OPSCT) greatly improves sensitivity, with some tumors as small as 4 mm being seen (21). Rapid injection of high concentration of contrast medium in the arterial phase ensures that the characteristic tumor blush is captured, whereas lesions may appear isodense on images acquired in the arterio-venous phase. In a recent series (22), pancreatic images acquired using 3 mm collimation in the arterial and arteriovenous perfusion phases following intravenous contrast medium administration identified six insulinomas in seven patients previously investigated using one or more other imaging modalities (endoscopic ultrasound, intraoperative ultrasound, CT, MRI and arteriography). All six tumors were identified on the early (arterial) phase, two of which would not have been detected by scanning in the arteriovenous phase only. No tumor was visible only in the arteriovenous phase in the series, although in one case conspicuity was improved. Occasional cases have been reported in which images acquired in the arterial phase have failed to demonstrate a lesion seen on images during the arteriovenous phase (21), suggesting that scanning should, ideally, be done in both phases. However, if a single phase only is used, the images should be acquired early in the arterial phase to maximize the detection rate.

CT also provides valuable information about local lymph node and hepatic metastases. Again, pre and post-intravenous contrast scans are necessary, as previously hypodense hepatic lesions on an uncontrasted scan may become isodense with the surrounding liver after contrast administration. However, most hepatic metastases from any islet cell tumor (insulinoma, gastrinoma, non-functioning or carcinoid) appear hyperdense after intravenous contrast, due to the increased vascularity. Distinguishing a solitary metastasis from a hemangioma may be impossible, although delayed scans and the characteristic centripetal enhancement of hemangioma may help in this regard.

C. Magnetic Resonance Imaging (MRI)

In recent years, the development of techniques that overcome the problems of motion artifact caused by bowel peristalsis, respiratory movement and vascular motion have significantly improved the quality of MR imaging of the pancreas. The diversity of imaging sequences available not only permits delineation of the anatomy of pancreatic lesions, but provides additional information about their nature. The rate of change of the techniques used means that there are few comparative studies that evaluate the role of MR in pancreatic imaging, although most authorities accept that it is now at least the equal of dynamic spiral CT in this regard.

Normal pancreas has medium signal intensity similar to that of liver on TI- weighted images. This is secondary to the presence of aqueous protein in the acini of normal pancreas (19). Islet cell tumors, which lack aqueous protein, are of low signal intensity compared to normal pancreas on TI-weighting (Figures 3C, 4C). Occasional tumors may be isointense. On T2-weighted images, islet cell tumors, most notably gastrinomas, appear hyperintense (Figure 2D), compared to normal pancreas, which, again, has a signal intensity similar to that of the liver. The vascular nature of most islet cell tumors means that they enhance markedly after intravenous gadolinium. Insulinomas usually show uniform enhancement whereas gastrinomas typically exhibit ring enhancement (Figure 4D) with a central area of low signal intensity (19).

A variety of techniques exist that may, in certain circumstances, improve the quality of the images acquired by MR and provide information about the nature of any underlying lesions. Fat suppression is a commonly used technique that enhances the information gained during TI-weighted imaging, removing the artifact generated by the high signal intensity of fat seen on spin echo sequences. With the signal generated by the fat effectively removed, the different signals generated by tumor and normal pancreas can be accentuated by increasing the receiver gain. In our experience, this has proved to be the single most valuable sequence in the imaging of pancreatic neuroendocrine tumors (23).

The different patterns of vascularity of tumor and normal pancreas give rise to different signal intensities on imaging, although with time, as contrast medium dissipates, this difference becomes less marked. Hence, the potential value of intravenous contrast medium in MR imaging is limited by the length of time taken to acquire the images. Recent improvements in optimizing breath-hold imaging sequences have allowed the acquisition of multiple images in a single breath hold and during the time that the concentration of contrast agent, such as gadolinium, remains sufficiently high (typically about 90 seconds).

A combination of different imaging sequences and variation in the quality of equipment between centers makes comparison of MR with other cross-sectional imaging techniques difficult. In one series (24) T1 -weighted fat- suppressed spin-echo (FSSE) and gradient-echo MR imaging demonstrated 11 islet cell tumors in ten patients, whereas dynamic contrast-enhanced CT identified only seven. The tumors not seen on CT were all 2.5 cm or less. In our own series, CT identified only 19 of the 27 lesions shown on MRI (23).

Conclusions

The detection of pancreatic neuroendocrine tumors and carcinoids remains a challenge for the radiologist and endocrinologist. Different centers develop various levels of expertise with each imaging modality, such that the literature contains levels of sensitivity and specificity with a given technique that other centers are unable to reproduce. To some extent, the choice of imaging modality depends on the question being posed and careful discussion with clinical colleagues is essential in this regard. Factors that need to be considered should include the cost of the technique and the known accuracy of each modality in detecting such small tumors. Irrespective of the modality chosen, the conduct of the investigation always requires extraordinary attention to detail as the tumors are often small, do not distort the pancreatic contour and can be extremely difficult to identify. Correlation with functional studies are often essential. More than one imaging modality is frequently needed in order to provide sufficient diagnostic certainty on which to base management decisions. In specialist centers with experience of imaging pancreatic neuroendocrine tumors, a combination

of endoscopic ultrasound and MR scanning probably provides the best sensitivity for the tumor detection. Where such expertise is not available, dual phase spiral CT is often the first imaging modality used and its sensitivity is slightly less than MRI or EUS. In the case of non-secreting tumors, the main role of imaging is in staging, particularly in the case of carcinoid tumors, where the presence of hepatic metastases dictates the management strategy. MR offers little advantage over TAUS and CT in this regard, both of which are widely available.

References

1. Fraker DL, Norton JA. Localization and resection of insulinomas and gastrinomas. J A M A. 1988;259:3601.
2. Service FJ, Dale AJD, Elveback LR, et al. Insulinoma: clinical and diagnostic features of 60 consecutive cases. Mayo Clin Proc. 1976;51: 417.
3. Howard TJ, Zinner MJ, Stabile BE, et al. Gastrinoma excision for cure. A prospective analysis. Ann Surg. 1990;211:9.
4. King CMP, Reznek RH, Dacie JE, Wass JAH. Review: imaging islet cell tumours. Clin Radiol. 1994;49:295.
5. Buetow PC, Parrino RV, Buck JL, Pantongrag-Brown L, et al. Islet cell tumors of the pancreas: pathologic-imaging correlation among size, necrosis and cysts, calcification, malignant behavior and functional status. Am J Roentgenol. 1995;:1175.
6. Gunther R W, Klose KJ, Ruckert K, et al. Islet-cell tumors: detection of small lesions with computed tomography and ultrasound. Radiology 1983;148:485.
7. Galiber AK, Reading CC, Charboneau JW, et al. Localization of pancreatic insulinoma: comparison of pre- and intraoperative US with CT and angiography. Radiology 1998;166:405.
8. Gorman B, Charboneau JW, James EM et al. Benign pancreatic insulinoma: preoperative and intraoperative sonographic localization. Am J Roentgenol. 1986;147:929.
9. London JF, Shawker TH, Doppman JL, et al. Zollinger-Ellison syndrome: prospective assessment of abdominal US in the localization of gastrinomas. Radiology 1991;178:763.
10. Stabile EE, Morrow DJ, Passaro E Jr. The gastrinoma triangle: operative implications. Am J Surg.1984;147:25.
11. Howard TJ, Zinner MJ, Stabile BE, et al. Gastrinoma excision for cure. A prospective analysis. Ann Surg. 1990;211:9.
12. Glover JR, Shorvon PJ, Lees WR. Endoscopic localisation of islet cell tumours. Gut 1992;22:108.
13. Rosch T, Lightdale CJ, Botet JF, et al. Localization of pancreatic endocrine tumours by endoscopic ultrasonography. N Engl J Med. 1992;326:1721.
14. Pitre J, Soubrane O, Palazzo L, Chapuis Y. Endoscopic ultrasonography for the preoperative localization of insulinomas. Pancreas 1996;I3:55.
15. Norton JA, Cromack OT, Shawker TH et al. Intraoperative ultrasonographic localisation of islet cell tumors. Gut 1992;33:108.
16. Gooding GAW. Adrenal, pancreatic and scrotal ultrasound in endocrine disease. Radiol Clin North Am. 1993;31:1069.
17. Imhof M, Frank P. Pancreatic calcifications in malignant islet cell tumors. Radiology 1977,122:333.
18. Sohaib SAA, Reznek RH, Healy JC, Besser GM. Cystic islet cell tumors of the pancreas. Am J Roentgenol. 1998;170:217.
19. Semelka RC, Cumming MJ, Shoenut JP, et al. Islet cell tumors: comparison of dynamic gadolinium enhancement and fat suppression. Radiology 1993;186:799.
20. Angeli E, Vanzulli A, Castrucci M et al. Value of abdominal sonography and MR imaging at 0.5T in the preoperative detection of pancreatic insulinoma: a comparison with dynamic CT and angiography. Abd Imag. 1997;22:295.
21. Van Hoe L, Gryspeerdt S, Marchal G, Baert A, Mertens L. Helical CT for the preoperative localization of islet cell tumors of the pancreas: value of arterial and parenchymal phase images. Am J Roentgenol.1995;165:1437.
22. King AD, Ko GTC, Yeung VTF, Chow CC, Griffith J, Cockram CS. Dual phase spiral CT in the detection of small insulinomas of the pancreas. Br J Radiol.1998;71:20.

23. Owen N, Peppercorn PD, Reznek RH, et al. MRI of neuroendocrine tumors. Am J Roentgenol. 1998;170 (Suppl.4):74.
24. Semelka RC, Cumming MJ, Shoenut JP, et al. Islet cell tumors: comparison of dynamic contrast-enhanced CT and MR imaging with dynamic gadolinium enhancement and fat suppression. Radiology 1993;186:799.

12
SCINTIGRAPHY OF PANCREATIC NEUROENDOCRINE TUMORS AND CARCINOIDS

Dik J. Kwekkeboom, M.D.
Wouter W. de Herder, M.D.
Eric P. Krenning, M.D.
University Hospital Rotterdam
Rotterdam, the Netherlands

INTRODUCTION

In diagnosing or staging cancer, conventional imaging techniques like CT scanning or MRI usually seem adequate in detecting tumor localizations. Difficulties are encountered, however, when patients harbor small tumors, especially in the abdomen, a site notorious for the lack of sensitivity that is achieved with even the most refined imaging modalities. For the localization of for instance neuroendocrine gastroenteropancreatic (GEP) tumors, like carcinoids, insulinomas, and gastrinomas, sensitivities of CT and MRI are at most 50%, depending on the size and localization of the lesions. Therefore, much effort has been put into developing other means to visualize such tumors. Because neuroendocrine tumors possess peptide hormone and/or growth factor receptors, radiolabeled compounds that bind to such receptors may be of potential use to be applied in tumor imaging and staging. Examples of such an approach are the application of the radiolabeled somatostatin analog, [^{111}In-DTPA-D-Phe^{1}]octreotide, and radioiodinated vasoactive intestinal peptide, ^{123}I-VIP. Other tumor characteristics that can be used to differentiate tumors from surrounding tissue are their metabolic behavior, used in ^{18}F-fluorodeoxyglucose positron emission tomography (FDG-PET), and the chromogranin-A (CgA) content of neuroendocrine tumor cells, used in an avidin-biotin three-step scintigraphic method with an anti-CgA monoclonal antibody.

Although it is true that these *in vivo* nuclear medicine imaging methods may be useful as tumor localizing techniques in a variety of diseases where they may detect tumor localizations prior to or in addition to conventional imaging, they will by their nature never be competitive with for instance CT or MRI in anatomical delineation of these disease sites. The physiologic nature of these methods, however, may offer complementary and advantageous information in several instances: 1) enlargement of tissues (like for instance lymph nodes) is in itself not indicative of spread of the investigated disease in that tissue. The appearance of certain peptide receptors in such tissue, a different glucose utilization, or a different CgA content, could be more indicative; 2) likewise the absence or disappearance during treatment of anatomical imaging modalities does not preclude the presence or persistence of foci of disease. Monitoring the peptide receptor status, the glucose utilization, or the CgA content with scintigraphic techniques could provide essential information in this respect; 3) the scintigraphic features may be used to monitor the efficacy of therapy; 4) the presence or absence of pathological uptake may also be used in the clinical decision how to treat the investigated disease, either because this uptake is linked to the differentiation state of the tumor or, in case of peptide receptor scintigraphy, because effective treatment with peptide analogs binding to that receptor are available; 5) lastly, the development of peptide analogs coupled to ß-emitting radiopharmaceuticals may lead to a situation in which diagnostic peptide scintigraphy can be followed by radiotherapy.

Mechanism of uptake, procedure and normal distribution

Somatostatin receptor scintigraphy (SRS)

Somatostatin membrane-receptors have been identified on many cells and tumors of neuroendocrine origin, like the somatotroph cells of the anterior pituitary, and the pancreatic islet-cell tumors (1-3). Also cells and tumors not known as classically neuroendocrine of origin, such as activated lymphocytes, lymphomas and breast cancer, may possess these receptors (4-6).

The somatostatin analog octreotide, which is 8 amino acids long, has been shown to bind to somatostatin receptor subtypes sst_2, sst_3, and sst_5 on both tumorous and non-tumorous tissues. Because of its relatively long effective half-life, [^{111}In-DTPA-D-Phe^1]-octreotide is a radiolabeled somatostatin analog which can be used to visualize somatostatin receptor bearing tumors efficiently after 24 and 48 h, when interfering background radioactivity is minimized by renal clearance (7).

Normal scintigraphic features include visualization of the pituitary in part of the patients, of the thyroid, the spleen, liver, and kidneys. Also, the urine bladder and the bowel (to a variable degree) are usually visualized. The visualization of the pituitary, thyroid, and spleen is due to receptor binding, whereas the uptake in the liver and kidneys is for the most part due to metabolism, although somatostatin receptors have been demonstrated in renal tubular cells and vasa recta (8). There is a predominant renal clearance of the somatostatin analog, although hepatobiliary clearance into the bowel also occurs, necessitating the use of laxatives in order to facilitate the interpretation of abdominal images.

The scanning protocol should include a sufficient dose of [^{111}In-DTPA-D-Phe^1]octreotide (about 200 MBq), to enable SPECT imaging, which increases the sensitivity to detect octreotide receptor expressing tissues and gives a better anatomical delineation than planar views. The acquisition of sufficient counts per view and also obtaining spot images with a sufficient counting time instead of performing whole-body scanning with a too low count density, are other important points that may make the difference between a successful localizing study and a disappointing one. For a detailed scanning protocol see (9,10).

VIP receptor scintigraphy (VIPRS)

VIP is a 28 amino-acid hormone, which regulates water and electrolyte secretion in the gut, and has a function in immune regulation (11-13). VIP receptors are present, amongst others, on gut epithelial cells, lung tissue, and immune cells (14-16). They have also been demonstrated on colonic adenocarcinomas, exocrine pancreatic tumors, and neuroendocrine tumors (15,17-19). Radioiodinated VIP was shown to have a biological activity on tumor cells identical to that of unlabeled VIP (20).

The principal site of uptake during VIPRS are the lungs, whereas virtually no uptake is seen in the liver, spleen or bowel (20). As with SRS, the predominant route of clearance of ^{123}I-VIP is renal. Spot images and SPECT images are obtained after 2 to 4 h (21).

CgA immunoscintigraphy (CgAIS)

CgA is a protein present in neuroendocrine secretory granules, and is used as a serum and immunohistochemical marker for a variety of neuroendocrine tumors (22-24).

The three-step immunoscintigraphy with anti-CgA monoclonal antibody consists of the following: On the first day the biotinylated monoclonal antibody is injected (step one); after 1 to 2 days unlabeled avidin is injected in order to reduce circulating unbound antibody concentrations (step two); finally, one day later, ^{111}In-labeled biotin derivative is injected, which binds to the monoclonal antibodies present on the tumor-target (step three) (25-27).

The advantages of this three-step *in vivo* labeling procedure over the usual way of monoclonal antibody scintigraphy, i.e. after the injection of antibodies that have been radiolabeled *in vitro*, are that the background radioactivity is lower due to lower concentrations of circulating labeled antibodies, and that therefore target to background ratios are higher, resulting in improved tumor detection.

Normally, background radioactivity is low, except for accumulation of the radiotracer in the kidneys, which represents the principal route of clearance. Image acquisition is started 2 h after ^{111}In-labeled biotin derivative administration, which is 2 to 3 days after the antibody administration (25-27).

FDG-PET

^{18}F-FDG is a radiolabeled D-glucose, which is phosphorylated intracellularly, after which the product is trapped in the cells. Its increased accumulation in tumor tissue is based on an increased glucose metabolism associated with malignancy. Aggressive tumors show higher uptake of ^{18}F-FDG than do benign lesions (28-30). Sites of inflammation and infection may also show increased uptake of the radiotracer (31).

The normal distribution of ^{18}F-FDG includes the brain, heart, lungs, kidneys and urinary tract. Because of the short half-life of cyclotron-derived ^{18}F (110 min), ^{18}F-FDG has to be prepared near to the site where the patient is investigated. Imaging is usually performed 40 to 60 min after injection, and requires a dedicated PET scanner. A newly developed way of scintigraphy is based on a modified gamma-camera with a coincidence detection system. Systematic comparison with PET scanning is being performed, and although image quality is less than with PET scanning, this type of coincidence scanning, because of the wide availability of conventional gamma-cameras which can be used to more purposes and the cost-saving aspect, may give ^{18}F-FDG scintigraphy a new impulse.

Patient preparation includes a several hour fast (preferably 12 h), in order to reduce serum glucose levels.

Results in pancreatic neuroendocrine tumors and carcinoids

SRS

Most peptide hormone-producing endocrine tumors stem from the islet-cells of the pancreas, but they may also occur elsewhere in the gastrointestinal tract. These tumors are named after the hormone(s) they secrete, e.g. gastrinomas, insulinomas, glucagonomas. Octreotide is of special benefit in the treatment of the clinical syndromes caused by hypersecretion of these hormones (32,33). Surgery is the treatment of choice in most patients, but the localization of the primary as well as metastatic tumors may prove very difficult or even impossible with conventional imaging means (34).

The majority of the endocrine pancreatic tumors can be visualized using SRS. Therefore, SRS can be of great value in localizing tumor sites in this type of patients, also in those cases where surgery is indicated but no tumor localization can be found with conventional imaging modalities. Reported data on the sensitivity of SRS in patients with gastrinomas vary from about 60 to 90% (35-39), and part of the discrepancy in results is likely due to insufficient scanning technique (especially short acquisition time), not performing SPECT studies, or injection of relatively low doses of [^{111}In-DTPA-D-Phe^{1}]-octreotide, all of which may lead to poorer performance of SRS.

Using ultrasound, CT, MRI, and/or angiography, endocrine pancreatic tumors can be localized in about 50% of cases (40,41). Endoscopic ultrasound has been reported to be very sensitive in detecting endocrine pancreatic tumors, also when CT or transabdominal ultrasound fail to demonstrate the tumor (42). Studies comparing the value of endoscopic ultrasonography with SRS in the same patients point to more favorable results for SRS (37,39). Recently, Gibril and coworkers. (38) published the results of a prospective study in 80 patients with Zollinger-Ellison syndrome, comparing SRS with a variety of other imaging techniques as well as angiography. Although whole-body scintigraphy with a total acquisition time of only 30 min. was used, SPECT of the upper abdomen was performed in every patient. They found that SRS was as sensitive as all of the other imaging studies combined and advocated its use as the first imaging method to be used in these patients because of its sensitivity, simplicity, and cost-effectiveness. In a cost-effectiveness study in our own institute (43) we found that the combination of SRS and CT scanning of the upper abdomen had the highest sensitivity in demonstrating gastrinomas. The relative high cost of this imaging regime was thought to be outweighed by demonstrating potentially resectable tumors.

Lebtahi and coworkers. (44) reported that the results of SRS in 160 patients with GEP tumors modified patient classification and surgical therapeutic strategy in 25% of patients. However, results in patients with insulinomas are disappointing, possibly because part of these tumors may either be somatostatin receptor negative or contain somatostatin receptors that do not bind octreotide (45).

In a study comprising 33 patients with carcinoids, 92% of lesions in 96% of patients were found with SRS, counting results of conventional imaging and SRS together as 100%. If results of only conventional imaging were analyzed, additional, unexpected localizations were detected with SRS in a considerable number of patients (46). Known liver metastases were not distinctly visualized with planar SRS in 12 of 24 patients. In all but 2 of these, an homogeneous distribution of radioactivity in the liver was observed. This is most probably due to the fact that these liver metastases accumulated about as much radioactivity as does normal liver tissue. Substraction techniques and/or SPECT studies might be useful in this respect, as an irregular distribution of radioactivity on the SPECT images was observed in several patients in whom planar images showed an even uptake of liver radioactivity.

Others have also reported high percentages of patients with carcinoids whose tumors were visualized with SRS. Reported values vary from 80 to nearly 100% (47-50). Also, several investigators report the detection of unexpected tumor sites, not suspected with conventional imaging (Figures 1-3)(49,50).

Treatment with octreotide may cause a relief of symptoms and a decrease of urinary 5-HIAA levels in patients with the carcinoid syndrome (51,52). In patients with the carcinoid syndrome, SRS, in consequence of its ability to demonstrate somatostatin receptor positive tumors, could therefore be used to select those patients who are likely to respond favorably to octreotide treatment. On the other hand, only for those patients who have somatostatin receptor negative tumors, chemotherapy is effective (53).

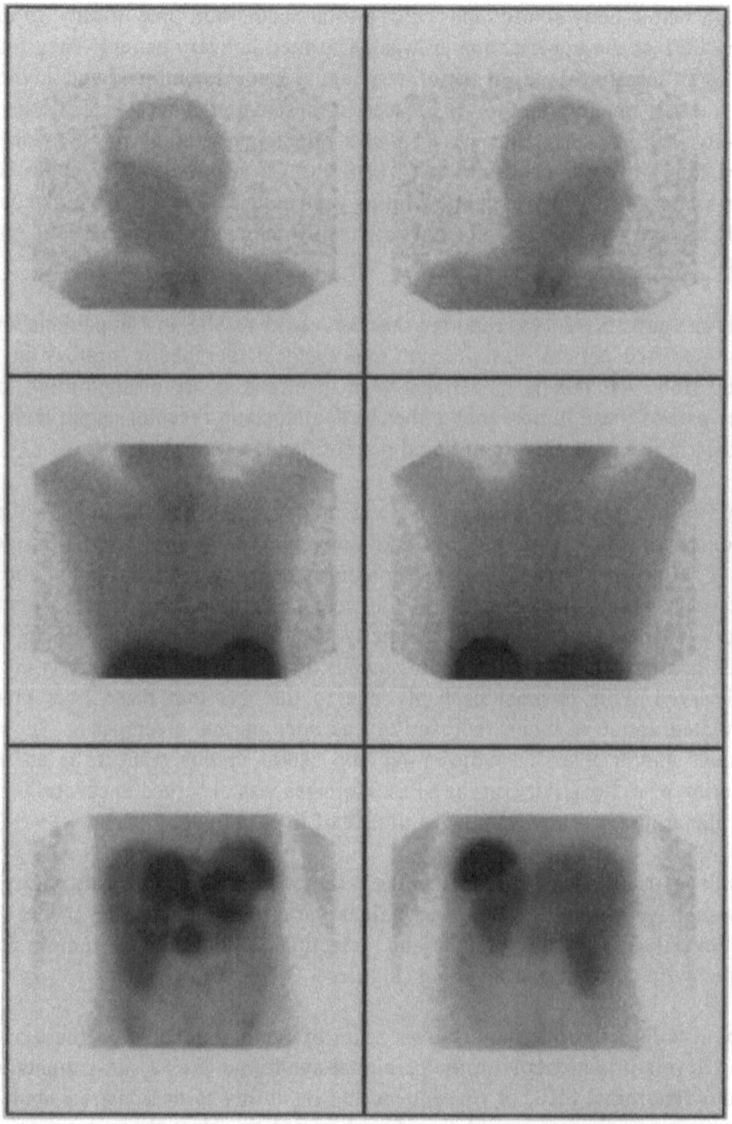

Figure 1. Somatostatin receptor scintigraphy, 24 h pi, in a patient with liver metastases from a neuroendocrine tumor from unknown origin. Spot images of the head (upper row), thorax (middle row; anterior is left, posterior right), and abdomen. Normal uptake in the thyroid, spleen, and kidneys. There is an enlarged liver with multiple sites of high accumulation of the radiopharmaceutical. The lowest lesion is located outside the liver, as demonstrated with additional SPECT studies (not shown).

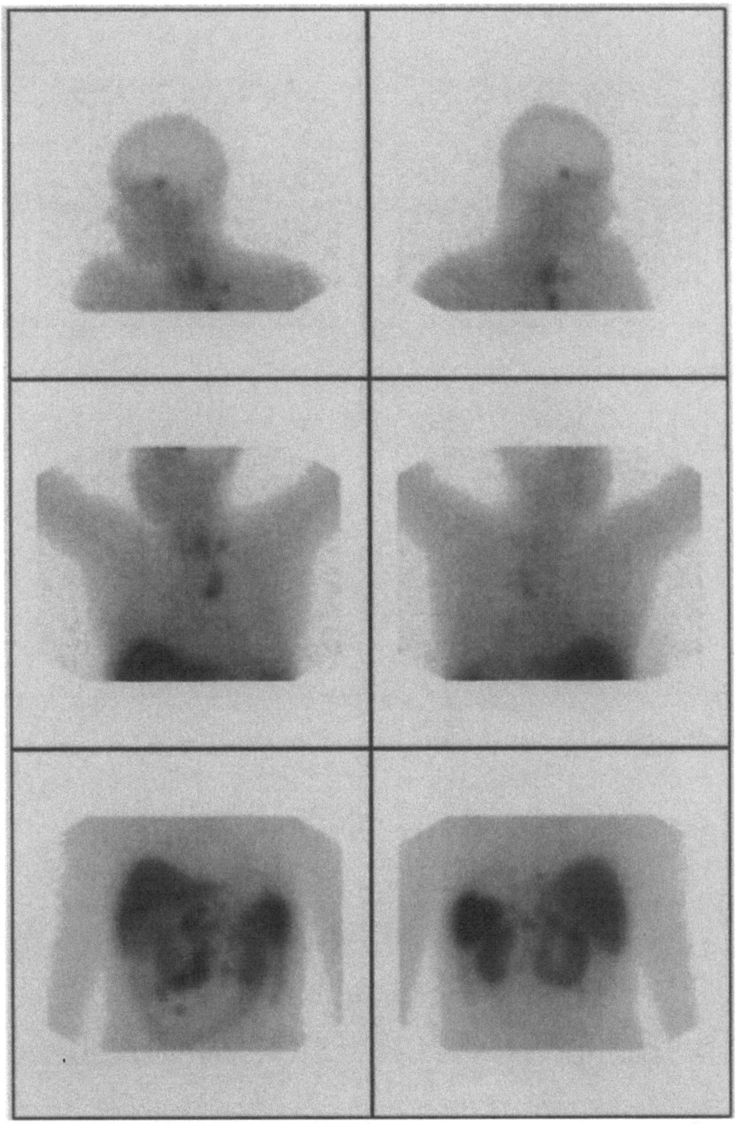

Figure 2. Somatostatin receptor scintigraphy, 24 h pi, in a patient with a metastasized carcinoid. Image arrangement as in Figure 1. Note the (normal) uptake in the pituitary, which varies between patients. There is a status after hemithyroidectomy. There is pathological uptake in the left supraclavicular lymphnode, the thorax, and the abdomen.

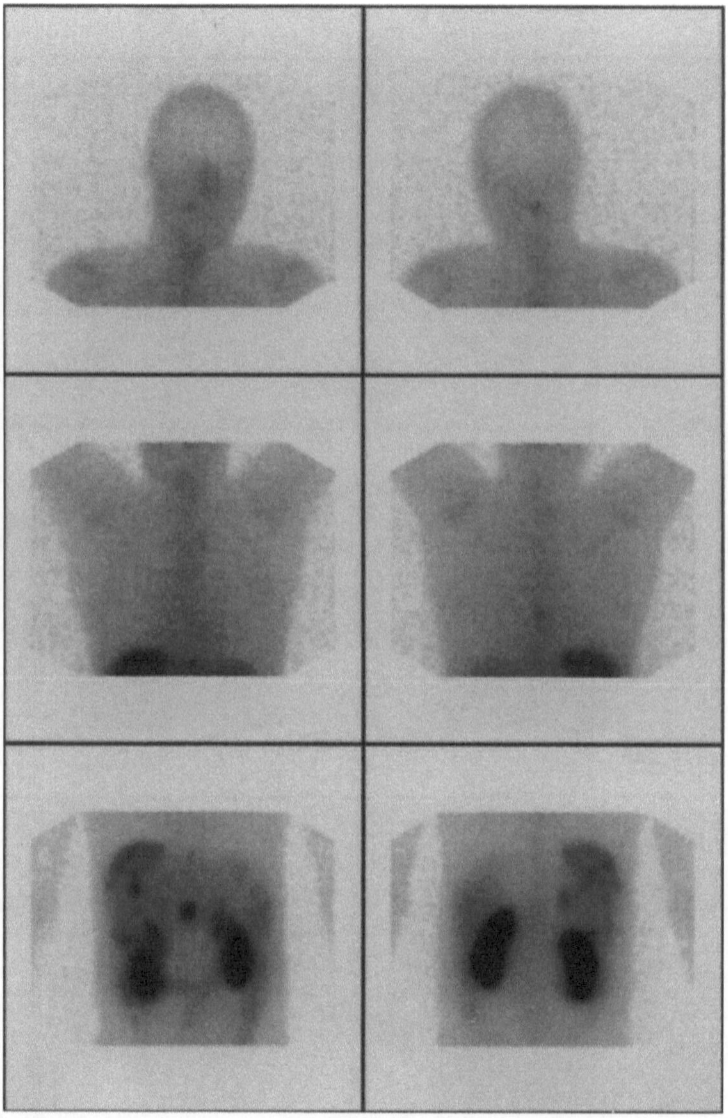

Figure 3. Somatostatin receptor scintigraphy, 24 h pi, in a patient with a metastasized carcinoid, under continued octreotide medication (500 μg, tid). Image arrangement as in Figure 1. Visualization of skeletal metastases at C2 and the thoracic spine. There is diffuse uptake in multiple ribs. Also visualization of multiple liver metastases, of which the most cranial one shows central necrosis. Reduced uptake in the spleen due to continued octreotide medication.

In a cost-effectiveness study (43), we found that the detection of more tumor sites in patients who are known to have one tumor localization with conventional imaging may be essential when deciding whether to perform surgery. The impact on patient management is fourfold: SRS may detect resectable tumors that would be unrecognized with conventional imaging techniques; it may prevent surgery in patients whose tumors have metastasized to a greater extent than can be detected with conventional imaging; it may direct the choice of therapy in patients with inoperable tumors; and it may be used to select patients for radionuclide therapy.

VIPRS

In 1994, Virgolini and coworkers (20) reported the successful visualization of colonic and pancreatic adenocarcinomas with VIPRS. Also, positive scans were obtained in 9 of 10 patients with carcinoids and 4 of 4 patients with insulinomas. The results were confirmed by *in vitro* binding studies on tumors from 10 patients. In some of the patients, SRS was performed as well; this investigation was positive in 8 of 9 patients with carcinoids and 2 of 2 patients with insulinomas. In a later update by the same group (54), the localization of intestinal carcinoids in 15 of 17 patients (88%) and of insulinomas in 8 of 10 patients (80%) was reported.

A relative drawback in VIPRS for neuroendocrine tumors, in comparison to SRS, are the low tumor to background ratios, and the high uptake of radioactivity in the lungs.

CgAIS

The first reports on the use of a three-step CgAIS by the group from the University of Milan, dealt with the detection of pituitary tumors (25,27,55). Most pituitary tumors, and especially the clinically nonfunctioning ones, were found to be positive.

In a more recent publication (26), the same group reported their results in neuroendocrine tumors other than pituitary adenomas. Positive scintigrams were obtained in all of 5 insulinomas, 6 of 8 carcinoids, 1 of 1 gastrinoma, and 1 of 1 glucagonoma (26). In most patients, conventional imaging methods and/or subsequent histology confirmed the results (Figure 4).

FDG-PET

Few reports on the value of FDG-PET in patients with pancreatic neuroendocrine tumors or carcinoids are available. Pasquali and coworkers. (56) recently reported an interesting comparison between FDG-PET and SRS in the same 16 patients with neuroendocrine tumors. ^{18}F-FDG uptake was increased in all 8 aggressively growing tumors, whereas it was slightly increased in only 1 out of 8 slowly growing tumors. SRS was performed in 13 patients. It was positive in all 6 patients with slowly growing tumors, but failed to demonstrate any lesion in 2 of 7 patients with aggressive tumors (56).

Adams and coworkers (57) have also compared FDG-PET with SRS in 15 patients with neuroendocrine tumors. Amongst these were 7 patients with GEP tumors. In 2 patients with less-differentiated GEP tumors associated with high proliferative activity and increased FDG uptake, SS-R failed to detect any lesion. In comparison, in four patients with well-differentiated GEP tumors showing low proliferative activity, SS-R localized four primary tumors, 22 lymph node metastases and 18 malignant liver lesions, whereas ^{18}F-FDG PET demonstrated normal distribution. In one patient with a metastasizing carcinoid (medium proliferative activity) SS-R localized multiple metastases, whereas PET demonstrated low FDG uptake in all known metastases.

Thus it seems that FDG-PET is complementary to SRS, in that aggressive tumors that are negative on SRS, may be detected with FDG-PET. Therefore, FDG-PET should best be reserved for those patients with neuroendocrine tumors who have a negative study with SRS.

Summary and perspective

At this moment, the radiopharmaceuticals for only 2 of the 4 nuclear medicine techniques that were discussed, namely SRS and FDG-PET, are commercially available in most countries. Because most neuroendocrine tumors are slow growing and have a relatively low grade of malignancy, the role of FDG-PET in this type of tumors is limited. SRS, on the other hand, has a high sensitivity for detecting neuroendocrine pancreatic tumors (save insulinomas) and carcinoids, and is therefore the imaging technique of first choice. If SRS is negative, PET-FDG could be tried. VIPRS and CgAIS have also been reported to be sensitive in detecting localizations of neuroendocrine tumors and carcinoids. A limitation to their widespread use at this moment is that the radiopharmaceuticals are not commercially available or government approved. For VIPRS additional drawbacks are the cumbersome peptide labeling of VIP with ^{123}I, and the relatively high background radioactivity, especially in the thorax. However, the development of chelated VIP analogs, which can be labeled with ^{111}In, might change this.

Apart for diagnostic purposes, radiolabeled peptides and monoclonal antibodies may be used for radiotherapy. Radionuclide therapy with high doses of [^{111}In-DTPA-D-Phe^{1}]-octreotide is now being performed in a phase-1-study. The initial evaluation in 6 end-stage patients with neuroendocrine tumors, treated up to a cumulative dose of 53GBq per patient, showed impressive results on hormone production and a likely anti-proliferative effect (58). A recent update in 16 patients with progressive tumor growth before the start of the therapy, and who were treated with a cumulative dose of at least 20 GBq, showed documented tumor regression in 5 patients, stable disease in 5 patients, and tumor progression in the other 6 patients. The observed tumor regression in part of the patients may either be ascribed to Auger- or to conversion-electrons.

^{111}In-coupled peptides, because of their small particle range, and therefore short tissue penetration, are not the ideal radiopharmaceuticals for radionuclide therapy. Recently, another somatostatin analog, [DOTA0, D-Phe^{1}, Tyr^{3}]-octreotide (DOTATOC) was developed, to which the ß-emitter ^{90}Y can be linked in a very stable manner (59,60). In a study in patients, the uptake of radioactivity in known somatostatin receptor positive organs and tumors was higher after ^{111}In-DOTATOC than after [^{111}In-DTPA-D-Phe^{1}]-octreotide (61). A recent preliminary study by Otte and coworkers. (62) showed favorable results of ^{90}Y-DOTATOC treatment in five patients with neuroendocrine tumors. Also, a study comparing both the uptake of ^{111}In-DOTATOC and 86Y-DOTATOC, as well as the effects of treatment with ^{90}Y-DOTATOC in the same patients has started in our hospital.

For as yet, treatment with native VIP, labeled with ^{131}I, does not seem feasible, because of the high uptake in the lungs. Unless VIP analogs that are fit for therapeutic use show considerably less thoracic uptake, the prospects for VIP analogs for therapeutic purposes are poor.

In their paper on CgAIS for endocrine tumors, Siccardi and coworkers. (26) report an experimental treatment in a patient with an ACTH-oma using the three-step CgAIS, in which the third step consisted of 3700 MBq ^{90}Y-biotin. The treatment resulted in a transient but significant decrease of cortisol levels, without toxicity to bone marrow, liver, or kidneys.

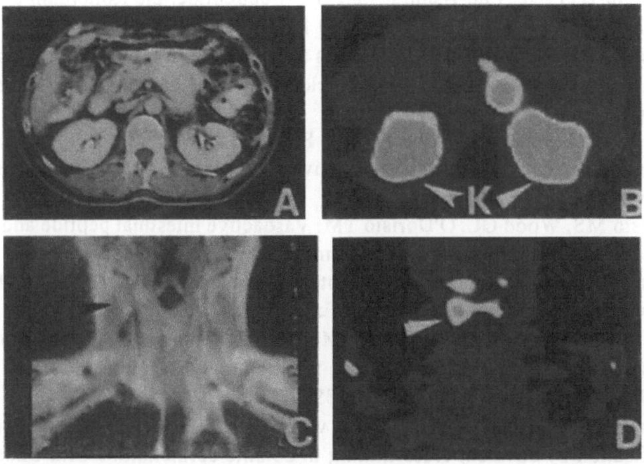

Figure 4: Comparison of CgAIS (B,D) with corresponding CT and MRI (A,C). A,B: Primary carcinoid of the pancreas ventral to the kidneys (K). C,D: Peritracheal lymph node metastases of a medullary thyroid carcinoma. Reproduced from Siccardi, et al. (26) with the permission of the publisher.

In conclusion, functional imaging based on the receptor status, metabolic behavior, or intracellular contents of neuroendocrine tumors may yield important information that influences therapy. A sequel to CgAIS and peptide receptor imaging may be three-step antibody therapy and peptide receptor radiotherapy.

REFERENCES

1. Patel YC, Amherdt M, Orci L. Quantitative electron microscopic autoradiography of insulin, glucagon and somatostatin binding sites on islets. Science 1982;217:1155.
2. Reubi JC, Maurer R. Autoradiographic mapping of somatostatin receptors in the rat CNS and pituitary. Neurosci 1985;15:1183.
3. Reubi JC, Kvols LK, Waser B, et al. Detection of somatostatin receptors in surgical and percutaneous needle biopsy samples of carcinoids and islet cell carcinomas. Cancer Res 1990;50:5969.
4. Sreedharan SP, Kodama KT, Peterson KE, Goetzl EJ. Distinct subsets of somatostatin receptors on cultured human lymphocytes. J Biol Chem 1989;264:949.
5. Reubi JC, Waser B, Foekens JA, et al. Somatostatin receptor incidence and distribution in breast cancer using receptor autoradiography: relationship to EGF-receptors. Int J Cancer 1990;46:416.
6. Reubi JC, Waser B, Vanhagen M, et al. *In vitro* and *in vivo* detection of somatostatin receptors in human malignant lymphomas. Int J Canc 1992;50:895.
7. Krenning EP, Bakker WH, Kooij PPM, et al. Somatostatin receptor scintigraphy with [^{111}In-DTPA-D-Phe^{1}]-octreotide in man: metabolism, dosimetry and comparison with [^{123}I-Tyr-3-]-octreotide. J Nucl Med 1992;33:652.
8. Reubi JC, Horisberger U, Studer UE, Waser B, Laissue JA. Human kidney as target for somatostatin: high affinity receptors in tubules and vasa recta. J Clin Endocrinol Metab 1993;77:1323.
9. Krenning EP, Kwekkeboom DJ, Bakker WH, et al. Somatostatin receptor scintigraphy with [^{111}In-DTPA-D-Phe^{1}]- and [^{123}I-Tyr-3-]-octreotide: the Rotterdam experience with more than 1000 patients. Eur J Nucl Med 1993;20:716.
10. Krenning EP, Kwekkeboom DJ, Pauwels S, Kvols LK, Reubi JC. Somatostatin receptor scintigraphy. In: Freeman LM (Ed). Nuclear Medicine Annual 1995. Raven Press, New York, p. 1.
11. Schwartz CJ, Kimberg DV, Sheerin HE, Field M, Said SI. Vasoactive intestinal peptide stimulation of adenylate cyclase and active electrolyte secretion in intestinal mucosa. J Clin Invest 1974;54:536.
12. O'Dorisio MS, Wood CL, O'Dorisio TM. Vasoactive intestinal peptide and neuropeptide modulation of the immune response. J Immunol 1985;135 (suppl):792.
13. Ottaway CA. *In vitro* alteration of receptors for vasoactive intestinal peptide changes the *in vivo* localization of mouse T cells. J Exp Med 1984;160:1054.
14. Blum AM, Mathew R, Cook GA, Metwali A, Felman R, Weinstock JV. Murine mucosal T cells have VIP receptors functionally distinct from those on intestinal epithelial cells. J Neuroimmunol 1992;39:101.
15. Couvineau A, Laburthe M. The human vasoactive intestinal peptide receptor: molecular identification by covalent cross-linking in colonic epithelium. J Clin Endocrinol Metab 1985;61:50.
16. Paul S, Said SI. Characterization of receptors for vasoactive intestinal peptide solubilized from the lung. J Biol Chem 1987;262:158.
17. Sreedharan SP, Robichon A, Peterson KE, Goetzl EJ. Cloning and expression of the human vasoactive intestinal peptide receptor. Proc Natl Acad Sci USA 1991;88:4986.
18. El Battari A, Martin JM, Luis J, et al. Solubilization of the active vasoactive intestinal peptide receptor from human colonic adenocarcinoma cells. J Biol Chem 1988;263:17685.
19. Svoboda M, De Neef P, Tastenoy M, Christophe J. Molecular characteristics and evidence for internalization of vasoactive-intestinal-peptide (VIP) receptors in the tumoral rat-pancreatic acinar cell line AR 4-2 J. Eur J Biochem 1988;176:707.

20. Virgolini I, Raderer M, Kurtaran A, et al. Vasoactive intestinal peptide-receptor imaging for the localization of intestinal adenocarcinomas and endocrine tumors. N Engl J Med 1994;331:1116.
21. Raderer M, Kurtaran A, Hejna M, et al. ^{123}I-labelled vasoactive intestinal peptide receptor scintigraphy in patients with colorectal cancer. Br J Cancer 1998;78:1.
22. O'Connor DT, Deftos LJ. Secretion of chromogranin A by peptide-producing endocrine neoplasms. N Eng J Med 1986;314:1145.
23. Deftos LJ. Chromogranin A: its role in endocrine function and as an endocrine tumour marker. Endocr Rev 1991;12:181.
24. Nobels FRE, Kwekkeboom DJ, Coopmans W, et al. Chromogranin A as serum marker for neuroendocrine neoplasia: comparison with neuron-specific enolase and the α-subunit of glycoprotein hormones. J Clin Endocrinol Metab 1997;82:2622.
25. Colombo P, Paganelli G, Magnani P, Songini C, Fazio F, Faglia G. Immunoscintigraphy with anti-chromogranin A antibodies in patients with endocrine/neuroendocrine tumors. J Endocrinol Invest 1993;16:841.
26. Siccardi AG, Paganelli G, Pontiroli AE, et al. *In vivo* imaging of chromogranin A-positive endocrine tumours by three-step monoclonal antibody targeting. Eur J Nucl Med 1996;23:1455.
27. Colombo P, Siccardi AG, Paganelli G, et al. Three-step immunoscintigraphy with anti-chromogranin A monoclonal antibody in tumours of the pituitary region. Eur J Endocrinol 1996;135:216.
28. Gupta NC, Frank AR, Dewan NA, et al. Solitary pulmonary nodules: detection of malignancy with PET with 2-[F-18]-fluoro-2-deoxy-D-glucose. Radiology 1992;184:441.
29. Patz EF, Lowe VJ, Hoffman JM, et al. Focal pulmonary abnormalities: evaluation with F-18 fluorodeoxyglucose PET scanning. Radiology 1993;188:487.
30. Strauss LG, Ponti PS. The application of PET in clinical oncology. J Nucl Med 1991;32:623.
31. Kubota R, Yamada S, Kubota K, Ishiwata K, Tamahashi N, Ido T. Intratumoral distribution of fluorine-18-fluorodeoxyglucose *in vivo*: high accumulation in macrophages and granulation tissues studied by microradioautoradiography. J Nucl Med 1992;33:1972.
32. Maton PM, O'Dorisio TM, Howe BA. Effect of a long-acting somatostatin analogue (SMS 201-995) in patients with pancreatic cholera. N Eng J Med 1985;312:17.
33. Wood SM, Kraenzlin ME, Adrian TE, Bloom SR. Treatment of patients with pancreatic endocrine tumours using a new long-acting somatostatin analogue SMS 201-995: symptomatic and peptide responses. Gut 1985;26:438.
34. Moertel CG. An odyssey in the land of small tumors. J Clin Oncol 1987;5:1503.
35. Kwekkeboom DJ, Krenning EP, Oei HY, van Eyck CHJ, Lamberts SWJ. Use of radiolabeled somatostatin to localize islet cell tumors. In: Mignon M, Jensen RT, eds. Frontiers of gastro-intestinal research, Vol 23. Endocrine tumors of the pancreas. New York: Karger, 1995, p. 298.
36. Cadiot G, Lebtahi R, Sarda L, et al. Preoperative detection of duodenal gastrinomas and peripancreatic lymph nodes by somatostatin receptor scintigraphy. Gastroenterology 1996;111:845.
37. De Kerviler E, Cadiot G, Lebtahi R, Faraggi M, Le Guludec D, Mignon M. Somatostatin receptor scintigraphy in forty-eight patients with the Zollinger-Ellison syndrome. Eur J Nucl Med 1994;21:1191.
38. Gibril F, Reynolds JC, Doppman JL, et al. Somatostatin receptor scintigraphy: its sensitivity compared with that of other imaging methods in detecting primary and metastatic gastrinomas. A prospective study. Ann Intern Med 1996;125:26.

39. Zimmer T, Stolzel U, Bader M, et al. Endoscopic ultrasonography and somatostatin receptor scintigraphy in the preoperative localisation of insulinomas and gastrinomas. Gut 1996;39:562.
40. Lunderquist A. Radiologic diagnosis of neuroendocrine tumors. Acta Oncol 1989;28:371.
41. Doherty GM, Doppman JL, Shawker TH, et al. Results of a prospective strategy to diagnose, localize, and resect insulinomas. Surgery 1991;110:989.
42. Rösch T, Lightdale CJ, Botet JF, et al. Localization of pancreatic endocrine tumors by endoscopic ultrasonography. N Engl J Med 1992;326:1721.
43. Kwekkeboom DJ, Lamberts SWJ, Habbema JD, Krenning EP. Cost-effectiveness analysis of somatostatin receptor scintigraphy. J Nucl Med 1996;37:886.
44. Lebtahi R, Cadiot G, Sarda L, et al. Clinical impact of somatostatin receptor scintigraphy in the management of patients with neuroendocrine gastroenteropancreatic tumors. J Nucl Med 1997;38:853.
45. Lamberts SWJ, Hofland LJ, Van Koetsveld PM, et al. Parallel *in vivo* and *in vitro* detection of functional somatostatin receptors in human endocrine pancreatic tumors. Consequences with regard to diagnosis, localisation and therapy. J Clin Endocrinol Metab 1990;71:566.
46. Kwekkeboom DJ, Krenning EP, Bakker WH, et al. Somatostatin analogue scintigraphy in carcinoid tumors. Eur J Nucl Med 1993;20:283.
47. Kalkner KM, Janson ET, Nilsson S, Carlsson S, Oberg K, Westlin JE. Somatostatin receptor scintigraphy in patients with carcinoid tumors: comparison between radioligand uptake and tumor markers. Cancer Res 1995;55(suppl 23):5801.
48. Anthony LB, Martin W, Delbeke D, Sandler M. Somatostatin receptor imaging: predictive and prognostic considerations. Digestion 1996;57(suppl 1):50.
49. Westlin JE, Janson ET, Arnberg H, Ahlstrom H, Oberg K, Nilsson S. Somatostatin receptor scintigraphy of carcinoid tumours using the [^{111}In-DTPA-D-Phe^{1}]-octreotide. Acta Oncol 1993;32:783.
50. Schillaci O, Scopinaro F, Angeletti S, et al. SPECT improves accuracy of somatostatin receptor scintigraphy in abdominal carcinoid tumors. J Nucl Med 1996;37:1452.
51. Kvols LK, Moertel CG, O'Connell MJ, et al. Treatment of the malignant carcinoid syndrome. N Eng J Med 1986;315:663.
52. Vinik AI, Tsai ST, Moattari AR, et al. Somatostatin analogue (SMS 201-995) in the management of gastroentero-pancreatic tumors and diarrhea syndromes. Am J Med 1986;81(suppl 6B):23.
53. Kvols LK. Medical oncology considerations in patients with metastatic neuroendocrine carcinomas. Semin Oncol 1994;21(suppl 13):56.
54. Virgolini I, Raderer M, Kurtaran A, et al. ^{123}I-vasoactive intestinal peptide (VIP) receptor scanning: update of imaging results in patients with adenocarcinomas and endocrine tumors of the gastrointestinal tract. Nucl Med Biol 1996;23:685.
55. Magnani P, Paganelli G, Siccardi AG, et al. Combined use of ^{111}In-labeled pentetreotide and three-step immunoscintigraphy with antichromogranin A monoclonal antibody in the diagnosis of pituitary adenomas. Cell Biophys 1994;24/25:307.
56. Pasquali C, Rubello D, Sperti C, et al. Neuroendocrine tumor imaging: can ^{18}F-fluorodeoxyglucose positron emission tomography detect tumors with poor prognosis and aggressive behavior? World J Surg 1998;22:588.
57. Adams S, Baum R, Rink T, Schumm-Drager PM, Usadel KH, Hor G. Limited value of fluorine-18 fluorodeoxyglucose positron emission tomography for the imaging of neuroendocrine tumours. Eur J Nucl Med 1998;25:79.
58. Krenning EP, Kooij PP, Pauwels S, et al. Somatostatin receptor scintigraphy and radionuclide therapy. Digestion 1996;57(suppl 1):57.

59. Moi MK, Meares CF, DeNardo SJ. The peptide way to macrocyclic bifunctional chelating agents: synthesis of 2-(p-Nitrobenzyl)-1,4,7,10-tetraazacyclododecane-N,N',N",N"'-tetraacetic acid and study of its Yttrium(III) complex. J Am Chem Soc 1998;10:6266.
60. Otte A, Jermann E, Behe M, et al. DOTATOC: a powerful new tool for receptor-mediated radionuclide therapy. Eur J Nucl Med 1997;24:792.
61. Kwekkeboom DJ, Kooij PPM, Bakker WH, Mäcke HR, Krenning EP. Comparison of Indium-111-DOTATOC and Indium-111-DTPA-octreotide in the same patients: biodistribution, kinetics, organ and tumor uptake. Submitted.
62. Otte A, Mueller-Brand J, Dellas S, Nitzsche EU, Herrmann R, Maecke HR. Yttrium 90-labelled somatostatin-analogue for cancer treatment. Lancet 1998;351:417.

INDEX

MIX
Papier aus verantwortungsvollen Quellen
Paper from responsible sources
FSC® C105338

If you have any concerns about our products,
you can contact us on
ProductSafety@springernature.com

In case Publisher is established outside the EU,
the EU authorized representative is:
Springer Nature Customer Service Center GmbH
Europaplatz 3, 69115 Heidelberg, Germany

Printed by Libri Plureos GmbH
in Hamburg, Germany